D1531887

DISCARD

# Progress in Chemical Toxicology

VOLUME 1

# Progress in Chemical Toxicology

*Edited by*

## ABRAHAM STOLMAN

*Toxicological Services Section*
*Laboratory Services Division*
*Connecticut State Department of Health*
*Hartford, Connecticut*

VOLUME 1

 1963

ACADEMIC PRESS · New York and London

ACADEMIC PRESS, INC.
111 Fifth Avenue, New York, New York 10003

*United Kingdom Edition published by*
ACADEMIC PRESS, INC. (LONDON) LTD.
Berkeley Square House, London W1X 6BA

LIBRARY OF CONGRESS CATALOG CARD NUMBER: 63-22331

*Second Printing, 1971*

PRINTED IN THE UNITED STATES OF AMERICA

# Contributors

Numbers in parentheses are the page numbers on which the author's contribution begins.

*ELVERA J. ALGERI (157), *Department of Legal Medicine, Harvard University Medical School, Boston, Massachusetts*

A. S. CURRY (135), *Forensic Science Laboratory, Harrogate, Yorkshire, England*

ABEL M. DOMINGUEZ (11), *Toxicology Laboratory, Armed Forces Institute of Pathology, Washington, D. C.*

CHARLES G. FARMILO (199), *Organic Chemistry and Narcotic Section, Food and Drug Directorate, Department of National Health and Welfare, Ottawa, Ontario, Canada*

MILTON FELDSTEIN (297, 317), *Bay Area Air Pollution Control District, San Francisco, California*

ROBERT B. FORNEY (53), *School of Medicine, Indiana University, Indianapolis, Indiana*

HENRY C. FREIMUTH (1), *Chief Medical Examiner's Office, State of Maryland, Baltimore, Maryland*

K⁻LAUS GENEST (199), *Organic Chemistry and Narcotic Section, Food and Drug Directorate, Department of National Health and Welfare, Ottawa, Ontario, Canada*

LEO R. GOLDBAUM (11), *Toxicology Laboratory, Armed Forces Institute of Pathology, Washington, D. C.*

ROLLA N. HARGER (53), *School of Medicine, Indiana University, Indianapolis, Indiana*

†ARTHUR J. McBAY (157), *Chemical Laboratory, Massachusetts State Police and Department of Legal Medicine, Harvard Medical School, Boston, Massachusetts*

FREDRIC RIEDERS (191), *Division of the Medical Examiner, Department of Public Health of the City of Philadelphia, Pennsylvania*

---

* Present address: Department of Biological Chemistry, Harvard University Medical School, Boston, Massachusetts.

† Present address: Law-Medicine Research Institute, Boston University, Boston, Massachusetts.

EUGENE L. SCHLOEGEL (11), *Toxicology Laboratory, Armed Forces Institute of Pathology, Washington, D. C.*

ARTHUR E. SCHWARTING (385), *School of Pharmacy, University of Connecticut, Storrs, Connecticut*

VARRO E. TYLER, JR. (339), *College of Pharmacy, University of Washington, Seattle, Washington*

# *Preface*

This volume is one of a continuing series covering developments in toxicology. Since the publication of the treatise "Toxicology: Mechanisms and Analytical Methods," new literature has appeared containing much valuable information for toxicologists and scientists in allied fields.

"Progress in Chemical Toxicology" will provide source material on selected subjects in which the most information is available. Each subject area selected is reviewed and discussed by experienced workers. The objectives are to report on the usefulness of the newly developed techniques and methods with necessary modifications for toxicological studies and to supply related information for the proper evaluation of the results obtained.

This book maintains the aims of the original treatise. Information on the main topics such as isolation procedures, alcohol, barbiturates, and narcotics and related bases is developed further. Knowledge accumulated on other subjects including ataraxics, air pollutants, mushrooms, opium, and poisonous seeds and fruits has developed to a stage where separate chapters are required for each subject. Stress is laid on details of practical analytical significance and those which may be of importance in arriving at a decision as to the toxic effects of drugs.

The Editor wishes to express his sincere thanks to the authors for their patience, their cooperation, and the willingness with which they shared their experiences and accomplished their tasks. He also acknowledges gratefully the assistance and guidance of his associate, Dr. C. P. Stewart. Finally, the publishers of the book deserve special recognition and thanks for their tireless cooperation.

ABRAHAM STOLMAN

*August, 1963*

# Contents

POISONOUS SEEDS AND FRUITS
*Arthur E. Schwarting*

# Isolation and Separation Techniques for Identification of Poisons

### by HENRY C. FREIMUTH

*Office of the Chief Medical Examiner, State of Maryland, Baltimore, Maryland*

## I. Acetone Extraction of Organic Substances

The classical Stas–Otto procedure for the isolation of nonvolatile organic substances from tissues has been found, through the years, to have many shortcomings. To cite only two of these, there may be mentioned the relative lack of purity of the extracted compounds and the poor yields of many of these compounds. Because of these factors, various modifications of the Stas–Otto technique have been proposed (F2). A further modification has been suggested by Alha and Lindfors (A2) in which acetone has been used, instead of ethanol, as the protein precipitant and solvent for the organic substances. This procedure was first employed by Chéramy and Lobo (C1, C2) for the isolation of barbiturates from biological material.

The procedure developed by Alha and Lindfors uses 100 gm of minced tissue which is made acid (pH 4) with aqueous tartaric acid. To this, there is then added 200 ml of 70% acetone. The mixture is heated on a water bath at 60°C, using a reflux condenser, for ½ hour. It is then allowed to stand at room temperature for several hours and preferably overnight. The acetone is filtered and the residue washed with 70% acetone with the washings being added to the original acetone filtrate.

The acetone is then distilled from the filtrate by vacuum distillation until approximately 50 ml of liquid remains in the distilling flask. After cooling, the residue in the distilling flask is rinsed into a beaker with water, made alkaline with ammonia, and then reacidified with tartaric acid. The precipitate formed at this point is removed by filtration and the residue is washed with water which is added to the filtrate.

Approximately 400 ml of acetone is added gradually to the aqueous filtrate and the mixture is allowed to stand at room temperature until the precipitate formed has settled to the bottom of the container. The mixture is filtered and the residue is washed with acetone. The filtrate (plus the washings) is subjected to vacuum distillation until 10–15 ml of liquid remain in the distilling flask. After cooling, another precipitation is carried out with 400 ml of acetone. The precipitate is allowed to settle and the mixture is filtered as before. The filtrate (plus washings) is again distilled until 10–15 ml remain. To this, 50 ml of hot water is added and, after cooling, the aqueous solution is filtered and the filtrate, which should still be acidic, is subjected to extraction procedures with immiscible solvents. The separation of four fractions is accomplished: (1) substances soluble in ether from acid solution; (2) substances soluble in chloroform from acid solution; (3) substances soluble in ether from NaOH solution; and (4) substances soluble in a mixture of $CHCl_3$ containing 10% $CH_3OH$ from a solution which is alkaline with $NaHCO_3$.

The authors report that the solvent-extraction steps are most efficiently accomplished by using liquid-liquid extractors with a capacity of 100 ml of aqueous solution. In each group, 75 ml of solvent is used. However, the authors also used a simple shaking procedure employing three 25-ml portions of solvent. The latter procedure did not give as good recovery as the former.

Alha and Lindfors (A2) also used a simplified acetone extraction procedure in which the acidified minced tissue is treated with undiluted acetone, heated, and filtered as in the procedure described above. The filtrate is treated with 25 gm of anhydrous sodium sulfate, shaken mechanically for ½ hour, allowed to stand several hours at room temperature, and then filtered. The residue is washed with acetone and the combined filtrate and washings are then vacuum distilled until 10–15 ml of solution remains in the distilling flask. The flask is rinsed with hot water to make 50 ml of solution. After cooling, this solution is filtered and extracted with immiscible solvents as above.

Using these procedures, the authors report recoveries ranging from approximately 40% for morphine to 95% for carbromal plus phenobarbital.

## II. Separation of Alkaloids from Tissue

### A. Cation-Exchange Columns

Tompsett (T1) has reported a technique for separating morphine and other alkaloids from tissue using a cation-exchange column. The procedure uses 100 gm of minced tissue to which are added 500 ml of water and 100 ml of 10 $N$ HCl. This mixture is heated to boiling and maintained in a boiling water bath for 1 hour. It is then cooled, diluted to 1000 ml with water, and filtered. The residue is washed with 500 ml of 1 $N$ HCl and the washings are added to the filtrate which is then passed through a cation-exchange column. The latter is 140 mm long and 15 mm in diameter and contains Dowex 50 $\times$ 12, 200–400 mesh. After the filtrate has passed through the column, the latter is washed with 500 ml of 1 $N$ HCl followed by 500 ml of water. The column is then eluted with 300 ml of 6 $N$ ammonia. This eluate constitutes the morphine fraction.

The column is next washed with 200 ml of water and 200 ml of 1 $N$ HCl. The more basic alkaloids are then eluted with 200 ml of 8 $N$ HCl.

Tompsett's data show morphine recovery in a concentration of 4 mg% to be quantitative as well as that of codeine, brucine, and strychnine.

## B. Acetonitrile Extraction

A method for isolating organic bases from tissues using acetonitrile and ether has been suggested by Abernathy *et al.* (A1). They have applied the method to liver, bile, and urine and have used it for the isolation and identification of morphine, nalorphine, codeine, meperidine, Methadone, amphetamine, quinine, caffeine, quinidine, colchicine, and phenothiazines. Recoveries of 75–80% were reported for codeine, morphine, strychnine, meperidine, and Methadone. Caffeine, amphetamine, and promazine were recovered in amounts in excess of 50%

The standard procedure results in the separation of two fractions, i.e., a "standard basic fraction" and a fraction designated as "solvent soluble salts." The latter contains Methadone, caffeine, and colchicine. The procedure, in detail, follows:
*Reagents:*
  (1) A-E Solvent: 1 volume acetonitrile and 2 volumes ethyl ether.
  (2) Alcoholic chloroform: 1 volume ethanol and 9 volumes chloroform.
  (3) Salt buffer: 20 gm sodium borate and 200 gm sodium chloride made up to 1 liter with water.
*Unhydrolyzed Tissue:* 100 gm of liver are homogenized with 50 ml of salt buffer. This is extracted with 500 ml of A-E solvent, in three portions, by mixing in the same homogenizer. It is suggested that a rheostat control on the homogenizer will prevent spilling of solvent into the motor. The extracts are decanted into a beaker to allow further settling of the aqueous phase, after which the solvent is decanted into a separatory funnel. The solvent is washed twice with one-twentieth of its volume of salt buffer. One fourth volume of petroleum ether is added and the mix-

ture is extracted twice with one-twentieth of its volume of $1\,N$ $H_2SO_4$. The combined acid extracts are washed with 2 volumes of A-E solvent and once with 2 volumes of chloroform. The original A-E solvent and the two solvent washes are combined and reserved for later extraction of the "solvent soluble salt" fraction. The aqueous phase above is adjusted to pH 8.6 and extracted twice with 3 volumes of alcoholic chloroform. The combined solvent phase is filtered, a few drops of HCl are added, and the solvent is evaporated using an air jet and mild heat. The residue is the "standard basic fraction."

The "solvent soluble salt" fraction is obtained by adding to the combined solvent one-twentieth of its volume of saturated sodium bicarbonate solution. The mixture is shaken and the aqueous layer is discarded. The solvent is decanted into a beaker and evaporated to near dryness in the presence of an excess of dilute HCl, using an air jet and mild heat. The residue is rinsed into a separatory funnel with 50 ml of water and 50 ml of ether. This is shaken and the ether phase is discarded. If necessary, any emulsion at this stage is broken by centrifuging. The ether wash is repeated after which excess sodium carbonate is added. The mixture is extracted twice with three times its volume of chloroform. The combined chloroform extract is filtered and, after addition of a slight excess of dilute HCl, the solvent is evaporated to dryness using an air jet and mild heat.

Urine samples may be extracted by first saturating 50 ml of urine with sodium chloride, adjusting to pH 8.6, and extracting twice with 3 volumes of A-E solvent. Thereafter, the procedure for tissue is followed beginning with the salt buffer washing.

For morphine and other conjugated compounds, hydrolysis is first carried out with sulfuric acid, with this procedure varying somewhat with the type of sample used. For tissues, 100 gm of homogenized tissue are treated with $18\,N$ sulfuric acid until the mixture is $1\,N$ in sulfuric acid. This is autoclaved for 15 minutes at 20 lb pressure. Urine samples of 50 ml are treated in the same way. Bile, which is used primarily for morphine, is treated by adding 5 ml of $2\,N$ sulfuric acid to 5 ml of bile and autoclaving in the same manner as tissue. After cooling, the hydrolyzed bile is filtered and the residue is boiled briefly with 5 ml of $1\,N$ sulfuric acid. This is cooled and filtered into the first filtrate.

To the hydrolyzate or filtrate obtained above, a few crystals of sodium sulfite are added to prevent oxidation of morphine. The mixture is then adjusted to pH 8.6 and extracted twice with three times its volume of A-E solvent. The solvent layer is washed twice with one-twentieth of its volume of $1\,N$ $H_2SO_4$. The acid layer is washed once with 2 volumes of A-E solvent and once with 2 volumes of chloroform.

One milligram of sodium sulfite is added to the aqueous phase and the pH is adjusted to 7.0 with 50% NaOH. Five drops of NaOH are added in excess and the mixture is extracted twice with 3 volumes of chloroform. The latter is filtered, and, after addition of a few drops of hydrochloric acid, evaporated to dryness, using an air jet and low heat. The residue is the basic fraction.

The aqueous phase remaining after the chloroform extraction is brought to pH 8.6 and extracted twice with 3 volumes of alcoholic chloroform. The extract is filtered and evaporated as above, leaving morphine in the residue.

## III. Two-Stage Extraction

### A. Acid Spot Extraction—Paper Chromatography

An elegant method for the rapid isolation and detection of organic bases in urine has been described by Morgan (M1). The method is especially suited for use with paper chromatographic methods of identification. In applying the method, oxygen-free nitrogen is used in both the extraction and isolation procedures. The apparatus used is shown in Fig. 1.

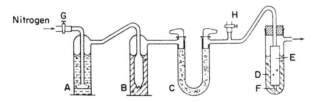

FIG. 1. Diagram of acid spot extraction apparatus.
A = Washing bottle containing chromous sulfate solution
B = Washing bottle containing concentrated sulfuric acid
C = U-tube containing self-indicating silica gel
D = Solvent extract
E = Paper strip with acid spots
F = Tip of gas delivery tube
G = Screw clip
H = By-pass to flowmeter

The chromous sulfate solution is prepared in the gas-washing bottle by mixing 12 gm of powdered chromic potassium sulfate, 50 ml of water, and 5 ml of concentrated sulfuric acid. When the solid has completely dissolved, the solution is cooled by the addition of 10–15 gm of crushed ice and the mixture is poured into 6 gm of zinc dust contained in the bottom of the gas-washing bottle. The inlet tube is immediately inserted and air is expelled by passing a small stream of nitrogen through the bottle. Complete reduction is indicated by a pale blue solution which will darken as oxygen is absorbed.

For extraction, the urine sample is first adjusted to a pH of 9 by adding 20% sodium hydroxide. One-fifth of the volume of chloroform is introduced into a separatory funnel and the urine is carefully poured onto the chloroform so that no emulsification occurs. A slow stream of nitrogen (less than 50 ml/minute) is then passed into the chloroform layer and the rate of gas flow is adjusted so that the coarse emulsion which forms at the interface does not extend to the tip of the gas-delivery tube. After 20 minutes the gas supply is shut off and any residual emulsion that does separate on standing is broken up as far as possible by gentle stirring of the chloroform layer. The latter is filtered through a dry filter paper into a test tube of such diameter that the height of the liquid is 5–7 cm.

A strip of Whatman 3MM filter paper 7 cm by 1.5 cm is spotted with drops of 0.25 and 0.5 N sulfuric acid, 2 cm from one end of the paper. Morgan indicates that it is advantageous for the sulfuric acid to contain thymol blue indicator. Such solutions can be prepared by dissolving separate 4-mg portions of thymol blue in 0.5 gm and 1.0 gm of concentrated sulfuric acid, respectively, in 50-ml stoppered flasks. These solutions are set aside overnight and diluted to 40 ml with distilled water. These are then used for spotting the filter paper as indicated above. It should be mentioned that the filter paper should first be washed chromatographically with chloroform followed by water before it is cut into strips. The acid spots can be applied with a loop of platinum wire adjusted to produce spots 3–5 mm in diameter.

Immediately after the paper has been spotted with the acid, the strip is placed in the chloroform extract so that the spots, and preferably the entire strip, are completely immersed. The extract is agitated with a stream of dry oxygen-free nitrogen flowing at a rate of 100 ± 50 ml/minute/20 ml of solvent. The gas passes into the test tube through a glass delivery tube whose lower end is below the acid spots. The latter should not come into contact with the delivery tube or the walls of the test tube.

After some minutes, the spots will become transparent owing to loss of water. If a high concentration of basic substances is expected the strip may be removed from the chloroform at this point. In any event, 15 minutes of agitation is sufficient to extract alkaloids which were originally present in the urine sample in a concentration of 1 ppm. Morgan indicates that lower concentrations can be detected after longer agitation or by simply immersing the paper strip in the chloroform extract overnight without passing nitrogen through it.

After the gas flow has been stopped, any part of the paper strip not immersed in the solvent is rinsed with the extract by shaking for a few minutes. Excess chloroform is removed by shaking the strip and exposing to a current of air. The dried strip is then suspended in a flask over a few drops of concentrated ammonia until the spots change from pink to yellow or blue. This will take about 15 minutes.

The ammonia vapor is removed from the paper in a current of air and the resulting mixture of the sulfates of organic bases extracted from the urine is developed on the paper strip as a paper chromatogram by any convenient ascending solvent technique.

### B. Protein-Free Filtrates—High Temperature Chromatography

A method for the simultaneous detection of alkaloidal, neutral, and acidic poisons in human tissues has been described by Street (S1). This procedure involves the separation of various toxic substances by the use of high temperature, reversed phase paper chromatography. The chief advantages for such a system are: (1) the use of a single solvent system and the same paper for the separation of a mixture of compounds having widely different properties; (2) the time required for chromatography is only 20 minutes rather than hours; (3) the chromatographic spots show little diffusion, (4) the solvent, which is $M/15$ phosphate buffer pH 7.4, is more stable than the usual organic solvents used in chromatography.

In the procedure described, a protein-free filtrate of blood or tissue is prepared by adding to 10 ml of blood (or 10 gm of tissue) 63 ml of distilled water and 20 ml of 10% (w/v) sodium tungstate. The mixture is homogenized and 7 ml of 10% (v/v) sulfuric acid are added while stirring vigorously. The acidified homogenate is placed in a boiling water bath for 15 minutes and then filtered while hot through Whatman No. 1 filter paper on a Buchner funnel using gentle suction.

The cooled filtrate is then treated as outlined in Fig. 2. This results in five fractions, each of which is dissolved in 2–3 drops of ethyl alcohol.

Each of these solutions is applied to a 6¼ by 7 inch sheet of Whatman No. 1 filter paper which has previously been dipped in 10% glycerol tributyrate (tributyrin) in acetone and dried. Suitable marker solutions are also applied as separate spots adjacent to the appropriate fraction extract.

In preparing the paper, an even distribution of the ester over the paper is obtained by placing the treated sheet between several sheets of filter paper immediately after it is removed from the ester solution and then pressing the top sheets with a 10-inch rubber roller. In cutting the paper, a portion is left at one corner to form a tongue which is used in clipping the paper in cylindrical form for chromatography.

The paper cylinder with the various fractions is then placed in a

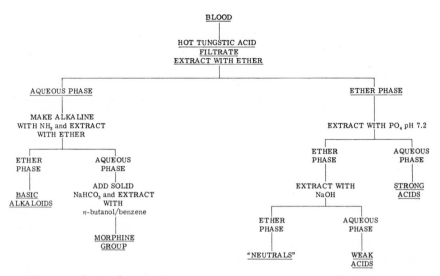

Fɪɢ. 2. Scheme showing the treatment of the protein-free filtrate in order to produce the various fractions for application of high temperature, reversed phase paper chromatography.

cylindrical jar fitted with a ground glass lid. Silicone grease is used to seal the lid of the jar. The jar is slightly larger in diameter than the paper cylinder and contains $M/15$ phosphate buffer, pH 7.4. The jar and solvent are maintained in an oven at 86°C before introducing the paper cylinder. Ascending chromatography is then carried out at 86°C for 20 minutes.

After chromatography, the wet paper is examined under ultraviolet light at 2540 Å. Any absorbing or fluorescent spots and their colors are noted. The paper is then exposed to ammonia gas and any additional absorbing spots are noted. The paper is subsequently dried with a hair dryer and re-examined in ultraviolet light. After this examination, the paper is cut into strips, thus isolating the various fractions.

The basic alkaloids and the morphine group of alkaloids are developed by dipping the appropriate strips in the iodoplatinate reagent of Farmilo and Genest (F1). The strips containing the neutral fraction may be treated with 0.1% potassium permanganate which will develop ethinamate (Valmid) as a yellow spot on a pink background. The same permanganate solution may also be used to locate those barbiturates having unsaturated groups in the side chain on the strip containing the weak acids. A typical chromatogram produced by this procedure is shown in Fig. 3.

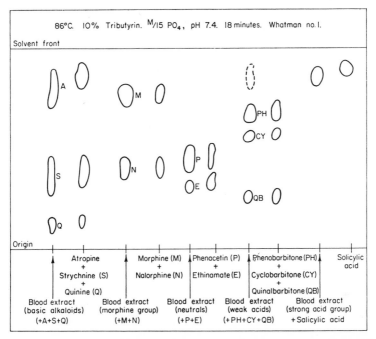

86°C.   10% Tributyrin.  M/15 PO₄ ,  pH 7.4.  18 minutes.  Whatman no. I.

Fɪɢ. 3. Tracing of composite chromatogram obtained by chromatography of various fractions isolated from blood to which the compounds referred to on the chromatogram had been added. The dotted area in the weak acid fraction is due to a trace of salicylic acid, present because of incomplete extraction by the phosphate buffer at pH 7.2. Tributyrin-impregnated Whatman No. 1 paper; solvent, $M/15$ phosphate buffer, pH 7.4, temperature, 86°C; time, 18 minutes.

## Rᴇғᴇʀᴇɴᴄᴇs

(A1) Abernethy, R. J., Villaudy, J., and Thompson, E. *J. Forensic Sci.* **4**, 486 (1959).

(A2) Alha, A. R., and Lindfors, R. O. *Ann. Med. Exptl. Biol. Fenniae (Helsinki)* **37**, 149 (1959).

(C1) Chéramy, P., and Lobo, R. *J. Pharm. Belg.* **20**, 400 (1934).

(C2) Chéramy, P., and Lobo, R. *J. Pharm. Belg.* **20**, 461 (1934).

(F1) Farmilo, C. G., and Genest, K. *In* "Toxicology, Mechanisms and Analytical Methods" (C. P. Stewart and A. Stolman, eds.), Vol. 2, p. 576. Academic Press, New York, 1961.

(F2) Freimuth, H. C. *In* "Toxicology: Mechanisms and Analytical Methods" (C. P. Stewart and A. Stolman, eds.), Vol. 1, pp. 293–302. Academic Press, New York, 1960.

(M1) Morgan, P. J. *Analyst* **84**, 418 (1959).

(S1) Street, H. V. *J. Forensic Sci.* **7**, 222 (1962).

(T1) Tompsett, S. L. *Acta Pharmacol. Toxicol.* **18**, 414 (1961).

# Application of Gas Chromatography to Toxicology

*by* Leo R. Goldbaum, Eugene L. Schloegel,
and Abel M. Dominguez

*Toxicology Laboratory, Armed Forces Institute of Pathology, Washington, D. C.*

## I. Introduction

The analytical problems confronting the toxicologist are first, that the quantity of sample is always limited, second, that the presence or absence of a large number of chemical agents must be determined, and finally, that these chemical agents when present are in low concentrations. With the present toxicologic procedures, the analysis for the presence of even a limited number of chemical agents requires a great expenditure

11

of man hours and equipment and is very costly. Therefore the toxicologist must direct his effort to the analysis of a selected number of chemical agents, a selection which is based upon his judgment and experience. A constant search is being made by the toxicologist for improved techniques and newer instruments to increase his capabilities by including the determination of a greater number of chemical agents. Of the newer techniques, gas chromatography has the potential of analyzing rapidly a wide variety of chemical agents including gases, liquids, and solids in extremely low concentrations and in complex mixtures. The technique and operation of this equipment is relatively simple and inexpensive.

Gas chromatography provides a physical method of separation in which a solute is distributed between a phase of large surface area and a mobile gas phase flowing over the stationary phase. The technique differs from other forms of chromatography in that only the mobile phase is a gas and the solutes are separated as vapors. The instrument consists of a sample inlet, a column, and a detector for the column effluents, along with a means of heating all three (Fig. 1).

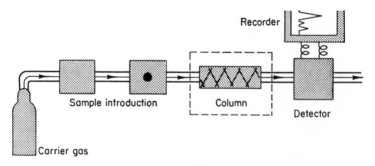

FIG. 1. Schematic diagram of gas chromatography.

## II. Columns

The column is where the actual separation occurs and is the heart of the technique. Therefore the first step is the selection of chromatographic columns. The names gas-solid chormatography (GSC), gas-liquid chromatography (GLC), and capillary chromatography (CC) are derived from the constituents of the columns (Fig. 2).

### A. Gas-Solid Chromatography Columns

Gas-solid chromatography (GSC) covers all gas chromatography methods in which the fixed phase is an active solid. Molecular sieve, silica gel, and activated charcoal comprise the active ingredients of most gas-solid columns. Table I shows the application of gas-solid chromatog-

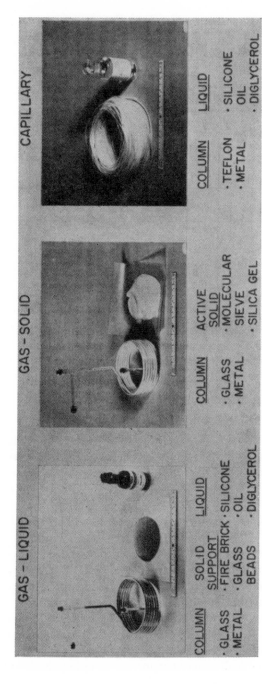

Fig. 2. Types of chromatographic columns. (Photograph reproduced with permission of Armed Forces Institute of Pathology, Washington, D. C.)

TABLE I
ACTIVE SOLIDS IN GAS-SOLID CHROMATOGRAPHY

| Active solid | Temperature range | Applications |
|---|---|---|
| Molecular sieve 4A, 5A, or 13X | Room to 300°C | Excellent resolution of light inorganic gases<br>Separates $O_2$ from $N_2$. Irreversibly absorbs $CO_2$ at temperatures below 160°C |
| Silica gel | Room to 225°C | Excellent for light inorganic gases and hydrocarbons up to $C_3$. Separates $H_2$, $N_2$, CO, $CO_2$. Does not separate $N_2$ from $O_2$ |
| Activated charcoal | −80 to +225°C | Light inorganic and organic gases |

raphy. The GSC column is usually ¼- to ⅛-inch tubing of glass, stainless steel, or copper either bent in a U or coiled. The length is usually from 4 to 10 ft but may be as long as 50 ft. The packing and activating of the column is relatively simple. There are several ways of packing a column. One way is by utilizing a vacuum pump on one end of the tubing and pouring the active solid into the open end while tapping lightly to prevent the formation of cavities. An advantage of using a glass column is to insure an evenly packed column. Before the column is used, it is activated by applying heat and a flow of carrier gas to carry off the interfering compounds which affect column efficiency.

## B. Gas-Liquid Chromatography Columns

Gas-liquid chromatography (GLC) is the method in which the fixed phase is a liquid distributed on a solid support which in turn is packed in a column of desired length and diameter. The solid support is normally an inert porous solid which is covered with a liquid phase. Occasionally, an active solid is used as a solid support to achieve special separation effects. The particle size range of the support should be specified because it affects column efficiency and the pressure differential necessary to achieve a given flow rate. Solid support material exert considerable influence on the elution of various compounds (B1, E3).

The general requirements for the solid support used in gas-liquid partition chromatograph (J2) are: (1) the material must have high surface area; (2) it must not break up under reasonable compaction or under the handling procedure required to prepare the material and fill the chromatographic column; (3) it must pack uniformly in the column; (4) it must be chemically inert toward the samples which are to be put through the column; (5) it must not be appreciably adsorptive. If columns with reasonably reproducible elution times and resolution are to be made, the particle size must be controlled as closely as possible. A particle size of about 30–70 mesh gives the most efficient compromise. Table II shows a partial list of commonly used solid supports.

TABLE II
SOLID SUPPORT MATERIALS

| | |
|---|---|
| Chromosorb P | Glass beads |
| Chromosorb | Teflon |
| Chromosorb W | Celite |
| Firebrick | |

The liquid phase is a compound which is nonvolatile at the operational temperature of the column. The solid support is coated with this liquid phase to bring about the separation of the sample components. The liquid phases commonly used are shown in Table III.

TABLE III
LIQUID PHASES COMMONLY USED IN TOXICOLOGY

| Phase | Temperature range | Applications |
|---|---|---|
| Silicone oil (P)[a] | Room to 175°C | Acetates |
| Apiezon "N" (P) | Room to 150°C | |
| Ucon 50 H.B. 2000 (P) | Room to 200°C | |
| Beckman column (I)[b] | Room to 150°C | Alcohols and aldehydes |
| Polyethylene glycol (N)[c] | Room to 140°C | |
| QF-1 (I) | Room to 225°C | Amines |
| SE-30 (I) | | |
| Glycerol (N) | Room to 70°C | Ammonia |
| Diglycerol (N) | Room to 110°C | |
| Ucon (P) | Room to 175°C | Aromatics |
| Apiezon "L" (P) | Room to 250°C | |
| SE-30 (I) | Room to 225°C | High boiling compounds, barbiturates, tranquilizers, and alkaloids |
| Silicone grease (I) | Room to 350°C | |
| Silicone rubber (I) | Room to 350°C | |
| QF-1 (I) | Room to 225°C | |

[a] P = polar.
[b] I = intermediate polarity.
[c] N = nonpolar.

A knowledge of the proper liquid substrate is essential to the intelligent solution of a specific analytical problem (T1). However, no single stationary liquid phase will solve all problems since it is rarely possible to separate all components of a complex mixture with the use of a single liquid substrate. Usually, several columns impregnated with different liquid phases are required to accomplish the separation of complex mixtures.

Liquid phases may be divided into three classes: (1) polar; (2) non-polar; and (3) intermediate polarity (Table III). There is no sharp line of demarcation between classes. These available liquid phases make possible a broad graduation of polarities. Although there are many known liquid phases or combinations of liquid phases (M1) which can resolve many classes of compound, trial and error is often required in the selection of the liquid phase to separate a particular mixture.

The column is usually $\frac{1}{4}$ to $\frac{1}{8}$-inch tubing of stainless steel, copper, or glass either bent in a U or coiled. The glass columns are usually treated with SC-01 (trimethylchlorisilane), 1–5%, or hexamethyldilazane to reduce the active sites on the walls of the column. This treatment results in less tailing and minimized catalytic effects and improves the results when low concentration of liquid phases are used on the inert supports.

The GLC column is prepared in three steps: first, the support is prepared; second, the support is coated with the phase; and third, the column is packed.

Most solid supports which do not require treatment are available commercially. The following procedure illustrates the preparation of an inert support.

The inert supports (Table II) are placed in a beaker and covered with sufficient concentrated hydrochloric acid to make a slurry which is easily stirred so that all particles are wetted. The slurry is continuously stirred for several minutes then allowed to settle for 2–5 minutes. The liquid including the fine particles in suspension is decanted. The solid is washed with several portions of distilled water using 3 volumes of water to 1 volume of solid for each washing. After settling for about 2 minutes, the water phases containing fine particles are decanted. The pH is adjusted to 7–8 using a solution of sodium hydroxide or ammonium hydroxide. The inert solid is spread in a thin layer on an evaporation dish and dried overnight in an oven at 120°C. When the support is used for preparation of a polar column, the complete covering of the active sites on the inert support is desirable. The dry support is added to a solution of 1–2% dichloro-dimethylsilane in toluene. For 1 part of solid 5 parts of solution are used. After 20 minutes the mixture is filtered over a Buchner funnel and washed with toluene followed by methanol. The vacuum is broken, and the suspension stirred with methanol and again filtered by suction. The support is spread on a sheet of filter paper in an oven and dried at 100°C for 2 hours.

The required amount of the liquid phase is weighed; this is usually 1–20% of the support. The liquid is dissolved in 10 volumes of a miscible volatile solvent such as acetone, petroleum ether, or ethyl ether. This solution of liquid phase is added to the inert support in a beaker. The beaker is transferred to a water bath and the slurry is stirred continuously as the solvent evaporates until the support appears dry. Then the treated solid is dried for over an hour with occasional stirring.

The treated support can be packed either into "U" tubes by gravity with slight tapping or in coiled columns with the aid of suction and slight vibration.

The prepared columns are then conditioned with the carrier gas flowing through the column at low pressure for several hours at 25–50°C below maximum operating temperature of the liquid phase before rising to its maximum operating temperature.

## C. Capillary Chromatography Columns

The CC is a GLC column in which the solid support is replaced by the wall of the capillary column (C6, G4). The advantage over the GLC is the long length which boosts the number of theoretical plates thereby increasing the separation and resolution of compounds.

The columns have inside diameters of 0.01 to 0.02 inches and are from 20 to 1000 ft in length. They are usually made of stainless steel, nylon, or glass. Only very small samples can be analyzed because of the reduced capacity of the columns. It is customary to introduce regular size samples but a splitter allows only a small percentage (0.10%) to enter the column. Because of the very small samples, it is necessary that the detectors be very sensitive, have small internal volume, and have a fast response time (discussed in detail in Section III, B).

The capillary column is cleaned with a solvent such as benzene or acetone by forcing it through the column with carrier gas before coating with the liquid phase. If the solvent of the coating is different from the cleaning solvent, several milliliters of this solvent should follow the cleaning solvent. The column is not allowed to dry before the addition of the coating solutions. With low pressure (6 psi) of the carrier gas, the solution is forced through the columns. The amount of the solution is about three times the volume of the capillary tubing. After all coating solution is in the capillary column, the gas pressure is increased gradually to about 15 psi and allowed to flow for 8 or more hours.

The column is conditioned at 25°C intervals for an hour until the maximum desired operation temperature is reached. If the prepared capillary column is not satisfactory, it can be reconditioned with a solution of 60% of the original coating solution.

## III. Detectors

The requirements of an ideal detector are:
(1) the signal should be linear with concentration;
(2) the response should be rapid;
(3) it should be sensitive to low concentrations of sample;
(4) it should be independent of fluctuation of flow rate, pressure, and temperature;
(5) the response should measure the amount of the component.

Although there are many detector systems, the most commonly used detectors are based on thermal conductors and ionization (J3).

### A. Thermal Conductors

Detection of gases by thermal conductivity is based on the principle that a gas surrounding a hot object conducts heat away from it at a rate which varies with the nature of the gas. The relative differences are usually measured since absolute measurements of thermal conductivity of gases are difficult. Thermal conductivity changes in the gas eluted from the column are detected with a sample cell having a thermistor or a filament wire located at the outlet of the column through which the carrier gas and the eluted sample pass. A matched cell, called a reference cell, is located in front of the injection site through which only a stream of pure carrier gas flows. A Wheatstone bridge balances the electrical resistance of the cells in each channel. The thermal conductivity is the same when pure carrier gas passes through both cells. Since both cells are at the same temperature the resistance is the same and so is the rate of current flow. Should a sample of different thermoconductivity than the carrier gas pass through one channel, the circuit becomes unbalanced because the temperature of the thermistor or wire changes. For the analysis of low boiling point compounds and permanent gases, the thermistor-type detector elements are recommended for they provide maximum sensitivity at low operational temperatures. The hot wire detector provides maximum sensitivity at high operational temperatures. Its performance at high temperature complements the superior characteristics of the thermistor detector at lower temperature ranges. This detector is used primarily for the analysis of liquids. Some of the disadvantages of thermal conductivity are that it is not independent of flow rate, pressure, or temperature.

## B. Ionization Detectors

One of the more important advances in gas chromatography has been the introduction of ionization detectors (C4, L4). Analysis of trace quantities in parts per billion range is possible with these detectors. The small sample loads used cause the efficiencies of the column to be greatly improved. There are many kinds of ionization detectors: argon detectors, flame detectors, electron mobility detectors, cross section detectors, and thermionic emission. The argon detectors are highly sensitive detectors and are used in those analyses where the sample size is extremely limited. Their use in conjunction with capillary columns allows the maximum column efficiency to be attained. They are responsive to most organic compounds and may be used with packed columns.

### 1. ARGON IONIZATION DETECTOR

The argon ionization detector is a simple but extremely sensitive detector for ionizable organic compounds (L3). It also combines small effective cell volume and rapid response to make it particularly well suited for use with high efficiency capillary columns as well as with packed columns.

The argon carrier gas, when exposed to a small radioactive source, is raised to a highly excited but unionized state (metastable atoms). Upon collision, these metastable argon atoms impart their excitation to the molecules of the sample. These molecules are then ionized:

$$\text{argon (metastable)} + \text{molecule} \rightarrow \text{argon} + \text{molecule} + e^-$$

A voltage is applied across the cell and the electrons formed are collected on the anode. This current is amplified and sent to the recorder.

### 2. FLAME IONIZATION DETECTOR

With the flame ionization detector (C4, L4), carrier gas from the column and hydrogen enter the detector and are mixed. The gas mixture is fed to a jet where it is burned in an atmosphere of air. The flame is ignited by a hot wire igniter. A potential is applied across the electrode and the resulting condition is suitably amplified and recorded.

Ionization phenomena in the flame detector are not yet fully understood. According to one explanation, small carbon aggregates are ionized rather than the organic molecules themselves. Ionization appears to be dependent on the work functions of carbon and not on the ionization potential of the organic molecules. The flame is insensitive to a large number of organic compounds and in general to inorganic compounds.

The detector is an extremely linear device with sample concentration below 0.1%. The insensitivity of the flame detector to the common inorganic gas enables a wide range of carrier gases to be used and renders unimportant the presence of inorganic contaminants.

This detector has an extremely wide linear range and thus may be used over a wide range of concentrations. It will accept higher flow rates than the argon detectors and thus it is possible to feed the effluent from a packed column directly into the detector. This detector is not entirely suitable for use with capillary columns since its sensitivity is often not great enough to allow full column efficiency to be achieved. It is equally as good as the argon detector in the analysis of hydrocarbons; it is sensitive to methane and ethane whereas the argon detector is not. The insensitivity of the flame detector to air and water is of great value in certain applications. The flame detector is particularly effective for the determination of compounds having retention times close to that of the water peak.

### 3. Electron-Capture Detector (C2, C4)

This detection system utilizes an ionizing radiation which provides a source of electrons for a small current between two electrodes when a low voltage is applied to the detector. With a carrier gas, such as nitrogen which has no affinity for electrons, the electron-capture detector current is at its maximum. The electron affinity of many organic compounds is determined primarily by the predominant functional group present in the molecule when this group contains atoms other than carbon or hydrogen. Thus, halogen- or oxygen-containing compounds may cause a significant decrease in the detector current while hydrocarbon components will capture weakly. By proper selection of the potential applied to the cell, classes of compounds may be selectively caused to give a detector response or become transparent to the detector system.

### 4. Cross Section Detector

The cross section detector (C4) is an ionization detector with another gas—hydrogen, helium, or nitrogen—replacing argon as the carrier gas. The detector's response to a particular component depends on the difference between the ionization cross sections of the sample and carrier gas. Thus, it will be insensitive to those compounds having cross sections similar to that of the carrier gas. There is a loss in sensitivity with this change in carrier gas. However, this detector has the advantage of measuring a greater range of sample concentration. Its response is linear from the minimum detectable concentration to 100% of sample vapor.

5. THERMIONIC EMISSION

The sample molecules passing through the detector are ionized by electrons that are emitted from a filament and accelerated across a potential. The bases for detection and determination of percentage concentration are due to the variation in the ionization potential between the sample and the carrier gas. The ionization energy of the electrons is maintained below the energy necessary for ionization of the carrier gas. When helium is used as the carrier gas, all compounds may be detected, since all compounds have ionization potentials below that of helium. Because of the ability to vary the ionization potential, it is possible to block out undesirable compounds. The detector (G5) is independent of temperature and flow and is linear over a large concentration range. A disadvantage is that it must be operated in a vacuum.

Thermionic emission has the advantage of not destroying the sample and, also, organic and inorganic compounds as well as fixed or permanent gases may be analyzed.

## IV. Carrier Gas

The choice of the carrier gas is determined by the type of detector used. Primarily helium is used with the thermal conductivity, thermionic emission, flame ionization, and cross section detectors. Argon is used for the argon ionization detector. Nitrogen is used on the electron-capture detector and may be used with thermal conductivity and cross section detectors. Hydrogen is used as the source along with air in the hydrogen flame detector. Hydrogen may be used with the thermal conductivity units for maximum sensitivity. The flow rates may be as low as fractions of a cubic centimeter per minute for a capillary column or as high as liters per minute for a preparative column. It is advisable that the carrier gas continually flow through the columns in order to maintain stability, prevent contamination, and save reconditioning time.

## V. Sample

The sample can be introduced into the chromatograph in either the gas, liquid, or solid state. Ideally the sample should reach the column in a plug flow. This is defined as occurring when the sample reaches the column undiluted with carrier gas. When dilution of sample with carrier gas occurs lateral tailing may appear. This is in contrast with the Gaussian-type peaks from the plug flow. Maximum efficiency comes from using a plug-type injector with the smallest possible sample consistent with detector sensitivity. Liquid or vapor samples are injected by hypodermic syringe, vacuum extraction apparatus, or reaction chambers. Gas samples are injected with special airtight syringes, or sample valves. The solids are dissolved in a solvent which is then injected into the chromatograph. Solids can also be introduced into the instrument by the ampoule or capsule technique.

## VI. Chromatogram Records

A chromatogram (Fig. 3) is a plot of the detector response versus

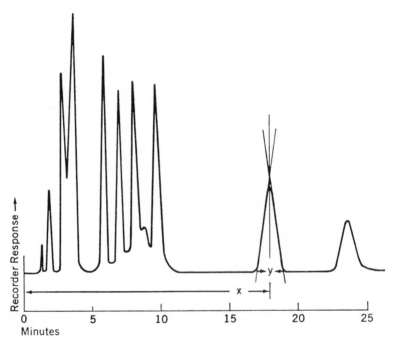

FIG. 3. Chromatogram. Retention volume = retention time × flow. Number of theoretical plates $(N) = 16\left( \dfrac{\text{retention volume}}{\text{peak width}} \right)^2$. $x$ = retention time; $y$ = peak width. (Photograph reproduced with permission of Armed Forces Institute of Pathology, Washington, D. C.)

time or volume of carrier gas. The horizontal direction of a chromatogram is its time axis corresponding to the recorder chart's line of travel. The vertical direction shows deflections of the recorder pen, usually scaled in millivolts, and represents a volume concentration. As carrier gas alone passes through the detector, there is no deflection of the pen from the baseline. But each component of the solute mixture is retarded in its travel through the column to an extent determined by the component's partition coefficient. Thus, the components appear at the detector after various lengths of time, each registering a signal on the detector and causing a deflection of the pen. The distance from zero time to the peak maximum is called the retention time and is characteristic for each solute under the condition of operation.

The chromatogram also supplies valuable information upon which calculation relative to column performance can be based. The column's efficiency can be expressed in terms of its number of theoretical plates and the height equivalent to a theoretical plate. Calculation of the number of theoretical plates makes use of the retention time, $x$, and the amount of band broadening, $y$. The latter is taken as the baseline width intercepted by tangents to the inflection points of the peak. The application of the calculation of column performance will determine the acceptance or rejection of a column to do specific analysis required. Usually 500 theoretical plates per foot is considered to be a usable column.

## VII. Basic Theory

A detailed discussion (B2, D1, G1, G2, G3) of the complex interaction of all the variables in gas chromatograph theory is neither possible nor desirable in a chapter of this type. However, a short presentation of the chromatographic concepts of retention behavior, column efficiency, and resolution is needed for proper utilization of gas chromatographic analysis.

### A. Retention Behavior

In a hypothetical isothermal GLC column with no pressure drop through the column, the characteristic retention volume of a solute at the column temperature is equal to the partition coefficient times the amount of liquid on the column support, plus the volume of gas in the column. The partition coefficient is the ratio of the solute concentration in the liquid phase to that in the gas phase. The gas volume of the column is the volume remaining in the column after the column has been packed. The gas volume of the column is usually small relative to the gas retention volume; consequently, the retention volume will primarily be determined by the partition of the liquid phase. Columns that have high liquid phase loadings will exhibit large retention values.

The partition coefficient varies exponentially with the absolute column temperature, and lower temperatures lead to increased retention. The separation between two peak maxima can be increased by lowering the temperature since the heat of solution is reasonably constant over a range of temperature. Consequently retention volumes may be expressed relative to the retention volume of a standard component on the same column at the same temperature. The relative retention time of any peak is obtained by dividing the retention time of the substance by the retention time of the standard. By utilizing relative retention time the change in retention time will be minimized due to changes in flow rate, temperature, column length, and age of column.

## B. Column Efficiency

Column efficiency is concerned with the retention volume and the shape of the peak eluted from the GLC column. This is commonly expressed in terms of theoretical plates. The number of theoretical plates, $N$, can be determined from measurements on the chromatogram (Fig. 3):

$$N = 16 \left( \frac{\text{retention volume}}{\text{peak width}} \right)^2$$

The peak width is the baseline width intercepted by tangents to the inflection points of the peak. $N$ values of 500 to 50,000 plates may be achieved with packed columns, and $N$ values approaching $10^6$ have been obtained with mile-long capillary columns. Ideally the solutes should elute in sharp narrow peaks; however, experimentally the peaks are spread or broadened because not all of the molecules in each peak move through the column at the same rate as they should if ideal conditions existed. Some molecules travel faster or slower than the average causing "tailing" of the peak. Gas chromatography columns usually operate in the concentration range where the partition coefficient is constant. Ideal conditions assume: (1) that the proportion of the gas and liquid phases are constant throughout the column; (2) that the flow of the moving phase is constant; (3) that the components are carried through the column only by the carrier gas; and (4) that there is instantaneous equilibrium. (Components go in and out of the two phases instantaneously.) The only above condition that can be approached experimentally is that the proportion of the liquid and gas phase is constant throughout the column. Van Deemter discusses the contribution to band-broadening by three other conditions: (1) eddy diffusion—nonuniform flow of moving phase through the column; (2) molecular diffusion—axial diffusion (up or down) of component molecules; (3) resistance to mass transfer—nonequilibrium conditions. The larger the above effects, the less efficient the column. The sum of these three effects is measured by the term height equivalent to one theoretical plate. The height equivalent to a theoretical plate, $H$, is obtained from $N$ and the length of the column, $L$,: $H = L/N$. The smaller the value of these terms, the more plates per column, the more efficient the column.

## C. Resolution

While $N$ is a measure of column performance with regard to the foregoing efficiency factors, the separation of two solutes depends also on their retention behavior, in which $N$ does not enter. Resolution is given for closely spaced peaks by

$$R = \sqrt{N}\left(\frac{x_2}{x_1} - 1\right)$$

where $R$ is the distance between peak maxima expressed as a multiple of the standard deviation of the first peak. The equation for $R$ contains an efficiency term $\sqrt{N}$ and the separation factor $x_2/x_1$. An equivalent expression given in terms of partition coefficient $K$ and the effect of the column characteristic $B$ ($B$ = volume gas/volume liquid) is:

$$R = \sqrt{N}\left(\frac{B + K_2}{B + K_1} - 1\right)$$

To double resolution the column length must be increased by a factor of 4 or $H$ reduced by a factor of 4. Further, the column characteristic $B$ = volume gas/volume liquid can be decreased by increasing the quantity of liquid phase in the column. The latter is more practical for packed columns, but increasing the column length is more practical for capillary columns. Conventional packed columns have $B$ equal to about 5, whereas for capillaries $B$ is greater than 100. Consequently, for any pair of $K$ values or solutes, more plates are required with the capillary column to obtain equivalent separation. For large values of $K$ and large retention, very few plates are required for either type of column. The effect of the column characteristic, $B$, becomes apparent for small $K$ values. This improved resolution is obtained from capillary columns operated at low temperature (increased $K$), whereas faster separations (higher temperatures, lower $K$) can be performed with packed columns. A large $B$ value implies a small amount of liquid phase and correspondingly small sample, as is usual with capillary column.

## VIII. Analytical Procedures

Gas chromatographic procedures furnish the toxicologist with a versatile approach to the solution of his analytical problems. Now it is possible to carry out complex analyses which were formerly difficult, time consuming, and in many instances insoluble by conventional methods. The sensitivity of these procedures provides for rapid screening and determination of specific compounds. This is especially desirable when the toxicologist must analyze a large number of samples for such poisons as alcohol and carbon monoxide. Gas chromatographic procedures increase the toxicologist's capability for screening many chemical agents with a single injection (sample). For example, in 15 minutes a single sample can be screened for the presence of volatile poisons such as ketones, aldehydes, and alcohols. The ability to resolve closely related compounds enables the toxicologist to quickly detect, separate, and identify either singly or in combination many closely related drugs in microgram quantities. The simplicity and rapidity of estimating poisons further affords him the opportunity to study their distribution in the various organs and body fluids. A general schematic approach for the determination of groups of poisons such as gases, volatiles, and drugs can be developed utilizing gas chromatography.

## A. Determination of Gases of Toxicological Significance

The following procedure represents an approach developed at the Armed Forces Institute of Pathology and will be used to illustrate the application of gas chromatography for the determination of gases in samples of toxicological interest. This procedure provides a simple technique for: (a) liberating any gas from biological material; (b) measuring the released gas; (c) introducing the released gas into the gas chromatograph; and finally (d) separating, identifying, and estimating the liberated gas by means of the gas chromatograph. The instruments for liberating gases are the Van Slyke or Natelson microgasometer with a gas-sampling chamber attached to the gas chromatograph by means of a special four-way stopcock illustrated in Figs. 4 and 5. The Van Slyke can be used with samples up to 20 ml whereas the Natelson can analyze samples as low as 0.01 ml.

## B. Determination of Carbon Monoxide in Blood and Tissues

### 1. Preparation of Sample

Blood is diluted 1:10 with distilled water. The dilution of blood yields a more uniform sample and permits identical aliquots to be removed for carbon monoxide content and carbon monoxide capacity. Blood, extracted from tissue, e.g., liver, lung, kidney, etc., also may be utilized. It is advisable to select the specimen containing the most blood. The external surfaces of the tissues should be removed and discarded to preclude contamination. The remaining tissue is diced and distilled water added to extract the blood from the tissue. The quantity of water depends on the amount of blood in the tissue. Ordinarily 20 ml of water produces a satisfactory extract although the final volume in some instances has been as high as 45 ml. The analysis for carbon monoxide is performed on this

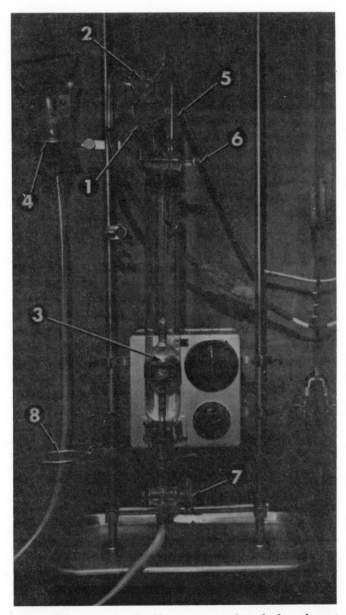

Fig. 4. Van Slyke apparatus for liberating gases from biological specimens and modified for introducing released gas into the gas chromatograph. Stopcock (2) of gas-sampling chamber (1) is a four-way stopcock, 2-mm bore, side arm 90° apart; bore configurations connect any two adjacent side arms (Kontes Glass Co.). (3) Extraction chamber; (5) intake cup; (6) and (7) stopcocks; (4) and (8) positions used during procedure (see text). (Photograph reproduced with permission of Armed Forces Institute of Pathology, Washington, D. C.)

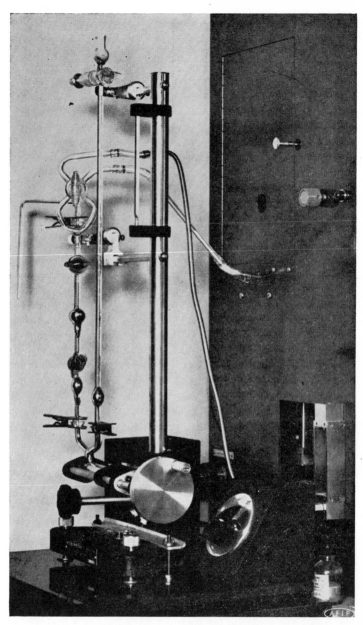

FIG. 5. Natelson Microgasometer for liberating gases from small amounts of biological specimens and modified for introducing released gas into gas chromatograph (see description and source for four-way stopcock of gas-sampling chamber listed in Fig. 4). (Photograph reproduced with permission of Armed Forces Institute of Pathology, Washington, D. C.)

extract. Aqueous tissue extracts prepared from decomposed cases should be examined for the presence of carbon monoxide as soon as possible after preparation because these diluted hemoglobin solutions will deteriorate rapidly, and thus make the results difficult to interpret.

## 2. LIBERATION OF CARBON MONOXIDE FROM SAMPLE

Figure 4 shows a modified Van Slyke apparatus utilized for liberating and introducing the gas sample for analysis. A gas-sampling chamber (1) with a special four-way stopcock (2) has been attached to the waste tube of the extraction chamber (3) of the Van Slyke apparatus. With the mercury reservoir bulb in position (4) the extraction chamber (3) and its bore are completely filled with mercury up to the bottom of intake cup (5). Stopcock (6) is closed and approximately 1 ml of caprylic alcohol is added to intake tube (5). Five to 20 ml of the sample to be analyzed are added to intake cup (5) and admitted into the extraction chamber (3) by opening stopcocks (6) and (7) after the mercury reservoir bulb is lowered to position (8). At this point the sample and about 0.5 ml of the caprylic alcohol have been drawn into the extraction chamber. In order to liberate carbon monoxide from carboxyhemoglobin, either 5 ml of 85% lactic acid *or* 4 ml of 10% $H_2SO_4$ may be used. Either of these solutions is added to intake tube (5) and then drawn into the extraction chamber (3) by turning stopcock (6), taking care not to introduce air. The sample, lactic acid solution, and mercury within the extraction chamber (3) are lowered to about the mid-level point of the extraction chamber. The oxygen normally present plus the added acid is sufficient to release the carbon monoxide from the carboxyhemoglobin. These solutions are preferred to the commonly used ferricyanide reagent for their ease of handling, preparation, and cleaning of the apparatus. The mixture which is under negative pressure is agitated for 2 minutes. The mercury reservoir is raised to position (4). The extracted gases and mixture in the chamber (3) are run up smoothly and when the upper meniscus of the solutions reaches the bifurcation of the gas-sampling chamber (1) it is stopped by turning off the stopcock (6). The recorder motor is turned on. Stopcock (2) is turned to allow the carrier gas (helium) to sweep the released gases present in the gas-sampling chamber (1) into the gas chromatograph. At this point and prior to the elution of the gases from the column, the recorder baseline is adjusted if necessary. After carbon monoxide has emerged from the gas chromatograph column and recorded, stopcock (2) of the gas sampling chamber (1) is turned, thus sealing this chamber from the flow of carrier gas. By the appropriate manipulation of the stopcocks, the solutions are removed first from the neck of the gas-sampling chamber (1) and lowered into the extraction chamber (3) and then ejected through intake cup (5). The system is rinsed with water to clean the apparatus to prepare for the introduction of the next sample.

### 3. MEASUREMENT OF CARBON MONOXIDE CAPACITY

The total quantity of hemoglobin in a specimen is determined by the maximum amount of carbon monoxide the blood or extract can bind. To establish the carbon monoxide capacity usually 5–10 ml of sample are placed in a 30-ml syringe and the remainder of the space filled with carbon monoxide gas. The syringe is then mechanically shaken for about 5 minutes. The unbound carbon monoxide is completely expelled from the syringe. The syringe is then filled with helium and again shaken for a few minutes. Following this, the gas is completely expelled. This procedure is repeated to remove all the physically dissolved carbon monoxide. A suitable aliquot, depending upon the hemoglobin concentration of the carbon monoxide–saturated sample, is transferred to the Van Slyke apparatus and the gas is liberated as described above and introduced into the gas chromatograph for analysis.

### 4. GAS CHROMATOGRAPH

The gas chromatograph routinely used at the Armed Forces Institute of Pathology for the determination of carbon monoxide employs a 8000-ohm thermister-type thermal conductivity unit as the detector and a 1-mv recorder. For the separation of carbon monoxide from other gases, a 2-meter partition column, $\frac{1}{4}$ inch in diameter, packed with Fisher molecular sieve type 5A $\frac{1}{16}$-inch pellets is used. When a new column is prepared and inserted into the instrument, it is activated by heating for several hours at about 190°C. For the routine determination of carbon monoxide, the column temperature is maintained at 75°C and helium employed as the carrier gas at a flow rate of 135 ml/minute. At this temperature and flow rate, carbon monoxide is separated within 5 minutes following introduction of the sample.

### 5. CALCULATION

The per cent carboxyhemoglobin in the specimen is derived by comparing the peak height reading of carbon monoxide content and carbon monoxide capacity. The fact that carbon monoxide content and carbon monoxide capacity are determined in an identical manner serves to nullify any inherent errors arising in the analysis. Therefore, the actual carbon monoxide content value is not necessary except in terms of peak height. The amount of carbon monoxide in the gas sample is calculated by measuring the peak height, i.e., the distance from the center of the base of the peak to its maximum height.

If $A$ = peak height measurement of unsaturated specimen (CO content),

$A_S$ = peak height measurement of saturated specimen (CO capacity),

$V$ = volume of unsaturated specimen, and

$V_S$ = volume of saturated specimen,

then the following formula may be used to establish per cent carboxyhemoglobin in a given specimen:

$$\frac{A \times V_S \times 100}{A_S \times V} = \text{per cent carboxyhemoglobin}$$

This method has been employed in over 2000 aircraft accident cases for the determination of carbon monoxide in specimens consisting of blood and blood extracted from tissue which have been exposed to varied environmental conditions. Blood extracted from tissue and containing as little as 0.5 mg of hemoglobin per ml and containing 10% carboxyhemoglobin has been analyzed satisfactorily. Samples containing concentration of less than 10% carboxyhemoglobin show an analytical error of less than 10% of the determined value, and samples containing carboxyhemoglobin concentrations greater than 10% have an analytical error of less than 5%. No interference from methane, ethane, hydrogen sulfide, acetylene, hydrogen, argon, carbon dioxide, or the products of putrefaction was observed. Although the described procedure is used for the determination of carbon monoxide in blood, it will serve to demonstrate an approach which may be employed to liberate other gases. Other investigators have developed similar procedures for the analysis of gases. Their approaches are summarized in Table IV.

## C. Volatile Poisons

### 1. Introduction

The procedure to be described is used at the Armed Forces Institute of Pathology for the determination of volatile compounds in biological samples. This procedure relies upon the rapid partition which takes place between a volatile compound in solution and the air above it. Harger and co-workers (H1) have demonstrated the feasibility of determining the alcohol concentration in the liquid phase from the analysis of an air sample. They have investigated the partition of alcohol between water, blood, urine, and air. The concentration of alcohol in the air phase is independent of the volume of the solution, but it is influenced primarily by temperature and salt concentration. For alcohol, the partition ratio between blood and air at 37°C is approximately 2000 to 1. For most volatile compounds present in biological samples, the concentration in the

TABLE IV

Gas Chromatographic Procedures for Determination of Gases

| Gas | Sample | Volume of sample | Sample device | Carrier gas | Column | Detector system | References |
|---|---|---|---|---|---|---|---|
| Oxygen Nitrogen Carbon monoxide Carbon dioxide Nitrous oxide | Respiratory | 2–10 ml | Loop | Helium | 5A molecular sieve, charcoal | Thermal conductivity | J1 |
| Oxygen | Water Plasma Blood | 1 ml | Modified Van Slyke | Helium | 5A molecular sieve | Thermal conductivity | R1 L7 |
| Carbon monoxide | Blood | 0.01 ml | Loop | Helium | 5A molecular sieve | Thermal conductivity | D2 |
| Oxygen Nitrogen Methane Carbon monoxide Carbon dioxide | Water | 1–2 ml | Special sample chamber | Helium | Dual column: 30% HMPA, 13X molecular sieve | Double thermal conductivity | S3 |
| Nitrogen Nitrous oxide Nitric oxide (NO) Carbon monoxide Carbon dioxide | Gas | 0.01 ml | Special stopcock | Helium | Silica gel and iodine pentoxide | Thermal conductivity | S1 |
| Carbon monoxide Methane | Gas | 10 $\mu$l | Syringe | Helium Hydrogen | Silocel Firebrick (nickel nitrate) | Flame ionization | P5 |

| | | | | | | | |
|---|---|---|---|---|---|---|---|
| Illuminating gas (natural) Cyclopropane Hydrocarbons | Alveolar air | 5 ml | Syringe | Helium | Di-*N*-maleate and silicone 550 5A molecular sieve | Thermal conductivity | K1 |
| Mercaptans | Water | 1 ml | Loop | Helium | Silicone 200 Tetraisobutylene | Thermal conductivity | L1 |

air phase also is low. However, the capability of gas chromatography to rapidly analyze compounds in parts per billion concentrations makes this technique ideally suited for the analysis of the equilibrated air above the sample. Because of the low concentration of water vapor in the injection samples, there is no interference with the analysis of volatile compounds utilizing the argon ionization detector. Thus, the toxicologist has a method for rapidly screening volatile poisons by simply analyzing a small volume of air removed from the confined space above the sample.

## 2. DETERMINATION OF VOLATILES

### a. General

(1) *Apparatus and operating conditions.* The instrument used at the Armed Forces Institute of Pathology is a Chromalab, Glowall Corporation, gas chromatograph. It is equipped with a beta ionization (radium 226) microdetector. The carrier gas used is argon. A full-scale Leeds and Northrup Speedomax H, 0–50 mv/sec response recorder, with a chart speed of 20 inches/hr is used with the Chromalab. The chromatographic column is a borosilicate coiled glass tube of 5 mm internal diameter, 6 ft in length, and packed with a 42–60 mesh, C-22 firebrick impregnated with 28 gm of liquid to 100 gm of firebrick. The liquid used for impregnation was a mixture of 15 parts by weight of Flexol 8N8 [2,2′-(2-ethylhexamido)diethyldi(2-ethylhexoate)], 10 parts diiosodecylphthalate, and 3 parts polyethylene glycol 600. This column material is available commercially from Beckman Instruments Incorporated, Fullerton, California. The column was preconditioned for 4 hours at 120°C. For injecting samples into the column, a two-way surgical stopcock is attached with a 19-gauge needle penetrating the half-hole silicone rubber stopper at the top of the chromatographic column. This prevents damage to the stopper caused by repeated injections. The stopcock is turned to the closed position after the injection. The sample is injected with a gastight "Hypak" disposable syringe. These syringes have been found to be as satisfactory as the expensive airtight "Hamilton" syringes. Its low cost enables the analyst to discard the syringes when contaminated.

The operating conditions for the determination of volatile compounds were: column temperature 95° ± 5°C, flash temperature 105°C, detector temperature 150°C, high voltage 1.2 kv, relative gain 100, and inlet pressure of argon set at 16 lb at the pressure gauge.

(2) *Analytical procedure.* The samples should be collected in containers stoppered with a puncture-type rubber cap. A recommended container for blood is the "Vacu-tube" containing fluoride as a preservative. Post-mortem specimens such as liver, brain, or other organs can be placed in a small flask with a rubber cap. The unknown specimens and the

standards are put in a water bath until the temperature of the specimens
are at the temperature of the bath (25°C). An airtight syringe is filled
with 1 cc of air and the needle of the syringe is inserted through the
puncture-type rubber cap of the sample container. The barrel of the
syringe is moved up and down a few times to obtain an equilibrated air
sample of 1 cc. The needle is disengaged from the syringe and the
syringe is attached to the two-way stopcock on the top of the chromatograph. The two-way stopcock is opened and the sample is injected into
the flash area of the column. The two-way stopcock is closed. The air
sample which appears as a negative peak will mark the point from which
the retention times of the compounds are determined. A chromatogram
illustrating the capability of this technique to detect and separate five
commonly encountered volatile compounds is shown in Fig. 6.

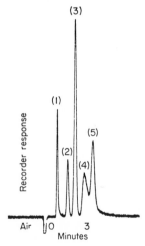

FIG. 6. Separation of five volatile compounds: chromatogram of 1 cc of injected
air sample from above a solution containing: (1) acetaldehyde, 0.04 mg/ml; (2)
formaldehyde, 0.33 mg/ml; (3) acetone, 0.19 mg/ml; (4) methanol, 0.79 mg/ml;
(5) ethanol, 0.79 mg/ml.

The relative retention times of compounds of toxicological interest are
listed in Table V. They are relative to the retention time (2.5 minutes) of
ethanol. In less than 30 minutes after the injection of an unknown air
sample it is possible to determine the presence or absence of those compounds listed in Table V as well as other compounds having boiling points
below 150°C. At the operating conditions described above, some compounds in Table V have almost similar retention times. It is possible to

TABLE V
RELATIVE RETENTION TIMES[a] OF VOLATILE COMPOUNDS STUDIED

| Compound | Relative retention time (min) | Compound | Relative retention time (min) |
|---|---|---|---|
| Acetaldehyde | 0.33 | n-Propanol | 2.25 |
| Ethyl ether | 0.33 | Chloroform | 2.53 |
| n-Hexane | 0.53 | Trichloroethylene | 2.59 |
| Formaldehyde | 0.56 | Propyl acetate | 2.64 |
| Acetone | 0.72 | Ethylene dichloride | 2.86 |
| Methyl alcohol | 0.89 | Isobutyl alcohol | 3.53 |
| Ethyl alcohol | 1.00 | Toluene | 4.19 |
| n-Heptane | 1.05 | Tetrachloroethylene | 4.41 |
| Isopropyl alcohol | 1.19 | n-Butyl alcohol | 4.86 |
| Methyl ethyl ketone | 1.44 | Paraldehyde | 4.97 |
| Ethyl acetate | 1.49 | Amyl acetate | 8.03 |
| Carbon tetrachloride | 1.61 | Xylene | 8.55 |
| Benzene | 2.08 | | |

[a] Relative to ethyl alcohol with a retention time of 2.5 minutes.

resolve these compounds by changing the temperature of the column. For example, to separate n-heptane from ethanol, the column temperature was lowered to 75°C. Now the retention time of ethanol is 8.5 minutes while the retention time of heptane is 7.6 minutes.

For the quantitative analysis of volatile compounds, standards are prepared by adding known amounts to blood containing the same amount of anticoagulant present in the unknown. For qualitative identification aqueous standards are satisfactory.

*b. Determination of Ethanol.* The detection and estimation of ethanol in blood illustrate one application of the above procedure. Standards containing anticoagulants, as in the unknowns, are prepared containing ethanol concentrations of 0.2 mg, 0.5 mg, 1.0 mg, 1.5 mg, etc., until 4.0 mg/ml. Before analyzing the unknown, 1 cc of equilibrated air above the blood standard containing 0.2 mg/ml is injected into the chromatograph to establish the retention time and sensitivity of the instrument. When only ethanol is to be determined, successive 1-cc equilibrated air samples of the unknowns are injected immediately at the end of the alcohol retention time. For those blood samples which show the presence of an ethanol peak, repeat injections are made. These are followed by an injection of air from blood ethanol standards whose peak heights are closest to the unknowns.

*c. Formation of Volatile Compounds.* It is also possible to identify compounds which yield volatile compounds by means of chemical reactions. For example, chloral hydrate is hydrolyzed quantitatively to chloroform in the presence of alkali. Chloroform is determined readily by the above procedure. Figure 7 shows a blood sample containing chloral

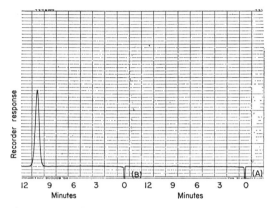

Fig. 7. Identification of chloral hydrate: chromatogram (A) of 1 cc of injected air sample from above a solution of chloral hydrate (1 mg/ml) and chromatogram (B) of 1 cc of injected air sample after the addition of a pellet of sodium hydroxide showing the appearance of chloroform (retention time 11 minutes).

hydrate before and after the addition of a pellet of sodium hydroxide. Likewise, paraldehyde is hydrolzed to acetaldehyde in an acid medium. Figure 8 shows a blood sample containing paraldehyde before and after the addition of 1 drop of concentrated sulfuric acid.

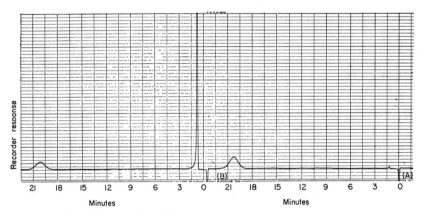

Fig. 8. Identification of paraldehyde: chromatogram (A) of 1 cc of injected air sample from above a solution of paraldehyde (1 mg/ml) showing the paraldehyde peak (retention time 20 minutes) and chromatogram (B) of 1 cc of injected air sample after the addition of concentrated sulfuric acid showing the appearance of acetaldehyde (retention time 0.8 minute) and the reduction of the paraldehyde peak (retention time 20 minutes).

*d. Complex Volatile Mixtures.* This procedure determines the retention volume and the relative quantities of each constituent in a complex mixture of volatile compounds. Thus, the injection of an equilibrated air above a sample containing jet fuel reveals each of the volatile constituents and their relative concentrations (Fig. 9). A specific identification of this

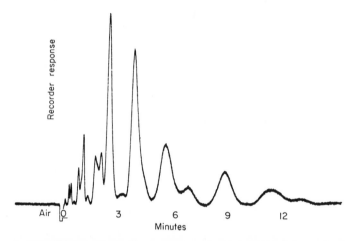

FIG. 9. Identification of complex mixtures: chromatogram of 1 cc of injected air sample from above a water solution of jet fuel showing the separation and peak heights of the volatile components.

fuel can be made by comparing not only the components present but their relative concentrations.

For the identification of vaporizable materials in arson cases, equilibrated air above samples of liquid, cloth, wood, etc., readily can be analyzed and compared with air samples from known fuels.

### 3. REMARKS

The procedure described for the determination of volatile poisons has the following advantages:

(1) There is only one easily measured sample—air. This eliminates errors due to pipetting, contaminating, and mislabeling that can occur in other procedures;

(2) It provides for the analysis of alveolar air samples either from living individuals or at the post-mortem examination;

(3) The quantity of the sample employed in the analysis is extremely small, enabling the analyst to make many duplicate determinations. The sample is still available for quantitative analysis by other chemical methods;

(4) The ease, rapidity, and sensitivity of the procedure makes possible the screening of a large number of samples in a relatively short time. The toxicologist can screen routinely all samples for volatile poisons;

(5) Mixtures of volatile compounds present in the sample can be separated, identified, and quantitatively determined. This is a distinct advantage over some of the nonspecific tests used for the determination of volatile compounds. For example, in this chromatographic procedure, aldehydes and ketones which reduce oxidizing reagents in the determination of ethanol are readily separated from ethanol (Fig. 6);

(6) The chromatogram provides a permanent record of each sample analyzed. This is important for medical legal purposes.

(7) The cost of analysis is reduced because of the saving in man hours, glassware, chemicals, and equipment.

## 4. Procedures of Other Investigators

The procedures used by other investigators for the determination of volatile compounds are summarized in Table VI.

## D. High Molecular Weight Compounds

### 1. Introduction

Considerable progress has been made in the separation and identification of high molecular weight compounds by gas chromatography. This was brought about through the use of columns packed with silicone polymers as substrates and the development of highly sensitive detector systems. Lloyd and co-workers (L2) first demonstrated the feasibility of gas chromatography for isolating, separating, and identifying alkaloids. Since then, other investigators have reported separation and identification of barbiturates, tranquilizers, and other drugs (Table VII). The application of gas chromatography to the analysis of drugs and other high molecular weight compounds will be illustrated by the procedure developed by Kazyak (K2) at the Walter Reed Army Institute of Research using an argon ionization detector.

### 2. Determination of Compounds of Toxicologic Interest

*a. Argon Ionization Detector.* The instrument used is the Barber-Coleman, Model 15, gas chromatograph with a $Sr^{90}$ ionization detector with a 50-mv recorder and argon as the carrier gas. The columns are constructed of U-shaped borosilicate glass, 4 mm ID, 6 ft in length, packed with either 1% SE-30, siloxane polymer substrate, or 3% QF-1-0065(FS

TABLE VI

Gas Chromatographic Procedures for Determination of Volatile Compounds

| Compounds | Technique | Carrier gas | Column | Detector | Reference |
|---|---|---|---|---|---|
| Alcohols Aldehydes Ketones | Blood is extracted with n-propylacetate. 0.35 ml of n-propylacetate injected | Helium | Beckman alcohol column | T/C[a] | C1 |
| Alcohols | 5 ml. blood distilled and 0.1-ml to 0.05-ml aliquot of distillate injected | Helium | Glycerol–tricresyl phosphate mixture | T/C | F2 |
| Volatiles | Mixture of blood, water, and ethylacetate prepared. 1.0 μl of mixture injected | Nitrogen | Castor wax 40% | H$_2$ flame | P3 |
| Alcohol Turpentine Gasoline Kerosene | Direct injection of solvents | Helium | Silicone 550 Carbowax 600 | T/C | C3 |
| Petroleum products | Direct injection of solvents from 0.005 to 0.03 ml | Helium | Silicone | T/C | L6 |
| Volatile compounds | General discussion type paper on application of toxicology with different columns | Helium | Many | T/C | C2 |

[a] T/C, thermal conductivity.

1265) fluorosiloxane polymer on Chromosorb "W". This packing material is commercially available. Prior to its use the column is conditioned at 300°C for 8 hours. During the analysis the detector voltage is set at 1750 volts. The Hamilton microsyringe was used for injecting microliter samples.

(*1*) *Column performance.* The capability of the column to separate and identify compounds of toxicological interest is determined by inject-

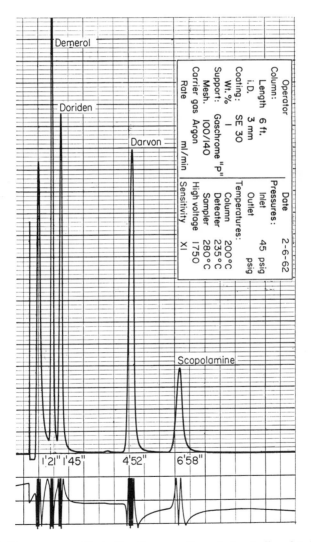

Fig. 10. Chromatogram illustrating the separation of chemically related drugs.

TABLE VII

GAS CHROMATOGRAPHIC PROCEDURES FOR THE DETERMINATION OF HIGH MOLECULAR WEIGHT COMPOUNDS

| Compounds | Technique | Carrier gas | Column | Detector | Reference |
|---|---|---|---|---|---|
| Alkaloids | 1–3 $\mu$l of a 0.5–1.0% solution of alkaloid in methanol, acetone, or chloroform is injected | Argon | SE-30, 2% | $\beta$-ray (Sr$^{-90}$) | L2 |
| Amines | The urine was adjusted to pH 14, extracted with ether, and the ether was re-extracted with a small volume of 1 $N$ hydrochloric acid. The acid extract was made basic with sodium hydroxide and the amines extracted into a small volume of chloroform. The extract was partially evaporated under a stream of nitrogen and an aliquot was injected into the apparatus | Argon | SE-30 $\frac{3}{4}$ or 4% | $\beta$-ray (Sr$^{-90}$) | F1 |
| Amines | Free bases and salts dissolved in ethanol or acetone to make concentration of 10 $\mu$g/$\mu$l 0.1–3 $\mu$g injected | Argon | Carbowax, 5% | $\beta$-ray (Sr$^{-90}$) | P2 |
| Barbiturates | 3–5 ml blood extracted with chloroform. Extract filtered, and a 35-ml portion of filtrate is extracted with 5 ml of 0.45 NaOH. This basic extract is brought to pH 4 with hydrochloric acid, re-extracted with three 15-ml portions of chloroform, and filtered. Concentrate by evaporation. The residue is desiccated *in vacuo* over alumina, washed into a 15-ml centrifuge cone with small portion of warm acetone, by alternate evaporating, and taken up into the micropipette. The entire residue is finally contained in a 50-$\mu$l volume. 1–5 $\mu$l of this solution is injected | Argon | SE-30, 5% | $\beta$-ray (Sr$^{-90}$) | P4 |

| | | | | | |
|---|---|---|---|---|---|
| Alkaloids | 80-mg samples of ground opium were refluxed 15 minutes with 50 ml of methanol, filtered through a sintered glass funnel, and the liquid concentrated in vacuum, dissolved in 1 ml of methanol. 2 μl of solution injected | Argon | SE-30, 1% | β-ray (Sr$^{-90}$) | E1 |
| Phenothiazines | 1-2 μl of a 0.5% solution of the free base in ethyl acetate injected | Argon | SE-30, 2% | β-ray (Sr$^{-90}$) | A1 |
| Tranquilizers | Fifty drugs studied: 1–8 μg of a sample of free compound or its salt in acetone or ethyl alcohol solution were injected into the instrument | Argon | SE-30 | β-ray (Sr$^{-90}$) | P1 |
| Aspirin | Pulverize the tissue extract with 25 ml hot anhydrous methanol. Add 20 ml of 20% boron trifluoride methylating reagent and reflux. Cool and transfer to 50-ml volume flask. Bring to volume and inject 5 μl into instrument | Helium | Carbowax | Thermal conductivity | C7 |
| Pyrolysis products of substituted barbituric acid | A few tenths of a milligram of sample are placed in a platinum vessel and inserted into the pyrolysis chamber. After the argon flow is turned on and the recorder registers a steady baseline, the sample is heated to a high temperature electrically. Free barbituric acids, sodium salts of barbituric acids, and a mixture of a free barbituric acid and anhydrous potassium carbonate were injected | Argon | Silicone 500, 5% | β-ray (Sr$^{-90}$) | N1 |
| Alkaloids and steroids | A peak-shift technique for gas-liquid chromatography is described whereby derivatives are formed directly on the column by following the injection of the parent compound with one injection of either acetic or propionic anhydride | Argon | SE-30, 2% | β-ray (Sr$^{-90}$) | A2 |

TABLE VIII
1% SE-30 Column[a]

| | | 115 | 130 | 150 | 165 | 180 | 200 | 210 | 225 | 250 |
|---|---|---|---|---|---|---|---|---|---|---|
| Conditions | Temperature (°C) | 115 | 130 | 150 | 165 | 180 | 200 | 210 | 225 | 250 |
| | Inlet pressure (psig) | 19 | 20 | 21 | 21 | 26 | 33 | 36 | 39 | 42 |
| | Flow rate (ml/min) | 50 | 50 | 60 | 60 | 65 | 65 | 70 | 80 | 80 |
| Compound | | | | | Retention time (min) | | | | | |
| Ethchlorvynol (Placidyl) | | 1.4 | 1.2 | — | — | — | — | — | — | — |
| Phenethylamine | | 2.1 | 1.7 | — | — | — | — | — | — | — |
| Amphetamine | | 2.4 | 1.9 | — | — | — | — | — | — | — |
| Desoxyephedrine (methamphetamine) | | 3.0 | 2.1 | 1.3 | — | — | — | — | — | — |
| Nicotine | | 6.7 | 4.1 | 2.2 | — | — | — | — | — | — |
| Ephedrine | | 7.5 | 4.2 | 2.3 | 1.2 | — | — | — | — | — |
| Ethynylcyclohexyl carbamate (Valmid) | | 9.5 | 4.9 | 2.5 | — | — | — | — | — | — |
| Warfarin | | — | — | — | 1.7 | 1.2 | 0.8 | — | — | — |
| Methyprylon (Noludar) | | — | 10.8 | 4.3 | 2.9 | 1.8 | — | — | — | — |
| Barbital | | — | — | 4.3 | 2.8 | 1.6 | — | — | — | — |
| Probarbital (Ipral) | | — | — | 5.6 | 3.5 | 1.9 | — | — | — | — |
| Acetophenetidin (Phenacetin) | | — | — | 8.6 | 5.7 | 2.6 | — | — | — | — |
| Meperidine (Demerol) | | — | — | 9.7 | 5.9 | 3.0 | 1.6 | — | — | — |
| Amobarbital (Amytal) | | — | — | 10.9 | 6.0 | 3.0 | — | — | — | — |
| Hydroxyphenamate (Listica) | | — | — | 11.3 | 6.5 | 3.2 | 1.6 | — | — | — |
| Pentobarbital | | — | — | 13.2 | 6.5 | 3.2 | — | — | — | — |
| Pheniramine (Trimeton) | | — | — | 13.0 | 7.5 | 3.6 | — | — | — | — |
| Caffeine | | — | — | 14.7 | 8.1 | 3.8 | — | — | — | — |
| Secobarbital (Seconal) | | — | — | 16.8 | 8.2 | 3.8 | — | — | — | — |
| Diphenhydramine (Benadryl) | | — | — | 16.9 | 9.3 | 4.2 | 1.9 | — | — | — |
| Glutethimide (Doriden) | | — | — | — | 9.1 | 4.2 | 2.0 | 1.6 | — | — |
| Meprobamate (Miltown) | | — | — | — | 10.4 | 4.4 | 1.8 | — | — | — |
| Lidocaine (Xylocaine) | | — | — | 18.0 | 9.9 | 4.5 | 2.1 | — | — | — |
| Prominal (Mebaral) | | — | — | 23.1 | 11.2 | 5.2 | — | — | — | — |
| Antipyrine | | — | — | 20.8 | 11.8 | 5.3 | 2.3 | 1.9 | — | — |
| Aminopyrine | | — | — | — | 12.0 | 5.7 | 2.6 | — | — | — |
| Tripelennamine (Pyribenzamine) | | — | — | — | 14.7 | 6.7 | 3.0 | — | — | — |

| | | | | | | |
|---|---|---|---|---|---|---|
| Methapyrilene (Histadyl) | 14.8 | 6.8 | 3.0 | — | — | — |
| Chlorpheniramine (Chlor-Trimeton) | 16.3 | 6.8 | 3.0 | — | — | — |
| Phenobarbital | 19.2 | 7.8 | 3.3 | — | — | — |
| Procaine | 18.6 | 7.9 | 3.4 | — | — | — |
| Methadone (Dolophine) | — | 12.1 | 4.9 | 3.3 | 2.0 | 2.0 |
| Bromodiphenhydramine (Ambodryl) | — | 12.3 | 4.7 | 3.3 | — | — |
| Propoxyphene (Darvon) | — | 13.8 | 5.5 | 4.0 | — | — |
| Atropine | — | 14.0 | 5.6 | 4.0 | 2.3 | 2.3 |
| Thonzylamine (Anahist) | — | 14.7 | 5.7 | 4.0 | 2.3 | 2.3 |
| Chlorcyclizine (Perazil) | — | 15.5 | 6.3 | 4.4 | 2.4 | 1.3 |
| α-Cyclohexyl-α-phenyl-1-piperidinepropanol (Artane) | — | 16.4 | 6.5 | 4.3 | — | — |
| Tetracaine (Pontocaine) | — | 17.2 | 6.4 | 4.2 | — | — |
| Promazine (Sparine) | — | — | — | 5.5 | 3.0 | 1.6 |
| Librium | — | — | — | 5.6 | 3.0 | 1.6 |
| Scopolamine | — | — | 8.1 | 5.7 | 3.1 | 1.6 |
| DDT (dichlorodiphenyltrichloroethane) | — | 26.0 | 8.5 | 5.5 | — | — |
| Antazoline (Antistine) | — | 20.3 | 8.6 | 6.0 | 3.2 | 1.6 |
| Codeine | — | — | 9.2 | 6.8 | 3.5 | 1.8 |
| Ethylmorphine (Dionin) | — | — | 10.7 | 7.4 | 3.8 | 2.0 |
| Diphenylhydantoin (Dilantin) | — | — | — | 9.0 | 3.9 | 1.9 |
| Chlorpromazine (Thorazine) | — | — | — | 9.7 | 4.6 | 2.2 |
| Morphine | — | — | — | 9.9 | 4.7 | 2.3 |
| Cinchonine | — | — | — | 13.6 | 6.2 | 2.8 |
| Cinchonidine | — | — | — | 14.6 | 6.4 | 2.8 |
| Diacetylmorphine (heroin) | — | — | — | 14.5 | 6.9 | 3.0 |
| Chloroquine | — | — | — | 14.7 | 6.9 | 2.6 |
| Dibucaine (Nupercaine) | — | — | — | 20.9 | 9.1 | 3.1 |
| Quinidine | — | — | — | — | 11.0 | 4.4 |
| Quinine | — | — | — | — | 11.2 | 4.4 |
| Anileridine (Leritine) | — | — | — | 32.2 | 13.9 | 4.4 |
| Meclizine (Bonamine) | — | 20.3 | — | — | 20.3 | 6.2 |
| Strychnine | — | — | — | — | 23.7 | 8.7 |

[a] Injection port and detector were maintained at temperatures higher than that of the column by 50°C and 25°C respectively.

ing into the gas chromatograph 3 $\mu$l of a chloroform solution containing 10 $\mu$g/$\mu$l of the various drugs. The retention times of these compounds are determined at different temperatures and inlet pressures using a SE-30 column (Table VIII) and a QF-1 column (Table IX). Figure 10 illus-

TABLE IX

3% QF-1-0065 (FS 1265) Column[a]

| Conditions | Temperature (°C) | 200 | 240 |
|---|---|---|---|
| | Inlet pressure (psig) | 25 | 30 |
| | Flow rate (ml/min) | 80 | 95 |

| Compound | Retention time (min) | |
|---|---|---|
| Hydroxyphenamate (Listica) | 1.6 | — |
| Warfarin | 2.2 | — |
| Propoxyphene (Darvon) | 2.6 | — |
| Pheniramine (Trimeton) | 2.6 | — |
| Diphenhydramine (Benadryl) | 2.8 | — |
| Barbital | 3.4 | — |
| Methyprylon (Noludar) | 4.0 | — |
| Acetophenetidin (Phenacetin) | 4.4 | — |
| Caffeine | 5.3 | — |
| Amobarbital | 5.6 | — |
| Pentobarbital | 5.8 | — |
| $\alpha$-Cyclohexyl-$\alpha$-phenyl-1-piperidine-propanol (Artane) | 5.9 | — |
| Chlorcyclizine (Perazil) | 6.6 | — |
| Secobarbital | 6.7 | — |
| Thonzylamine (Anahist) | 6.8 | — |
| Aminopyrine | 8.5 | — |
| Procaine | 9.3 | — |
| Glutethimide (Doriden) | 9.3 | — |
| Atropine | 10.8 | — |
| Lidocaine (Xylocaine) | 11.0 | — |
| Phenobarbital | 13.3 | — |
| Librium | 13.5 | — |
| Promazine (Sparine) | 13.6 | — |
| Tetracaine (Pontocaine) | 14.2 | — |
| Antipyrine | 17.3 | — |
| Antazoline (Antistine) | 18.6 | — |
| Scopolamine | 30.1 | — |
| Chlorpromazine (Thorazine) | — | 4.9 |
| Morphine | — | 7.0 |
| Cinchonidine | — | 8.6 |
| Cinchonine | — | 8.7 |
| Chloroquine | — | 10.7 |
| Heroin | — | 12.2 |

[a] Injection port and detector were maintained at temperatures higher than that of the column by 50°C and 25°C respectively.

trates the separation of some related drugs. The determination of retention times at more than one temperature and inlet pressure as well as on two different packed columns provides for a more specific identification of a compound.

(2) *Isolation procedure.* A number of procedures for the isolation of drugs from biological specimens are described in Stewart and Stolman (S2).

The following procedure was used by Kazyak for the gas chromatographic separation and identification of compounds from biological materials. The quantity of specimen should be such that the final residue of the evaporated solvent contains at least 25 $\mu$g of the drug. Initially, a chloroform extraction of body fluids or tissue homogenates at a pH within the range of 4.0–7.5 is made for the isolation of weak acids and neutral and weakly basic compounds. The solvent is filtered through Whatman 41 paper, washed with phosphate buffer pH 7.4, and refiltered through Whatman 41 paper again. This filtration removes small amounts of water which usually contain interfering substances. The solvent is then evaporated to dryness at 55° with a stream of air and the residue is retained for subsequent gas chromatographic analysis. For strong acidic and strong basic compounds, the specimen is adjusted to a pH below 3 for the acidic drugs and above 9 for the basic drugs. The extraction is performed as described above except for the substitution of an appropriate buffer wash. Conjugated basic and amphoteric compounds such as morphine are isolated after an acid hydrolysis. The hydrolyzate is adjusted to pH 8.5–9.0 and extracted with 20% isobutanol in chloroform. The solvent extract is washed with a pH 9 buffer and evaporated to dryness. The residues from the above fractions are taken up in 50 $\mu$l of chloroform. The final solution should contain not less than 25 $\mu$g of the drug.

(3) *Gas chromatographic analysis:*

(*i*) Operating Conditions. Prior to the analysis of an unknown it is desirable to determine the operating conditions of the gas chromatograph. For this purpose, a test solution is prepared containing compounds having early, medium, and late retention times. For example, a suitable mixture is a solution containing 10 $\mu$g/$\mu$l of ephedrine, glutethimide, and phenobarbital in chloroform. The column temperature is set at 165°C and the pressure gauge of the argon tank is set at 21 lb. Three microliters of the mixture are injected and the retention times are recorded and compared with the retention times listed in Table VIII. If they are within 30 seconds, the operating conditions are suitable for the determination of those compounds listed in Table VIII. If they are not within 30 seconds, the pressure is changed so that the retention times are brought into line. Occasionally the temperature of the column is changed to adjust the retention times.

(*ii*) Analysis of the Extract. The presence or absence of any of the drugs listed in Table VIII is determined by injecting three 10-$\mu$l aliquots of the dissolved residue into the gas chromatograph at the column temperatures of 130°C, 165°C, and 225°C. The retention times of any eluted compounds are determined at these three temperatures. The identification of the compound is made from the retention times listed in Table VIII. Even at different temperatures some of the compounds in this table cannot be separated on the 1% SE-30 column. Methyprylon and barbital, antipyrine and aminopyrine, and several other pairs of compounds have similar retention times. Separations of some of these compounds can be made by injecting another aliquot on the 3% QF-1 column (Table IX).

In some instances, quantitative analysis is possible as, for example, the quantitative estimation of glutethimide and meprobamate in serum and urine. For these determinations standard solutions are chromatographed alternately with the extracts of the specimens and the resultant peak areas are compared.

(*iii*) Collection of Eluents. (*a*) Split flow arrangement. Eluents can be collected for subsequent confirmation by ultraviolet spectral analysis or some other suitable method. By means of a split flow arrangement, the effluent gas is divided partly to the detector and partly to a heated collection port which passes out of the apparatus. The emergent gas is bubbled through a small test tube immersed in an ice water bath. Depending on the nature of the eluent, a few milliliters of either dilute acid or alkali or alcohol are placed in the collecting tube to aid in the recovery of the material. If more than one compound is present, several tubes may be prepared, and each tube is held in place at the collection port for as long as the peak of a particular component is being recorded. With the collections complete, the solutions may be transferred to a cuvette and scanned in an ultraviolet spectrophotometer.

(*b*) Preparative gas chromatograph. Preparative gas chromatographic equipment is necessary to collect quantities larger than 0.5 mg of eluent. For this purpose the Beckman Megachrom equipped with eight 6 ft metal columns (⅝ inch ID) connected in parallel was used. In place of the thermal conductivity detector supplied with the instrument, a flame ionization detector was substituted for greater sensitivity. The column contained 1% SE-30 on Anakrom ABS (siliconized Chromosorb "W" supplied by Analabs, Inc.). With this equipment, eluted fractions were sufficiently large to enable melting point determinations and/or preparation of potassium bromide pellets for infrared spectral analysis.

(*iv*) Temperature Programming. The importance of temperature-programming lies in its capacity to separate complex mixtures containing compounds with widely differing boiling points. The column can be heated by passing a high current at low voltage directly through a stainless steel column, by a heater wrapped directly on the column, or by a rapidly circulating hot air oven.

The application of temperature programming in the analysis of high molecular weight compounds of toxicological interest is illustrated by the analysis of opium alkaloids (E1). When the temperature of the column was maintained at 200°C, morphine was poorly separated at this high temperature, while narcotine appeared with considerable tailing. When the temperature of the column was increased linearly with time by a temperature-programming device (F & M Scientific Corp.), e.g., the specimen was injected at 150°C and programming continued at 1.2°C per minute until an upper limit of 250°C had been attained, there was elimination of the tailing and more resolution and better quantification were obtained.

(*v*) Use of Pyrolysis. Pyrolysis with gas chromatography is a technique used to analyze materials which are nonvolatile. A few tenths of a milligram of sample are placed in a platinum vessel and inserted into the pyrolysis chamber. After the argon flow is turned on and the recorder registers a stall baseline, the sample is heated to a high temperature electrically.

This technique can be effectively employed for the determination of poisons. For example, a study of the pyrolysis products of twenty-seven substituted barbituric acids has been reported by Nelson and Kirk (N1). It appears that this technique offers a practical method for the identification of barbiturates and other drugs.

(*vi*) Beta Electron Affinity Detector. Lovelock and Lipsky (L4, L5) reported the development of a detection technique based on the electron affinity of molecular species. Its principal characteristic is variable sensitivity dependent upon the electron absorptivity of the sample molecule. Thus, the detector may be used qualitatively and quantitatively to identify compounds which are separated on a chromatographic column from a knowledge of their retention times and electron absorptivities. Traces of strongly absorbing compounds even in the presence of a large excess of materials having low electron absorptivities can be determined. Types of compounds particularly amenable to this approach include halogenated materials, nitro compounds, polycyclic hydrocarbons, and certain organometallic compounds.

*b. Determination of Pesticides.* The procedure developed by Clark (C5) for the separation and detection of pesticides will illustrate the application of this detector system. Solutions of pesticides of suitable concentration (usually 1 $\mu g/\mu l$) are prepared in ethyl acetate or acetone. One microliter of this solution is injected into a Jarrell-Ash Model 700 Universal Chromatograph equipped with an electron affinity detector. A 4-ft, $\frac{1}{4}$ inch in diameter, stainless steel column was packed with 5% DC-11 silicone grease on 80–100 mesh Chromosorb "W" and placed into the column oven maintained at 165°C. The temperature of the detector and flash was set at 220°C. The uncorrected carrier gas (nitrogen) flow rate was 80 ml/minute. The attenuator of the instrument was set at $3 \times 10^{-9}$ amperage and dc voltage at 12. Table X lists a number of selected chlorinated and phosphorous pesticides and the sensitivity of their detector. Limit of detection is approximately 0.01 ppm for the more highly chlorinated materials and approximately 1.0 ppm for the phosphorous materials such as methyl parathion and parathion.

TABLE X
PESTICIDES BY ELECTRON AFFINITY TECHNIQUE

| Chlorinated hydrocarbon | Detectable sensitivity (ppm) | Organic phosphorus | Detectable sensitivity (ppm) |
|---|---|---|---|
| Methoxychlor | 1.0 | Methyl parathion | 1.0 |
| DDT | 0.1 | Parathion | 1.0 |
| BHC | 0.1 | Trithion | 1.0 |
| Dieldrin | 0.01 | Ronnel | 1.0 |
| Aldrin | 0.01 | Diazinon | 1.0 |
| Metachlor | 0.01 | Malathion | 10.0 |
| | | Guthion | 100.0 |

REFERENCES

(A1) Anders, M. W., and Mannering, G. J. *J. Chromatog.* **7**, 258 (1962).
(A2) Anders, M. W., and Mannering, G. J. *Anal. Chem.* **34**, 730 (1962).
(B1) Bens, M. *Anal. Chem.* **33**, 178 (1961).
(B2) Brandt, W. W. *Anal. Chem.* **33**, 23A (1961).
(C1) Cadman, W. J., and Johns, T. "Gas Chromatographic Determination of Ethanol and Other Volatiles from Blood." Unpublished data present at the 9th Ann. Conf. on Anal. Chem. and Appl. Spectroscopy, Pittsburgh, March, 1958.
(C2) Cadman, W. J., and Johns, T. "The Analysis of Some Vaporizable Materials of Interest to the Laboratory of Criminalistics." Presented at the Symposium on Forensic Chemistry, Am. Chem. Soc., Cleveland, Ohio, April 1960.
(C3) Cadman, W. J., and Johns, T. *J. Forensic Sci.* **5**, 236 (1960).
(C4) Clark, S. J. "Ionization Detectors," Publ. No. 26-750 (A). Jarrell-Ash Co., Newtonville, Massachusetts.
(C5) Clark, S. J. "Gas Chromatographic Analysis of Pesticide Residues Using the Electron Affinity Detector." Jarrell-Ash Co., Newtonville, Massachusetts.

(C6) Condon, R. D. *Anal. Chem.* **31**, 1717 (1959).

(C7) Crippen, R. C., and Freimuth, H. Personal communication.

(D1) Dal Nogare, S., and Chiu, J. *Anal. Chem.* **34**, 890 (1962).

(D2) Dominguez, A. M., Christensen, H. E., Goldbaum, L. R., and Stembridge, V. A. *J. Toxicol. Appl. Pharmacol.* **1**, 135 (1959).

(E1) Eddy, N. B., Fales, H. M., Haahti, E., Highet, P. F., Horning, E. C., May, E. L., and Wildman, W. C. "Identification and Analysis of Opium Samples by Linear-Programmed Gas Chromatography." U.N. Document, ST/SOA/ SER.K/114 (October, 1961).

(E2) Electron Capture Detection. "Chromatofacts: New Developments in the Field of Gas Chromatography." Research Specialties Co., Richmond, California, 1962.

(E3) Ettre, L. S. *J. Chromatog.* **4**, 166 (1960).

(F1) Fales, H. M., and Pisano, J. J. *Anal. Biochem.* **3**, 337 (1962).

(F2) Fox, J. E. *Proc. Soc. Exptl. Biol. Med.* **97**, 236 (1958).

(G1) Golay, M. J. E. *Anal. Chem.* **29**, 928 (1957).

(G2) Golay, M. J. E. Theory of chromatography in open and coated tublar columns with round and rectangular cross-sections. *In* "Gas Chromatography: Proc. 2nd Symposium, Amsterdam, May, 1958" (D. H. Desty, ed.) Butterworths, London, 1958.

(G3) Golay, M. J. E. Theory and practice of gas-liquid partition chromatography with coated capillaries. *In* "Gas Chromatography" (V. J. Coates, H. J. Noebels, and I. S. Fagerson, eds.), p. 1. Academic Press, New York, 1958.

(G4) Golay, M. J. E., and Ettre, L. S. "Golay Column," 5th Anniversary Suppl., Perkin-Elmer Instrument News for Science and Industry, Vol. 13, No. 1a.

(G5) Guild, L. V., Lloyd, M. I., and Aul, F. Performance data on a new ionization detector. *In* "Gas Chromatography, Proc. 2nd Intern. Symposium, East Lansing, Michigan, June, 1959" (H. J. Noebels, N. Brenner, and R. F. Wall, eds.), p. 91. Academic Press, New York, 1960.

(H1) Harger, R. N., Raney, B. B., Bridwell, E. G., and Kitchel, M. F. *J. Biol. Chem.* **183**, 197 (1950).

(J1) Jay, B. E., and Wilson, R. H. *J. Appl. Physiol.* **15**, 298 (1960).

(J2) Johns, T. The behavior of the solid support in gas-liquid partition chromatography. *In* "Gas Chromatography" (V. C. Coates, H. J. Noebels, and I. S. Fagerson, eds.), p. 31. Academic Press, New York, 1958.

(J3) Johnson, R. E. "Gas Chromatography Detectors: Progress in Industrial Gas Chromatography," Vol. 1. Plenum Press, New York, 1961.

(K1) Kade, H., and Abernethy, R. *J. Forensic Sci.* **6**, 125 (1961).

(K2) Kazyak, L. (Walter Reed Army Institute of Research, Washington, D. C.) Personal communication (1963).

(L1) LeRosen, H. D. *Anal. Chem.* **33**, 973 (1961).

(L2) Lloyd, H. A., Fales, H. M., Highet, P. F., Vanden Heuvel, W. J. A., and Wildman, W. C. *J. Am. Chem. Soc.* **82**, 3791 (1960).

(L3) Lovelock, J. E. *J. Chromatog.* **1**, 35 (1958).

(L4) Lovelock, J. E. *Anal. Chem.* **33**, 162 (1961).

(L5) Lovelock, J. E., and Lipsky, S. R. *J. Am. Chem. Soc.* **82**, 431 (1960).

(L6) Lucas, D. M. *J. Forensic Sci.* **5**, 236 (1960).

(L7) Lukas, D. S., and Ayres, S. M. *J. Appl. Physiol.* **16**, 371 (1961).

(M1) McFadden, W. H. *Anal. Chem.* **30**, 479 (1958).

(N1) Nelson, D. F., and Kirk, P. L. *Anal. Chem.* **34**, 899 (1962).

(P1) Parker, K. D., Fontan, C. R., and Kirk, P. L. *Anal. Chem.* **34**, 757 (1962).
(P2) Parker, K. D., Fontan, C. R., and Kirk, P. L. *Anal. Chem.* **34**, 1345 (1962); **35**, 356 (1963).
(P3) Parker, K. D., Fontan, C. R., Yee, J. L., and Kirk, P. L. *Anal. Chem.* **34**, 1234 (1962).
(P4) Parker, K. D., and Kirk, P. L. *Anal. Chem.* **33**, 1378 (1961).
(P5) Porter, K., and Volman, D. H. *Anal. Chem.* **34**, 748 (1962).
(R1) Ramsey, L. H. *Science* **129**, 900 (1959).
(S1) Smith, N., and Lesninil, D. G. *Anal. Chem.* **30**, 1217 (1958).
(S2) Stewart, C. P., and Stolman, A., eds. "Toxicology: Mechanisms and Analytical Methods," Vol. 1. Academic Press, New York, 1960.
(S3) Swinnerton, J. W., Linnenbom, J. J., and Cheek, C. H. *Anal. Chem.* **34**, 483, 1509 (1962).
(T1) Tenney, H. M. *Anal. Chem.* **30**, 2 (1958).

# Aliphatic Alcohols

by Rolla N. Harger* and Robert B. Forney†

*Indiana University School of Medicine, Indianapolis, Indiana*

* Professor Emeritus of Biochemistry and Toxicology.
† Professor of Toxicology.

# I. Introduction

For the most part, this chapter will review publications on ethanol and its homologues of interest to toxicologists, which have appeared since 1954. However, in order to interpret some of the findings in these papers, it will occasionally be necessary to refer to earlier publications on the same phase of the subject. For the literature prior to 1954, the reader is referred to the excellent, comprehensive monograph, *Blutalkohol,* by Elbel and Schleyer (E4), and to briefer reviews by Muehlberger (M15), Harger and Hulpieu (H13), Friedemann and Dubowski (F15), and Harger (H9).

In this chapter the unmodified word *alcohol* refers to *ethanol.* To minimize the use of fractions, the concentration of alcohol will be expressed as *milligrams per cent* (mg%), which commonly means milligrams per 100 ml of fluid or per 100 gm of tissue. To convert mg% to ordinary per cent, divide by 1000; to convert mg% to parts per thousand (per mil, %o), divide by 100.

# II. "Endogenous" Alcohol

Beginning with Ford in 1858 (F4), many investigators have published results of analyses made on distillates of body materials which they interpreted as indicating the presence of traces of alcohol in normal body tissues and fluids and in concentrations ranging from 1 to 10 mg%. In 1932, Gettler *et al.* (G5) reported the isolation from 28 kg of pig's brain of a droplet of a clear fluid which exhibited typical physical and chemical properties of ethanol. In 1935, Harger and Goss (H12) reported that prolonged steam-distillation of very fresh body materials will continue to bring over dichromate-reducing material, in quantities which diminish very slowly. Thus, most of this volatile, reducing material is certainly not

preformed ethanol and the maximum figure for preformed alcohol should
be the difference between the "alcohol" in fraction 1 minus the "alcohol"
in fraction 2. This difference is further reduced by concentrating and
purifying the two fractions. On this basis, they reported maximum figures
for "normal" alcohol ranging from 0.004 to 0.227 mg%. In 1939, these
findings were confirmed by Gettler's pupil, Umberger (U1), using two
analytical methods which are more specific for ethanol. Since this part
of Umberger's study was published only in his thesis, we have sum-

TABLE I
EFFECT OF PROLONGED DISTILLATION ON YIELD OF "NORMAL ALCOHOL"[a,b]

| Fraction[c] | Liver[d] | Blood[e] | Blood[f] |
|---|---|---|---|
| No. 1 | 1.36 | 9.2 | 4.0 |
| No. 2 | 1.07 | 5.8 | 2.5 |
| No. 3 | 1.36 | 8.9 | 1.7 |
| No. 4 | 3.75[g] | 4.6 | — |
| No. 5 | — | 3.5 | — |
| No. 6 | — | 1.7 | — |

[a] Selected from data published by Harger and Goss (H12) and Umberger (U1).
[b] Results expressed as mg% "alcohol."
[c] The volume of distillate was: H. & G., 1 ml per gm of tissue; U., dichromate method, 8 ml per ml of blood; U., alkoxy method, blood heated to dryness in a stream of $CO_2$, then water added before the next analysis.
[d] Harger and Goss: $K_2Cr_2O_7$ in 17 $N$ $H_2SO_4$; excess $K_2Cr_2O_7$ titrated.
[e] Umberger: $K_2Cr_2O_7$ in 5 $N$ $H_2SO_4$; acetic acid formed distilled and titrated.
[f] Umberger: Alkoxy reaction with 70% HI; alkyl iodide → $HIO_3$; KI added and liberated iodine titrated.
[g] Very rapid distillation.

marized in Table I the results of two of his experiments and of one experiment by Harger and Goss. Umberger also steam-distilled 3 kg of
sheep's blood, discarded the first 3 liters of distillate, and concentrated
and purified the second 3-liter fraction of the distillate. The final concen-
trate of 2 ml yielded typical color reactions for ethanol.

In a 1954 publication (G14), Umberger stated:

> Experimental work on the so-called normal alcohol (U1) demonstrated that
> the ethyl alcohol isolated from normal tissue by Gettler *et al.* (G5) was
> produced in the tissue distillation process. The fact that the normal alcohol
> increased with the increase in ammonia liberated during the distillation led
> to the postulation that the alcohol was formed by hydrolysis of compounds
> containing the amino linkage.

From Table I, it is evident that one can increase the amount of "endogenous" alcohol several fold by simply increasing the volume of distillate per gram of body material analyzed.

With the advent of the alcohol dehydrogenase (ADH) enzyme method, which is almost specific for ethanol, the usual procedure yields a blank of zero. However, using up to one hundred times the usual aliquot of blood, the following findings of "endogenous" alcohol have been reported for blood: Bucher and Redetzki (B22), 0.24 mg%; Marshall and Fritz (M5), "a very small fraction of 1 mg. percent"; Redetzki and Johannsmeier (R5), 0.15 mg%; and Lundquist and Wolthers (L14), eighteen analyses with nine subjects, average, 0.12 mg%, range, 0.035–0.26 mg% (one sample, 0.55 mg%).

Much higher levels of "endogenous" alcohol have recently been reported by McManus *et al.* (M9), using a novel method of separating the volatile materials from tissues. They homogenized equal parts of the tissue and water and lyophilized (freeze-drying under high vacuum) the mixture, condensing the distillate at a low temperature. The distillate was then analyzed by an ADH method. By this procedure they found "endogenous" alcohol values ranging from 1.1 to 6.7 mg%, averaging 3.8 mg%. A product having the properties of ethyl-3,5-dinitrobenzoate was formed from an ingredient of the distillate. It would be interesting to see if further "alcohol" could be evolved by adding water to the freeze-dried residue and analyzing the second distillate, which is analogous to the procedure used by Harger and Goss and by Umberger.

In 1957, Plesso and Fuskov (P9) reported that the "endogenous" blood alcohol of schizophrenics may reach 21–41 mg%, as compared with 9 mg% for control subjects. They used an acid-permanganate method for their analyses.

A 1961 review paper by Lester (L2) gives a somewhat incomplete presentation of the published work on "endogenous ethanol." He was inclined to accept a figure of about 2 mg% as the normal level of endogenous alcohol. He even speculated on the hourly formation of ethanol in the body which will maintain this level in the blood, and calculated that it would be around 1.6 gm/hour for a 70-kg person, "accounting for some 14 to 20 per cent of the basal energy requirement." Lundquist and Wolthers made a similar calculation from their data and arrived at an hourly production in the body of only about 0.15 gm of ethanol, which they think may be due to intestinal fermentation. In the next issue of the journal, after the one which contained Lester's review paper, he published an account of his experimental study on this question of "endogenous" alcohol (L3). In this study he used a gas chromatograph fitted with a flame ionization chamber which, as mentioned in Section IX,E, he stated will detect as little as 0.002 $\mu$g of ethanol. With this instrument he analyzed 7-ml samples of alveolar air from twenty-five non-drinking subjects. The concentrations of "endogenous" alcohol which he found, calculated from the accepted 2100:1 blood:alveolar air ratio as blood alcohol level, were: ten subjects, none; seven subjects, 0.05 mg%; five subjects, 0.10 mg%; and three subjects, 0.15 mg%. Nitrogen, placed in the peritoneal space of nonalcoholic rats, was analyzed by this gas chromatograph method. The result indicated a body concentration of "endogenous" alcohol of 0.13 mg%. However, when a homogenate of rat liver was distilled and the concentrated distillate equilibrated with nitrogen, the gas chromatograph analysis indicated a concentration of 0.90 mg% alcohol in the liver tissue. This would seem to confirm the observations of Harger and Goss (H12) and Umberger (U1) that distillation of body tissues and fluids yields artifact "alcohol." In his second paper, Lester stated:

> It is concluded that ethyl alcohol may be present in humans in concentrations up to 1.5 mg. per liter (0.15 mg%) but whether this alcohol is of endogenous origin is unresolved; even if such formation were endogenous, its fraction of the basal metabolic rate would not exceed 1 per cent.

Lester's experimental findings for blood agree quite well with those of four earlier workers: Harger and Goss, 0.0–0.027 mg%; Marshall and Fritz, "a very small fraction of 1 mg. per cent"; Redetzki and Johannsmeier, 0.15 mg%; Lundquist and Wolthers, 0.035–0.26 mg%.

## III. Absorption of Alcohol

### A. Factors Affecting Speed of Absorption of Ingested Alcohol

While the blood alcohol peak may slightly precede complete alcohol equilibrium between stomach contents and the remainder of the body, published data indicate that absorption is practically complete when the blood alcohol maximum is reached.

### 1. Food in Stomach

Tuovinen's extensive studies with five subjects, published in 1930 (T6), still serve as a model for subsequent investigations of the effect of food on the blood alcohol curve. Tuovinen's subjects ingested 60 ml of alcohol (0.68–0.78 gm/kg), fasting, or immediately after eating. When they ate 610 gm of cooked beef, 132 gm of butter, or 1100 gm of boiled potatoes, the blood alcohol peak was usually delayed 1 or 2 hours and its height averaged only about half of that of the curve without food. Olive oil (50 gm) had little effect. However, the time for complete disappearance of the alcohol would seem to be about the same in the control and food experiments, although the analyses were not continued to zero blood alcohol.

Bayly and McCallum (B3) had subjects ingest, during 100 minutes, 1.65 gm/kg of alcohol as 5% beer, either fasting or after a "substantial meal." The results (Table VI, Section V) show that food somewhat shortened the time between the end of drinking and the blood alcohol peak and reduced the rise in blood alcohol after drinking ceased. As shown by Fig. 4, Section V, for a given dose of alcohol per kilogram, the blood alcohol peak tended to be slightly lower in the food experiments.

Cordebard (C16) has published urine alcohol curves for one subject who, without food, drank 0.5 gm/kg of alcohol either as rum diluted to 19%, 11% wine, or 6.8% beer. The three fasting curves, shown in Fig. 1(I), are almost identical, except that the peak of urinary alcohol was reached

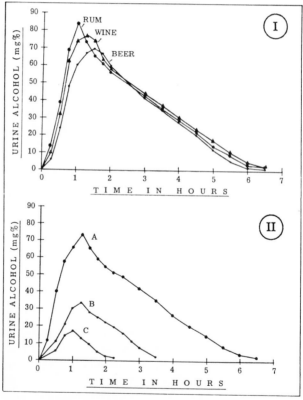

Fig. 1. Urine alcohol–time curves for a subject who ingested, during about 15 minutes, 0.5 gm/kg of alcohol. (I) Rum, wine, or beer; no food for 8 hours prior to drinking. (II) Wine: A, taken 8 hours after last meal; B, taken during a meal; C, taken just after a meal. Redrawn from Cordebard (C16).

slightly earlier after drinking rum. When the wine drinking was done during a meal, the urine alcohol maximum was only about half of that in the fasting experiments; and drinking just after a meal decreased the urine alcohol peak still more. The results are given in Fig. 1(II), and show that drinking just after a meal also very greatly reduced the duration of the urine alcohol curve as compared with the results without food. Cordebard calls this effect "fixation of alcohol." Alcohol ingestion with, or after, food caused a reduction in the total urinary excretion of alcohol, which was about parallel to the drop in the concentration of alcohol in the urine. With increase in the alcohol intake, the food effect was very much less. Bogen (B10), in discussing similar findings by earlier investigators, suggested that the more rapid disappearance of alcohol, when taken with food, may be due to destruction of alcohol within the gastrointestinal tract by certain microorganisms there, leaving less to be absorbed.

## 2. DILUTION

Bayly and McCallum's subjects who received the same dose of alcohol as whiskey diluted to 20% or as 5% beer had about the same average blood alcohol peaks from the two (see Fig. 4). Pihkanen (P7) gave twelve male subjects 1 gm/kg of alcohol as 32.6% brandy or 3.6% beer, in six equal doses during 1 hour. Blood alcohols at the end of the drinking period were generally definitely higher in the subjects receiving brandy. They were about the same 1, 2, and 3 hours later. In Tuovinen's experiments (T6) the blood alcohol peak from 5% or 20% alcohol was usually definitely higher than from 40% or 60% alcohol, probably due to the irritating effects of the last two. That ingestion of beer produces a lower blood alcohol curve than that from the same dose of alcohol as spirits has been reported by Haggard *et al.* (H3) and by Goldberg (G12). This may be due to the dextrins in beer, which would be analogous to the simultaneous ingestion of food and alcohol.

## 3. STRESS

Exercise delays the absorption of alcohol, according to experiments by Hebbelinck (H18) and by Garlind *et al.* (G1). Hebbelinck also reported that stress caused by solving problems in arithmetic and distaste due to ingestion of a warm solution of alcohol both retarded the absorption of alcohol.

## 4. HABITUATION

Troshina (T5) found that, with rats made very tolerant to alcohol by prolonged daily ingestion, the average fraction of administered alcohol remaining in the gastrointestinal tract 3 hours later rose from 17% at the start to 58%.

## B. Other Avenues of Absorption

### 1. THROUGH THE SKIN (Ludin, L12)

The backs of six nondrinking men were thoroughly rubbed for 15 minutes with 70–80% alcohol in the form of a camphor spirit or Cologne water. Blood alcohol determinations made before and 1–2½ hours after the treatment showed no change from the normal blank in six analyses and a rise of only 1–4 mg% in the remaining seven analyses.

### 2. BY INHALATION

Hogberg (H24) investigated the matter of three drivers who claimed that their blood alcohol levels of 144–176 mg% were due to inhalation of alcohol from shellac solutions used in their work. Tests at the end of a working day showed no accumulation of alcohol in their blood. Earlier, Lester and Greenberg (L4) reported that prolonged inhalation of air containing 0.9% alcohol vapor, which is very irritating, caused no significant accumulation of alcohol, except during very drastic hyperventilation, when the blood alcohol level rose to 45 mg% in 3–5 hours.

## IV. Distribution of Absorbed Alcohol

### A. Blood Source and Alcohol Level

In 1934, Haggard and Greenberg (H2) described an experiment with one dog, which received 3 gm/kg of alcohol by stomach tube, where they determined the alcohol level in heart blood and femoral vein blood during the following 5½ hours. They reported that 30 minutes after the alcohol was given, the level of alcohol in femoral vein blood was only 47% of that in heart blood, and that this lag persisted, in diminishing degree, for more than 1½ hours. Harger *et al.* (H14) and Forney *et al.* (F6) repeated this type of experiment using thirteen to seventeen dogs. They confirmed this lag in the alcohol level of peripheral venous blood during active absorption, but found somewhat higher venous/heart blood alcohol ratios, which approached unity in about 1 hour after alcohol administration. Table II presents the data from these three studies.

Haggard and Greenberg also reported that the alcohol level of jugular vein blood and of skin capillary blood did not lag significantly behind that of arterial blood during the rising blood alcohol phase. In the experiments by Forney *et al.*, where they sacrificed the dogs just 10 minutes after administering 3 gm/kg of alcohol, the alcohol level in heart blood paralleled

TABLE II
Ratio of Alcohol Levels in Heart Blood and Saphenous Vein[a]
Blood of Dogs at Various Intervals after Oral Administration[b,c]

| Number of dogs used | | | Saphenous blood/heart blood alcohol ratio | | |
|---|---|---|---|---|---|
| | | | | F. *et al.* & H. *et al.* (F6, H14) | |
| H. & G. (H2) | H. *et al.* & F. *et al.* (H14, F6) | Time after administration | H. & G. (H2) | Average | Range |
| — | 13 | 10 min | — | 0.71 | 0.52–1.02 |
| — | 17 | 15 min | — | 0.83 | 0.67–0.96 |
| 1 | 17 | 30 min | 0.47 | 0.91 | 0.79–1.02 |
| 1 | 17 | 1 hr | 0.73 | 0.99 | 0.87–1.11 |
| 1 | — | 1½ hr | 0.89 | — | — |
| — | 17 | 2 hr | — | 1.01 | 0.97–1.10 |
| 1 | — | 2½ hr | 0.95 | — | — |
| — | 17 | 3 hr | — | 0.99 | 0.88–1.04 |
| 1 | — | 3½ hr | 0.94 | — | — |

[a] Haggard and Greenberg used femoral vein blood. With some of their dogs, Harger *et al.* used both saphenous and femoral vein blood, and found them to have practically the same alcohol levels.

[b] Data tabulated from Haggard and Greenberg (H2); Harger *et al.* (H14) (15-minute to 3-hour experiments); and Forney *et al.* (F6) (10-minute experiments).

[c] Dosage: Haggard and Greenberg, 3 gm/kg; Harger *et al.*, 1–4 gm/kg; Forney *et al.*, 3 gm/kg.

that of the brain, while the level in saphenous blood lagged far behind (Fig. 2). Harger *et al.* (H10) analyzed sixty-nine pairs of simultaneously drawn samples of cubital vein and fingertip blood from twenty-seven human subjects, withdrawn within 2 hours after the end of drinking. The data are given in Fig. 3. Where the samples were taken less than 70 minutes after the last drink (thirty-four pairs) the fingertip blood alcohol level exceeded that of the cubital vein by an average of 7.5% and in seven of the thirty-four pairs the excess ranged from 15 to 22%. With these thirty-four pairs of blood, all, or most, of the drinking was finished 60 minutes before the time of taking the samples. Had most of the drinking been done within 15 to 30 minutes of drawing the blood samples, the capillary-venous differences would have been much greater.

An even greater lag in alcohol level occurs in the peripheral venous blood from the foot, according to McCallum and Scroggie (M8). They analyzed simultaneously drawn samples of blood from the cubital vein and from a vein in the foot at various intervals following a beer-drinking period lasting 54–150 minutes. In fourteen cases where the average interval between the end of drinking and withdrawal of blood samples was

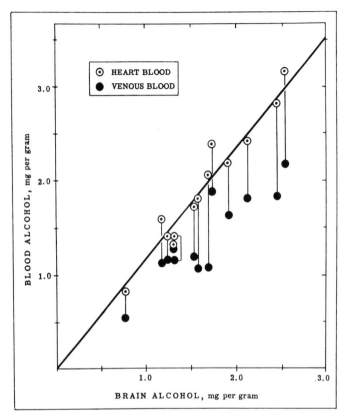

Fig. 2. Alcohol levels in heart blood, saphenous vein blood, and brain of thirteen dogs killed 10 minutes after receiving, by stomach, 3.0 gm/kg of alcohol. Each line indicates a pair of blood samples drawn simultaneously. From Forney, Hulpieu, and Harger (F6).

20 minutes (4–48 minutes), the alcohol level in the foot vein blood was 10–35% (average 20%) below that of the cubital vein blood.

Since the level of brain alcohol is controlled by that of arterial blood but, during active absorption, *not by that of cubital vein blood,* many published blood alcohol curves derived from analyses of cubital vein blood are erroneously low during the rising phase. Unfortunately, this holds for several of the recent studies which we will review in the following pages.

## B. Distribution within the Blood

### 1. Plasma/Whole Blood Ratio

Gruner (G18) analyzed whole blood, plasma, and serum from eight

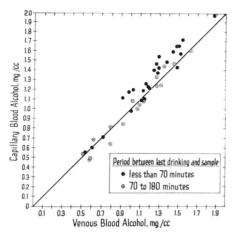

FIG. 3. Comparison of levels of alcohol in cubital vein blood and fingertip capillary blood. The data represent sixty-nine pairs of samples from twenty-seven human subjects. From Harger, Forney, and Baker (H10).

subjects, and also whole blood to which separated plasma had been added to give a lower hematocrit. Varying the hematocrit from 36.3 to 59.6 caused the plasma/whole blood ratio to increase from 1.18 to 1.26.

## 2. SERUM/WHOLE BLOOD RATIO

Three recent studies give the following serum/whole blood alcohol ratios: Gruner (G18), range, 1.13–1.17, average, 1.16; Illchmann-Christ (I1), Widmark method, $1.17 \pm 0.06$; Dotzauer *et al.* (D4), ADH method, $1.12 \pm 0.006$.

Krauland *et al.* (K19, K20) reported that long storage in sterile ampules of blood without added fluoride results in considerable hemolysis, although there is practically no drop in total alcohol present. This hemolysis makes a larger proportion of "serum" and, to calculate the whole blood level from the serum level, one should not divide by the usual factor of 1.2, but by a lower factor. A formula for the change of factor with time is given. On using this formula, they found practically no drop in whole blood alcohol during storage up to 600 days.

Hallermann *et al.* (H7) reported average clot/whole blood alcohol ratios of 0.75–0.79, with a rather wide range of variation. On rolling the separated clot over filter paper and analyzing the core and outside of the clot, the alcohol content of the outside portion tended to be a little higher than that of the core. From the wide range of clot/whole blood alcohol ratios which they found, Hallermann *et al.* question the reliability of estimating the level of alcohol in whole blood from analysis of the clot.

## C. Blood/Brain Ratio

### 1. ANIMAL EXPERIMENTS

Gettler and Freireich (G3), Harger *et al.* (H15), Gettler *et al.* (G4), and Forney *et al.* (F6) have conducted studies of the blood/brain alcohol ratio of dogs, which received various doses of alcohol, orally or intravenously, and were sacrificed for analysis at certain time intervals following alcohol administration. The data from these four studies, employing a total of 102 dogs, are presented in Table III.

It will be noted that, for the first four groups of dogs, there is good agreement as regards average blood/brain alcohol ratio and also the range of this ratio, except that the range for group 2 is narrower than the others. With the first three groups a period of 1–12 hours had elapsed between alcohol administration and death of the animal, so that there was no longer a lag in the alcohol level of the venous blood used with groups 1 and 2. With group 4 the time interval was only 10 minutes, but heart blood, drawn just before quickly killing the animal, was used. As mentioned earlier, heart blood is always in alcohol equilibrium with brain.

In group 5 the blood/brain alcohol ratio is distinctly below the ratios of groups 1–4. With these dogs, active absorption of alcohol was progressing and the venous blood used exhibited the usual lag in alcohol level for this period. Had we used skin capillary blood, or heart blood, the ratios would have been close to those of groups 1–4.

In group 6, on the other hand, the average blood/brain alcohol ratio is significantly higher than the ratios of groups 1–4, in spite of the fact that heart blood was used. To explain this apparent anomaly, we have suggested (H9) that the higher blood alcohol here is due to the manner of killing the dogs, which was by exposure to carbon monoxide. Here death is by no means instantaneous, and the peripheral circulation usually fails before the heart stops beating. If, during the last few heart beats, the blood entering the heart contained an abnormally high proportion of venous return from the viscera, which, during active absorption, has a higher alcohol level than blood in the rest of the body, this would leave blood in the heart containing a higher level of alcohol than that in the heart just prior to exposing the dog to carbon monoxide. With the animals in groups 1, 2, 4, and 5, the blood sample was drawn *just prior* to quickly killing them by a blow on the head.

The almost unbelievable speed with which brain tissue attains alcohol equilibrium with arterial blood and the lag in alcohol uptake by muscle tissue are strikingly demonstrated by experiments conducted by Hulpieu and Cole (H29). In these experiments, rabbits received 0.52 gm/kg of alcohol by injections in the ear vein during a period of 20 seconds

TABLE III

BLOOD/BRAIN ALCOHOL RATIO OF DOGS

| Investigators | Dog group | Number of dogs | Alcohol Given | | | | Blood/brain ratio | |
|---|---|---|---|---|---|---|---|---|
| | | | Route | Dosage (gm/kg) | Time interval[a] | Blood used | Average | Range |
| Harger et al.[b] | 1 | 30 | Oral | 1–3 | 1–12 hr | Venous | 1.17 | 0.83–1.48 |
| Harger et al. | 2 | 8 | IV | 3 | 2–3 hr | Venous | 1.20 | 1.13–1.36 |
| Gettler et al.[c] | 3 | 20 | Oral | 1–5.5 | 1–3½ hr | Heart | 1.19 | 0.77–1.45 |
| Forney et al.[d] | 4 | 13 | Oral | 3 | 10 min | Heart | 1.17 | 0.99–1.40 |
| Harger et al.[b] | 5 | 15 | Oral | 0.5–6.0 | 15–30 min | Venous | 1.03 | 0.86–1.31 |
| Gettler et al.[c] | 6 | 16 | Oral | 1–5 | 7–47 min | Heart | 1.38 | 0.95–2.09 |

[a] Time between alcohol administration and sacrifice of animal.
[b] Harger et al. (H15); peripheral venous blood, just ante mortem.
[c] Combined data from Gettler and Freireich (G3) and Gettler et al. (G4); heart blood, post mortem.
[d] Forney et al. (F6); heart blood, just ante mortem.

TABLE IV

AVERAGE ALCOHOL LEVELS IN BLOOD, BRAIN AND MUSCLE
AFTER INTRAVENOUS INJECTION; EFFECT OF ADRENALINE[a]

| Time after alcohol | | Alcohol only[b] | | | | Alcohol after adrenaline[c] | | |
|---|---|---|---|---|---|---|---|---|
| | Rabbits | Blood (mg%) | Brain (mg%) | Muscle (mg%) | Rabbits | Blood (mg%) | Brain (mg%) | Muscle (mg%) |
| 30 sec | 2 | 124 | 168 | 32 | 2 | 881 | 444 | 9 |
| 45 sec | 1 | 93 | 126 | 32 | 1 | 363 | 331 | 11 |
| 1 min | 2 | 104 | 133 | 42 | 4 | 510 | 529 | 7 |
| 2 min | 2 | 86 | 86 | 43 | 2 | 128 | 137 | 14 |
| 5 min | 3 | 79 | 75 | 51 | 3 | 101 | 100 | 36 |

[a] Condensed from data published by Hulpieu and Cole (H29).

[b] Alcohol dosage, 0.52 gm/kg, as 33% solution injected in ear vein over a period of 20 seconds.

[c] Adrenaline dose, 0.5 ml of 1–10,000 solution, IV during 11 seconds, followed by alcohol in 2 minutes.

and were decapitated at intervals ranging from 30 seconds to 5 minutes later. Drainage blood, brain, and muscle tissue were analyzed for alcohol. The results are given in Table IV. At alcohol equilibrium throughout the body, the level of blood alcohol from 0.52 gm/kg should have been about 70 mg%. Thirty seconds after the alcohol was given, the levels in blood and brain were about double this figure, but the muscle tissue had taken up only about half of its quota of alcohol. The blood, in fact, had already passed its peak alcohol level. Within 4½ minutes, blood and brain levels were close to equilibrium values, but the muscle alcohol level still lagged by about 30%. These results illustrate the "overshooting" of the blood alcohol curve often seen during rapid absorption. The blood alcohol curve then drops sharply from the peak, due to shift of alcohol from blood and brain to muscle. When Hulpieu and Cole gave adrenaline 2 minutes prior to the alcohol, this irregular distribution of alcohol was greatly accentuated, and equilibrium distribution was not yet attained at the end of 5 minutes. While the rabbits receiving alcohol alone showed only mild intoxication, the high brain level after adrenaline killed some of the animals.

Very different blood/brain alcohol ratios were reported by Meyer (M12) using rats. Alcohol, 3 gm/kg, was given intraperitoneally and the animals were decapitated 1 minute to 6 hours after the injection. The drainage blood and tissue from various areas of the brain were analyzed. The blood/brain alcohol ratios ranged from 1.45 for the forebrain to 2.35 for the medulla. He concluded that the alcohol level in various parts of the brain is controlled by the blood supply and not by the water content.

## 2. Analyses of Human Cadavers

Results of alcohol determinations made on human brain and blood, obtained at autopsy, continue to be published. A summary of the results reported in four papers since 1950, and two prior to that date, are collected in Table V.

TABLE V

BLOOD/BRAIN ALCOHOL RATIO OF HUMAN CADAVERS

| Investigators | Year | Number of cases | Blood alcohol range (mg%) | Blood/brain alcohol ratio | |
|---|---|---|---|---|---|
| | | | | Average | Range |
| Gettler and Freireich (G2) | 1931 | 3 | 21–78 | 2.29 | 0.69–4.33 |
| | | 12 | 103–475 | 1.04 | 0.63–1.47 |
| Ellerbrook and Van Gaasbeek (E5) | 1943 | 19 | 100–400 | 1.09 | 0.88–1.31 |
| Van Hecke *et al.* (V1) | 1951 | 1 | 193 | 5.10 | — |
| | | 47 | 74–268 | 1.44 | 0.74–2.68 |
| Hine (H22) | 1951 | 100 | 35–465 | 1.53 | 0.50–3.20 |
| Freireich (F14) | 1960 | 12 | 5–54 | 1.22 | 0.85–2.45 |
| | | 82 | 54–469 | 1.06 | 0.68–1.45 |
| Herold and Prokop (H21)[a] | 1960 | 1 | 160 | 4.00 | — |
| | | 35 | 110–460 | 1.45 | 0.77–2.65 |

[a] Cases where the blood alcohol level was above 100 mg%; brain alcohol levels are from analyses of frontal lobe.

The average blood/brain alcohol ratios reported by Ellerbrook and Van Gaasbeek (E5) and by Freireich (F14) are quite similar to the ratios for the first four groups of experimental dogs listed in Table III. The other human ratios given in Table V are much higher. Whether the proportionally higher blood alcohol levels may be due to post-mortem disappearance of alcohol in the brain, or perhaps to the post-mortem formation of volatile, dichromate-reducing material in the blood, remains to be investigated. Hine (H22) incubated weak alcohol solutions with slices of liver, brain, and diaphragm and reported considerable disappearance of the alcohol. He suggested that this destruction of alcohol may occur in cadavers between death and autopsy. On this point see Section VII,B,2 of this chapter.

Muehlberger (M15) has emphasized that, for living subjects, this matter of the blood/brain alcohol ratio is of academic interest only, because all of the studies on alcohol level and impairment have been based on analyses of blood, and not of brain.

## D. Saliva/Blood Ratio

Coldwell and Smith (C14) have reported a study of the correlation between the levels of alcohol in saliva and venous blood covering 244 saliva-blood pairs. Their results give a saliva/blood alcohol ratio of $1.12 \pm 7.5$ mg%.

## E. Urine/Blood Ratio

From analyses of ninety-one pairs of urine and blood samples taken very close together, Coldwell and Smith (C14) obtained a urine/blood alcohol ratio of $1.24 \pm 0.08$. Lundquist (L13) had subjects ingest 1 gm/kg of alcohol as wine or brandy and analyzed samples of urine and earlobe blood during several hours. He found the average urine/blood alcohol ratio to be 1.35, with a range of 1.12–1.51. The average ratio was practically identical for the rising and falling blood alcohol phases. Two tests on one subject gave an average urine/serum alcohol ratio of 1.07. Robljek-Priversek (R7) determined the urine/blood alcohol ratio for thirty subjects and reported the average to be 1.32.

## F. Spinal Fluid/Blood Ratio

Using the Widmark and ADH methods, Hebold (H20) analyzed simultaneous samples of spinal fluid and blood from twenty-two subjects. The spinal fluid/blood alcohol ratio varied from 0.93 to 1.40 in twenty-two subjects, and was 0.47 in one subject. In the absence of drinking, spinal fluid both from normal individuals and from persons with disease showed no alcohol whatever by the ADH method. Marcellini (M4) gave ten subjects 1 ml/kg of alcohol in 25% solution and determined the alcohol level in blood and lumbar spinal fluid during 6 hours. With eight of the ten subjects the peak of blood alcohol was reached within 90 minutes, while with nine of the ten, it took 180 minutes to reach the maximum spinal fluid alcohol level. In the elimination phase, the spinal fluid alcohol level was considerably higher than the blood level. Marcellini ascribed this lag in spinal fluid alcohol level to a hemoencephalic barrier, but the more probable cause is limited circulation to the spine, and is analogous to the normal lag in muscle alcohol during active absorption. Bladder urine shows the same phenomenon. That the level of spinal fluid alcohol changes more slowly than that of blood, during both the rise and decline, was pointed out in 1933 by Mehrtens and Newman (M11).

## G. Water–Alcohol Relationship

Further papers tend to confirm the generally accepted principle that the distribution of alcohol in the various body tissues and fluids is proportional to the distribution of water in these body materials. Gruner (G21) placed hashed portions of human tissues, containing alcohol, in dialyzing sacs and suspended the sacs in a certain volume of water. After equilibrium was reached, which took 24–56 hours, the ratio of alcohol concentration in the two phases, divided by the ratio of water concentration in the two phases, was found to be 0.993 ± 0.076. Gruner also used the dose of alcohol, its concentration in the blood, and the volume of water in the blood to calculate total body water. He reported that this procedure is as reliable as the common antipyrine method. In his study (G18) on the plasma/whole blood and serum/whole blood alcohol ratios, mentioned above, Gruner reported that these ratios are governed by the water content of the two phases. In another paper, Gruner (G22) reported figures for the distribution of alcohol between water and body fat. Using the Widmark method, the fat/water alcohol ratio which he obtained at 35–40°C was 0.0187, and with the ADH method it was 0.0234. At 0°C it was 0.0219. Thus, alcohol is about fifty times as soluble in water as in body fat.

Sachs (S2) produced a cantharides blister on the inner forearm of a subject and then administered 0.8–1.5 gm/kg of alcohol to the subject. The top of the blister was excised and a small funnel was fastened over the exposed area. Tissue fluid ("bloodless plasma") was then secured by gentle suction. Simultaneous samples of the subject's tissue fluid and blood were analyzed for alcohol. The alcohol level of the tissue fluid averaged about 50% lower than that of the blood, but the two curves were parallel. Sachs ascribed this difference to loss of alcohol from the tissue fluid due to reduced pressure from the suction applied.

## V. Fate of Body Alcohol

### A. The Blood Alcohol Curve; Back-Calculation of Alcohol Level

1. Nature of the Falling Blood Alcohol Curve—
   Linear or Exponential

Widmark (W11) stated that, after distribution equilibrium is complete, the descending alcohol curve is a straight line. This means that, for a given individual, alcohol disappears from the body at a constant rate per hour. According to Widmark, the hourly drop in blood alcohol for man (Widmark's $\beta$) averages about 15 mg%, with a range of about 10–20 mg%. Many subsequent investigators have published experimental data which seem to confirm Widmark's claims.

In 1953, Marshall and Fritz (M5) reported that with dogs the decline in blood alcohol level is a straight line until a level of about 20 mg% is reached, after which it follows an exponential curve, indicating a slower rate of fall from 20 mg% to zero. Lundquist and Wolthers (L14), using a modified ADH method which is said to correctly determine blood alcohol to less than 0.5 mg%, have reported blood alcohol analyses with ten human subjects which indicate that with humans too the blood alcohol drop becomes exponential below about 15 mg%.

Experiments with dogs or cats by some investigators, including ourselves (H9), indicate that doubling the alcohol level causes an increase in $\beta_{60}$ of 17–37%.

Elbel (E3) reported that with rats the drop in blood alcohol level after complete absorption follows an exponential curve, but that with dogs the drop is a straight line. He interprets this to mean that in dogs the supply of alcohol dehydrogenase in the liver is more limited than in the rat.

## 2. Correlation of Alcohol Dosage and Maximum Blood Alcohol Level

As mentioned in Section III,A,1, the speed of absorption of alcohol is reduced by food in the stomach. This would give a lower blood alcohol peak. A lower peak will also result by prolonging the drinking period for a given dose of alcohol, because some of the alcohol will be oxidized or excreted during this period.

Abele and Kropp (A4) compared the maximum blood alcohol level and the alcohol dose in ninety-one subjects, who during "less than 20 minutes to 60–100 minutes" drank brandy to furnish an alcohol dose of 0.5–1.8 gm/kg. Blood samples (blood source not given) were taken at frequent intervals from the start of drinking to 45 minutes after the blood alcohol peak was reached. For all the subjects, the ratio, maximum blood alcohol in mg% ÷ alcohol dose in gm/kg, was 118 ± 7. This ratio varied according to the time between the last meal and the start of drinking as follows: 6 hours, 138 ± 7; 3–6 hours, 108 ± 18; and 3 hours, 109 ± 9.3.

Bayly and McCallum (B3) have conducted a similar study using fifty-six subjects, most of whom drank 5% beer 3 hours after a light meal, at their "fastest possible rate." In one of the experiments nine of the subjects drank whisky diluted to 20% and in another seven subjects drank beer just after a "substantial" meal. The dosage of alcohol for all experiments varied from 0.43 to 2.03 gm/kg. In Table VI and Fig. 4, we have summarized Bayly and McCallum's data. As shown by Fig. 4, the maximum blood alcohol per gram of alcohol per kilogram averaged 114 mg% for all eighty-five experiments. It was 105 mg% for the group drinking beer just after a meal, and 118 mg% for the whisky group.

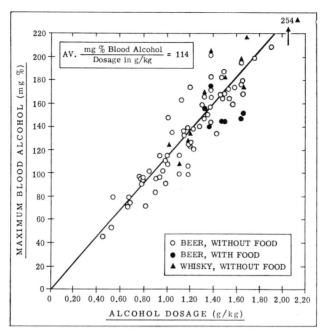

Fig. 4. Correlation between alcohol dosage in gm/kg and maximum blood alcohol level. From data in Tables I–IV of Bayly and McCallum (B3).

### 3. Time Interval and Alcohol Rise between End of Drinking and Blood Alcohol Peak

In the study by Abele and Kropp, mentioned above, the percentage of all subjects whose blood alcohol had reached its maximum, at various time intervals after the end of drinking, was: 30 minutes, 15%; 60 minutes, 40%; 90 minutes, 70%; 120 minutes, 90%; and 170 minutes, 100%. The rise in blood alcohol level between the end of drinking and blood alcohol peak is not given in Abele and Kopp's data.

The paper by Bayly and McCallum does present data on both time interval and increase in blood alcohol between end of drinking and blood alcohol peak. These data are summarized in Table VI. In the two beer experiments without food, the average time between end of drinking and blood alcohol peak was about 60 minutes, with a range of 20–118 minutes, and during this interval the blood alcohol level rose 3–83 mg%, with an average of 36 mg%. When the beer was consumed following a substantial meal, the average time interval to reach the blood alcohol peak was reduced to 39 minutes (0–55), and the blood alcohol rose only 15 mg% (0–27 mg%). With whisky the average time interval between end

TABLE VI

RISE IN BLOOD ALCOHOL LEVEL AFTER END OF DRINKING[a]

| Total subjects | Beverages | Food | Alcohol intake (gm/kg) | Drinking time (min) | End of drinking to maximum level | | | | | |
|---|---|---|---|---|---|---|---|---|---|---|
| | | | | | Time | | | Rise | | |
| | | | | | Average (min) | Range (min) | | Average (mg%) | Range (mg%) | |
| 56 | Beer, 5% (v/v) | None[b] | 0.43–2.03 | 20–103 | 62 | 20–114 | | 39 | 3–83 | |
| 13 | Beer, 5% (v/v) | None | 1.65 | 100 | 54 | 30–118 | | 28 | 10–54 | |
| 7 | Beer, 5% (v/v) | Substantial meal | 1.65 | 100 | 39 | 0–55 | | 15 | 0–27 | |
| 9 | Whiskey diluted to 20% | None | 1.32–1.65 | 55–60 | 31 | 0–45 | | 29 | 0–57 | |

[a] Condensed from four tables presented by Bayly and McCallum (B3).
[b] Three hours after a light meal.

of drinking and blood alcohol peak was 31 minutes (0–45) and the average blood alcohol rise was 29 mg% (0–57).

Cubital vein blood was used by Bayly and McCallum (personal communication), and it seems likely that it was also used by Abele and Kropp. Had they used capillary blood from the fingertip, the blood alcohol peak would have been reached much earlier and it would have been higher. This is shown by experiments conducted by Pihkanen (P7). His twelve subjects ingested brandy or beer to give an alcohol dosage of 1 gm/kg, taken in six equal doses over one hour. Capillary blood samples from the fingertip were drawn at the end of the drinking period and 1, 2, and 3 hours later. As shown by his tables and figures, at the end of the drinking period eleven of the twelve brandy drinkers and three of the twelve beer drinkers had already reached their blood alcohol peaks. One hour after the end of drinking the average blood alcohol level of the brandy drinkers had dropped 12%, and the level of the beer drinkers had reached, or passed, its peak. Abele and Kropp's subjects also drank brandy (0.5–1.8 gm/kg of alcohol in an average of about 30 minutes) but even 1 hour after the end of drinking only 40% had reached their blood alcohol peak. Bayly and McCallum's whisky drinkers took 0–45 minutes after the end of drinking (average, 31 minutes) to reach their blood alcohol peak.

Gerchow and Steigleder (G7) studied the blood alcohol curves of sixty subjects who ingested, during 50–55 minutes, 0.8, 1.2, or 1.6 gm/kg of alcohol (twenty subjects for each dosage; per cent of alcohol in drink not given). Blood samples were taken at the end of drinking and at 20-minute intervals for 4½ hours. Five of the subjects had atypical blood alcohol curves with plateau or secondary peaks. The remaining fifty-five subjects exhibited typical blood alcohol curves. With these fifty-five subjects, the distribution as regards the time interval within which the blood alcohol peak was reached was: 30 minutes, eight subjects; 30–60 minutes, twenty-three subjects; 60–90 minutes, fifteen subjects; 90–120 minutes, seven subjects; and 120–150 minutes, one subject (blood source not given). The nineteen subjects with the highest dosage all reached their maximum within 90 minutes. The blood alcohol rise between end of drinking and peak is not given. The results are much like those of Abele and Kropp and strongly suggest that cubital vein blood was used. Cubital vein blood, collected in sterile venules, is very commonly used in Germany.

Forster *et al.* (F11) followed the blood alcohol curves of ninety-two subjects. With two thirds of the subjects the maximum level was reached within 20–30 minutes after the end of drinking, and within 1 hour in all but nine subjects. In these nine there was a delayed peak due to vomiting or heavy food intake at the time of drinking (blood source not given).

4. FALLING PHASE OF THE BLOOD ALCOHOL CURVE;
   BACK-CALCULATION OF ALCOHOL LEVEL

When blood is employed in chemical tests for intoxication in traffic cases, there is always a delay between the time of the alleged offense and the time of withdrawing the blood sample. This time interval may vary from 15 minutes to 3 hours. Therefore, the alcohol level in the blood sample is usually not the same as the level in the subject's blood at the time of the alleged offense. While the difference is usually a lower level in the blood sample analyzed, this may not be true if the driving offense occurred during the rising phase of the blood alcohol curve. Much attention has recently been given to this question of back-calculation of the blood alcohol level.

*a. Rate of Fall of Blood Alcohol Level, Widmark's Factor $\beta$.* In his pioneer work on the disappearance of alcohol from the body, Widmark (W11) reported that, when the blood alcohol curve has reached its peak, it frequently falls rather rapidly, and perhaps irregularly, for $\frac{1}{2}$ to 1 hour, after which it then descends in a straight line to zero. This "overshooting" of the peak is due to lag in the storage of alcohol in the voluntary muscles, which constitute about 40% of the total body weight. If absorption is not too rapid this "overshooting" does not occur. The rate of fall of blood alcohol when the descending blood alcohol curve becomes linear is expressed by Widmark's factor $\beta$, which he defined as the drop in parts per thousand (pro mil, %) per minute. This gives a long decimal fraction and we prefer to use $\beta_{60}$, defined as mg% per hour. Widmark's results with men indicated an average $\beta_{60}$ of about 15 mg% per hour, with a range of 10–22. Since Widmark's time many investigators have reported determination of $\beta_{60}$ for humans. For the most part, their results agree quite well with Widmark's values. Reports prior to 1954 have been reviewed by Elbel and Schleyer (E4), Harger and Hulpieu (H13), and others.

Forster *et al.* (F11) determined the drop in blood alcohol of ninety-two subjects during a period of 4–8 hours after the peak was reached. They reported an average $\beta_{60}$ of 16.3 mg% with extremes of 11.6 and 27 mg%. Robljek-Priversek (R7) followed the blood alcohol curves of thirty male subjects who drank 0.2–2.4 liters of 10% wine during 30 minutes. Blood samples (blood source not given) were drawn hourly, beginning $\frac{1}{2}$ hour after the end of drinking. The average $\beta_{60}$ was 16, with a range of 11–21. The author reported that the blood alcohol curve was consistently around 30% lower than he calculated from the Widmark factor $r$, which is the ratio of alcohol concentration in the whole body to alcohol concentration in the blood. His average blood alcohol curve for the whole group does not look too low, if he used an average alcohol dosage of around 1 liter of the 10% wine which would furnish about 1 gm/ kg of alcohol. If he used a sweet wine the blood alcohol curve would be depressed, according to Goldberg (G12). Ponsold and Heite (P11) conducted alcohol analyses on two samples of blood drawn ½ hour apart from 1655 persons arrested for intoxication. Their blood alcohol levels ranged from below 50 mg% to above 250 mg%, and the time between the last drinking and the withdrawal of blood ranged from less than 30 minutes to 4 hours. From the drop in blood alcohol level during this 30-minute period, they calculated $\beta_{60}$ for these subjects. The average $\beta_{60}$ was 17 mg%. With about 2% of the subjects there was no change in blood alcohol level during the 30 minutes, with about 5% $\beta_{60}$ was less than 4 mg%, and with about 5% $\beta_{60}$ was around 34 mg%. The low figures for $\beta_{60}$ were probably due to a blood alcohol plateau at the maximum and the high results could have occurred following the "overshooting" phenomenon already mentioned (blood source not given). In Subsection A,1 of the present section, we reported on the work of Lundquist and Wolthers (L14) who found that, at blood alcohol levels below about 20 mg%, the curve becomes exponential making $\beta_{60}$ much lower. However, in the studies cited in the present paragraph, no attempt was made to determine $\beta_{60}$ where the blood alcohol was below 20 mg%. The change in $\beta_{60}$ in this range is of no practical importance in the usual forensic case.

b. *Back-Calculation of Blood Alcohol Level.* Schleyer (S6) determined the blood alcohol curves for 174 human subjects. He reported that 25% of the curves were atypical with plateaus and secondary peaks and advised against attempting back-calculation where the alcohol level is much above 100 mg% and the time interval is greater than 1–2 hours. On the other hand, Gerchow and Steigleder (G7) found only five atypical curves among sixty subjects, or an incidence of 8.3%. Ponsold and Heite (P11) felt that their average $\beta_{60}$ of 17 mg% is too high to be used forensically, because it would be unfair to subjects with a low $\beta_{60}$. Forster et al. (F11) stated that back-calculation using 10–11 mg% as the hourly drop in blood alcohol should be fair to practically all persons. Gerchow and Steigleder (G7) had no hesitation in saying that, for a period of 1–2 hours, no injustice will be done if one uses $\beta_{60}$ of 10 mg% for cases with blood alcohol below 100 mg% and $\beta_{60}$ of 12 mg% for persons with blood alcohol above 100 mg%. From their results, Bayly and

McCallum stated (B3) "an accurate assessment cannot be made of the blood alcohol concentration in an individual at some time prior to the taking of a blood sample."

The use of cubital vein blood by Bayly and McCallum and probably by all the other investigators quoted in this section, with the exception of Pihkanen, makes their results open to serious question. *Capillary blood from a fingertip should have been used in these studies.* Pihkanen, who did use fingertip capillary blood, found that all blood alcohol peaks occurred within 1 hour after the end of drinking, and by the end of the drinking period with practically all of his subjects who drank brandy. This indicates that back-calculation can usually be safely done within an hour after drinking, and perhaps much earlier. We have re-examined the data of Harger *et al.* (H10) where they analyzed both cubital vein blood and fingertip blood with twenty subjects 1 hour and 2 hours after drinking whisky to give an alcohol dose of 0.68–1.03 gm/kg.[1] With five of the subjects there was a rise in the cubital vein blood alcohol between hours 1 and 2 from 8 to 24 mg%. However, with nineteen of the twenty subjects the fingertip blood had reached its peak within the first hour, and with one it rose 9 mg% between hour 1 and hour 2. One of the authors of this chapter (H9) has recommended that, in performing back-calculation of blood alcohol level, we should not use just one value for $\beta_{60}$, but should give the average and the extremes. For the average we suggested 15 mg%, with 10–20 mg% for the extremes. Using this procedure for our twenty subjects, mentioned above, and employing capillary blood for all samples taken less than 70 minutes after drinking, we found that for nineteen of the twenty subjects calculation of the 1-hour blood level from the results at 2 hours and 3 hours were accurate within the $\beta_{60}$ limits of 10–20 mg% drop per hour.

Finally, some of the experimental conditions used by Bayly and McCallum, particularly where they had subjects drink beer "at their fastest possible rate" with consumption of four-fifths of a U. S. gallon of beer in 30–100 minutes, seem quite abnormal behavior for most people. Even here, the use of fingertip blood would probably have shown much earlier blood alcohol peaks.

## B. Factors Which Might Alter Rate of Alcohol Disappearance

Many attempts have been made to increase $\beta_{60}$. We will review only those studies which have been published since 1954.

### 1. DOSAGE AND MANNER OF ADMINISTRATION

Abele (A1) gave fourteen subjects 1.07–2.00 gm/kg of alcohol. Five

---

[1] The remaining eleven subjects drank again between hours 1 and 2 or 2 and 3.

subjects, who drank while fasting, had an average blood alcohol peak of 198 mg% and an average $\beta_{60}$ of 17.6. The other nine subjects drank soon after a meal and their average blood alcohol peak was 148 mg% and an average $\beta_{60}$ was 14.7. Abele also took two blood samples, 1 hour apart, from 922 drinking, arrested subjects. With 161 of these subjects, whose blood alcohol levels were 41–120 mg%, the average $\beta_{60}$ was 17, while with 166 subjects with blood alcohol above 200 mg% $\beta_{60}$ averaged 20.3. Schweitzer (S13) also concluded that $\beta_{60}$ increases with blood alcohol level. Harger and Hulpieu found that same result with dogs (H9).

Nelson and Kinard (N5) administered to dogs 20% alcohol in saline, intravenously, to give a dosage of 2 gm/kg, during 4–8 minutes, or 30 minutes. The two rates of administration caused no difference in $\beta_{60}$.

With Pihkanen's twelve subjects who received brandy or beer to give a dosage of 1 gm/kg of alcohol, brandy gave higher blood alcohol maxima, but the average blood alcohol levels 1, 2, and 3 hours after drinking were essentially the same for the two beverages, indicating no difference in $\beta_{60}$.

On the other hand, as shown by Fig. 1, Cordebard reported that food eaten during or shortly before wine drinking caused the blood alcohol curve to be much lower and of much shorter duration. However, as mentioned earlier, this difference may have been due to destruction of some of the alcohol in the alimentary tract. On the other hand, Fig. 1 indicates no variation of $\beta_{60}$ in one of Cordebard's subjects who ingested 0.5 gm/ kg of alcohol as rum, wine, or beer.

## 2. Physiological Factors

Willner (W13) had subjects drink 40–60 gm of alcohol as beer, when the air temperature was 40°C or 10°C. At the higher external temperature the resulting blood alcohol levels were higher and $\beta_{60}$ appeared to be smaller.

Gruner (G19) gave ten subjects 0.75 gm/kg of alcohol in 25% solution, during 15 minutes, and followed the blood alcohol for 5 hours. Between hours 3 and 4 the subjects were warmed with a heat lamp for about ½ hour. With seven of the ten subjects, the slope of the blood alcohol curve was definitely less during the period of heating, but returned to normal afterward. He ascribed this phenomenon to increase in plasma volume.

Gruner and Sattler (G24) gave fourteen subjects 1 gm/kg of alcohol and determined the alcohol curve for 3½ hours. At about 2¾ hours after drinking the subjects were required to stand rigidly erect for 15 minutes. This caused a sharp drop in the blood alcohol curve, averaging 9 mg%. The maximum drop was 25 mg%. After the drop, the blood alcohol level rose and the curve resumed its original course. Gruner and Sattler ascribed this drop to a temporary increase in the oxidation of alcohol. A more probable explanation would be increased production of adrenaline from the stress, with lessened circulation through the voluntary muscles (see Table IV). With most of the circulation serving only a portion of the total body tissues, the same rate of oxidation of alcohol would cause an abnormal drop in the alcohol level of the blood.

Apel (A13) found no change in $\beta_{60}$ of ten subjects during sleep, as compared with the value while awake.

Wilson *et al.* (W15) gave six persons a "priming" dose of alcohol (0.8 gm/kg) and then small, hourly doses for 36 hours, with frequent sampling of the blood. They reported a diurnal variation of $\beta_{60}$ in a pattern corresponding to the sleep habits of each subject. Among the subjects, the maximum 24 hour variation of $\beta_{60}$ was 25%.

## 3. BODILY INJURIES AND ILLNESS

In eight experiments by Rauschke (R3), alcohol was administered to a subject who could vomit at will. On each occasion emesis was followed by a rise of 9–35 mg% in the blood alcohol curve, either in the ascending or descending phase. Rauschke also followed the alcohol curve of rabbits which had received alcohol by stomach tube, and bled the animals during the experiment, removing 3.5–11% of the total blood. This caused an increase in blood alcohol level up to 31 mg%. He thought this was due to increase in the proportion of blood plasma, which has a higher concentration of alcohol than an equal volume of cells.

Newman (N6) found that emesis frequently occurs when the blood alcohol level reaches 120 mg%, regardless of whether the alcohol is received orally or by vein, and that a temporary rise in blood alcohol level results after emesis from either route of administration. This seems to rule out more rapid absorption as the cause of the blood alcohol rise associated with vomiting.

Beck (B5) found that, with rabbits given alcohol, both bleeding and transfusion with a plasma expander caused a rise in blood alcohol level. Gumbel (G25) reported no significant change in the blood alcohol level of humans after withdrawing 500 ml of blood.

Forster (F10) analyzed two samples of blood, taken ½ hour apart, from 112 alcoholic patients with brain concussion. With forty-six, who were in deep coma, the average $\beta_{60}$ was 18.5 mg%, and in another group, who had only light concussion, $\beta_{60}$ averaged 18.8. Since both of these values are normal, he concluded that traumatic coma does not affect the rate of fall of blood alcohol.

Bernstein and Staub (B8), Pietz *et al.* (P6), and others have employed the drop in blood alcohol following the administration of about

0.5 gm/kg of alcohol as a liver function test, with reasonably good results. On the other hand, Kulpe and Mallach (K22) used such an alcohol tolerance test on fifteen healthy subjects and fifteen cases of cirrhosis of the liver and reported no significant difference in the blood alcohol curves of the two groups.

4. Sugars and Amino Acids

Pletscher and colleagues have continued their studies on the effect of fructose in accelerating the disappearance of blood alcohol. A recent paper by them (B7) described studies with normal subjects and patients with hepatitis, who received 0.8 gm/kg of alcohol followed later by intravenous fructose in a dosage of 100 gm in 10% solution. They reported an increase of 24% in the rate of alcohol metabolism with the normal subjects, and 11–25% with the hepatitis subjects. Johannsmeier *et al.* (J3), using sheep and two human subjects, found no increased $\beta_{60}$ after fructose. The dose of fructose, given orally, was 1.2 or 0.8 gm/kg and this nauseated the human subjects. Using dogs, Clark and Hulpieu (C9) reported that intravenous fructose raised the alcohol $\beta_{60}$ from an average of 15.2 mg% to 22.8 mg%. Dextrose had no such effect. Lundquist and Wolthers (L15) gave five human subjects 0.5 gm/kg of alcohol. Two hours later they ingested 22 gm of fructose at ½-hour intervals. With four of the subjects $\beta_{60}$ increased 28–56%, and with one only 1.6%. Glucose was ineffective.

Schiller *et al.* (S5) had ten subjects drink 120 ml of 100-proof whisky in 20 minutes. At the end of drinking, the subjects were given by intravenous drip, during 75–90 minutes, 1 liter of solution containing 5% protein hydrolyzate plus 5% glucose. With all subjects the blood alcohol peak with the amino acids plus glucose was lower than the control tests and the zero level was reached somewhat sooner in four of the cases. Glucose alone was not effective.

5. Hormones and Vitamins

The effect of insulin on the rate of fall of blood alcohol in dogs has been tested by Kinard and Cox (K6) and by Newman *et al.* (N9). The dosages used were: alcohol, 2–3 gm/kg; and insulin, 1 unit/kg. Smith and Newman repeated the dose of insulin 3 hours after the first dose. Kinard and Cox reported no effect from the insulin, while Smith and Newman observed an average increase in $\beta_{60}$ of 27%, although one of their seven dogs showed no change in rate of alcohol metabolism.

Gruner (G20) had ten subjects ingest 0.75 gm/kg of alcohol, and after 3 hours they were given, subcutaneously, 1 ml of 1-1000 adrenaline. During ½ hour after the adrenaline, nine of the subjects exhibited a sharp drop in the blood alcohol curve, the greatest drop being 16 mg% in 15 minutes. The average drop was 8 mg%. After the fall the blood alcohol curve rose and resumed its previous slope. Gruner ascribed this fall to increase in circulating plasma. We feel that it could quite as well be due to lessened circulation to the voluntary muscle tissue (see Subsection B,2 of this section).

The possible effect of triiodothyronine (TIT) on the fall of blood alcohol has been tested on dogs by Newman and Smith (N8) and by Kinard *et al.* (K8), and with humans by Goldberg *et al.* (G13). Newman and Smith found an insignificant increase of $\beta_{60}$ of perhaps 2% after TIT, while Kinard *et al.* observed no change. Goldberg *et al.* used deeply intoxicated humans, who received by vein 200 mg of triiodothyronine; they reported that $\beta_{60}$ for twelve treated patients averaged 32 mg%, while eight equally intoxicated, untreated patients had an average $\beta_{60}$ of only 15 mg%.

That *glucagon,* the glucose-elevating hormone of the pancreas, will lower blood alcohol was reported by Nelson and Jensen (N4). They gave dogs alcohol, intravenously, to produce blood alcohol levels of about 250 mg%. At the end of the 3rd, 4th, 5th, and 6th hours the dogs were given glucagon, 0.05 mg/kg, iv. The control $\beta_{60}$ was 12.5–13.7 mg%, average, 13.1. After glucagon it rose to 16.2–23.7 mg%, average, 19.0. Since glucagon is said to increase liver blood flow, they thought this might explain the fall in blood alcohol. We doubt this because the supply of ADH in the liver, and not the blood flow, would seem to govern the rate of alcohol metabolism.

Smith *et al.* (S19) gave mice 500 mg of nicotinamide 6 hours prior to intraperitoneal injection of 4 gm/kg of alcohol. The $\beta_{60}$ was the same as that of untreated controls.

6. Drugs

The effect of chlorpromazine (Thorazine) on the blood alcohol curve of rabbits was tested by Tipton *et al.* (T4). When the drug dosage was 3 mg/kg 90 minutes before the alcohol (0.78–1.56 gm/kg orally), the blood alcohol levels averaged 52% above the controls 15 minutes after alcohol administration, and 22% higher at 40 minutes after the alcohol. Since chlorpromazine did not cause an elevation of orally administered salicylic acid or sulfamerazine, Tipton *et al.* concluded that the elevated blood alcohol level was due to retarded oxidation. Sutherland *et al.* (S23) gave nine human subjects 1 gm/kg of alcohol, orally during 6 minutes, and took samples of arterial blood for alcohol analysis 0, 15, 30, and 60 minutes afterward. During the following week, the subjects received daily doses of chlorpromazine, starting with 25 mg and ending with

400 mg, and the alcohol experiment was repeated. After chlorpromazine, the average blood alcohol level compared with that of the controls was +35% at 15 minutes after administration of alcohol, +40% at 30 minutes, and +10% at 1 hour.

Forney and Hulpieu (F5) reported no change in the blood alcohol curve of dogs which had received daily oral doses of carbutamide for periods up to 2 weeks.

Calcium chloride, administered to subjects in an oral dose of 2 gm, or an intravenous dose of 1 gm in 10% solution, had no effect on the blood alcohol curve of three human subjects receiving 1 gm/kg of alcohol orally, according to Alha (A9).

"Promill-Ex," an alleged sobering drug, was tested by Burger (B24), Gerchow and Sachs (G6), Gruner *et al.* (G23), Mallach (M2), and Wuermling *et al.* (W18). All reported that it did not alter the blood alcohol curve. It was said to be mostly caffeine.

"Contra," another alleged antidote for alcohol, was tried on subjects by Gumbel (G26). He reported that it did not hasten the disappearance of alcohol.

## 7. Acquired Tolerance

Kinard and Hay (K7) and Troshina (T5) studied the blood alcohol level of rats made tolerant to alcohol by prolonged feeding. Kinard and Hay found no change in the blood alcohol curve. On the other hand, Troshina reported that his rats, made alcohol-resistant by prolonged alcohol feeding, absorbed alcohol more slowly (see Section III,A,4) and also had higher levels of alcohol in the blood than did nonhabituated rats receiving the same dose of alcohol (111 mg% compared with 63 mg%, 3 hours after a given dose of alcohol). Troshina's results are contrary to the findings of many previous investigators and should be checked.

## C. Metabolism of Alcohol; Conversion to Body Tissues

Investigations during the past 75 years have conclusively demonstrated that over 90% of the alcohol taken into the body is oxidized to $CO_2$ and $H_2O$, the remainder being excreted in the urine, breath, and perspiration. Lundsgaard (L16) and later workers showed that the first step of this oxidation occurs mostly in the liver, where the enzyme *alcohol dehydrogenase* catalyzes the oxidation of alcohol to acetaldehyde. The resulting acetaldehyde is then metabolized in various body tissues.

Beginning with the work of Bartlett and Barnet in 1949, investigators have used alcohol containing radioactive $C^{14}$ to better ascertain the fate of administered alcohol and its oxidation products. In their 1949 paper Bartlett and Barnet reported (B1) that when alcohol, tagged by the addition of 1,2-$C^{14}$ ethanol, was administered by stomach tube to a rat, $C^{14}O_2$ quickly appeared in the breath. Within 5 hours the exhaled $C^{14}O_2$ accounted for 75% of the administered alcohol and in 10 hours it represented 90% of the alcohol fed. Habituated rats receiving the same dose of tagged alcohol exhaled $C^{14}O_2$ at the same rate. Experiments with rat tissue slices, incubated with $C^{14}$-tagged alcohol solutions, showed that liver and kidney tissue oxidized alcohol at a rapid rate, heart and diaphragm at a slower rate, and brain tissue very little, if any.

Lowenstein *et al.* (L11) obtained almost identical results with mice receiving $C^{14}$-tagged alcohol. Five mice, which drank water containing 5% $C^{14}$-tagged alcohol, were sacrificed 6 or 14 days later, and 12–72 hours after their last intake of alcohol. The tissues of the 6-day mice contained $C^{14}$ accounting for 3–4% of the total $C^{14}$ administered, and the tissues of the 14-day mice contained 1–1.5% of the $C^{14}$ they had ingested. In the 6-day rats, the greatest concentration of $C^{14}$ was found in the liver, while with the 14-day rats the adipose tissue contained the highest concentration of $C^{14}$. In all tissues most of the $C^{14}$ was in the lipids. Smith and Newman (S18) found that ethanol-1-$C^{14}$ and acetate-1-$C^{14}$ were equally incorporated into the lipids of mice.

The matter of the fixation of $C^{14}$ into the tissues of mice was investigated by Casier *et al.* (C3). They fed the same dose of 1-$C^{14}$ as alcohol, acetaldehyde, and acetate and found that alcohol and acetaldehyde produced about the same amount of tissue $C^{14}$, but acetate caused the formation of only about half this amount. From this, and other evidence, they concluded that the metabolism of alcohol does not go through the acetate stage, but goes through acetaldehyde to acetyl coenzyme A and then to cholesterol and other lipids.

Kulonen and Forsander (K21) fractionated the cellular parts of rat tissues after administration of ethanol-1-$C^{14}$ or -2-$C^{14}$, and found about 66% of the liver $C^{14}$ in the liver cytoplasm, 8–24% in the nuclear fraction, and 1–10% in the mitochondrial washings. With the brain, about one-third of the cytoplasm $C^{14}$ was in the protein.

# VI. Pharmacological and Toxicological Effects

## A. Alterations in Body Chemistry

### 1. BLOOD SUGAR

Eger and Ottensmeier (E1) reported that administration of alcohol caused a rise in blood sugar in guinea pigs and rats. Matsumoto (M7) found that alcohol caused an immediate, mild increase in blood sugar of rabbits. With humans, Forsander *et al.* (F8) reported that, after alcohol, the blood sugar rose to a maximum in 12 hours, returned to normal during 12–24 hours, and then was depressed for several days. Coulthard (C17) administered 20 gm of alcohol to human subjects who had fasted 8–17 hours and observed no change in blood sugar level. Kulpe and Mallach (K23) gave seventeen fasting humans 0.75 gm/kg of alcohol. The blood sugar rose from 97 to 102 mg% in ½ hour and then declined to 79 mg% by the 7th hour. Fasting controls showed no such change. Klingman and Haag (K12) administered by stomach tube 6.3 gm/kg of alcohol to seven dogs. The mean blood sugar rose from an initial value of 109 mg% to 243 mg% in 4 hours and then declined to about the initial level in 24 hours. After adrenalectomy, this change did not occur. An alcohol dose of 3.2 gm/kg caused a much smaller rise in blood sugar. Vartia *et al.* (V2) conducted blood sugar determinations on fifty-three subjects arrested for drunkenness, on the "morning after" the intoxication. The average blood sugar was 20% below that of controls. With those "hangover" subjects whose original blood alcohol averaged 321 mg%, the mean blood sugar level was 29% below that of controls. Forsander *et al.* (F8) gave each of ten fasting human subjects 150 ml of whisky. Their blood sugar increased during the first ½ hour and later declined to levels below those at the start. However, when 50 ml of whisky was administered to sixteen subjects who had been drinking heavily the night before, the reduced blood sugar of some of them was mildly increased. Forsander *et al.* suggested that this may explain why a small drink of an alcoholic beverage may help to relieve a "hangover." Clark *et al.* (C10) administered by stomach tube a daily dose of 4 gm/kg of alcohol to four dogs and took blood samples for sugar analysis 24 hours later. By the 11th day, the blood sugar had fallen to 52% of the initial level. Repeating the experiment with "Solox"[2] produced about the same blood sugar drop as with pure ethanol. The blood sugar level of fasted control dogs declined only 10% during the 11-day period.

## 2. Blood Acetaldehyde

One explanation for the very unpleasant reaction experienced by a person on Antabuse medication, who ingests a little alcohol, is that the Antabuse inhibits the oxidation of acetaldehyde formed from alcohol, and the elevated acetaldehyde causes the reaction. Hald *et al.* (H5) reported that a small dose of alcohol, given to rabbits following Antabuse medication, caused the normal level of blood acetaldehyde of about 0.3 mg% to rise to 2.45 mg%. Raby (R1) determined the blood acetaldehyde levels of twenty-seven human subjects, nine after alcohol only and eighteen who received 0.5–4.5 gm of Antabuse during 3 days prior to the

[2] A commercial solvent containing ethanol plus 4% methanol and 1% each of ethyl acetate, gasoline, and isobutyl ketone.

alcohol. With alcohol only, the blood alcohol levels were 26–334 mg%, and the blood acetaldehyde levels were 0.59–1.48 mg%. When alcohol ingestion followed Antabuse medication, the blood analyses showed 25–133 mg% alcohol and 0.016–2.51 mg% acetaldehyde. Raby used the method of Stotz (S21) to determine acetaldehyde.

Hulpieu *et al.* (H28) gave 1 gm/kg of alcohol to normal dogs and to dogs pretreated with Antabuse and determined the blood acetaldehyde level for 6½ hours after the alcohol administration. Using the method of Stotz, they found a normal acetaldehyde level of about 0.001 mg%, which did not change by giving the animals alcohol alone. Alcohol administered to dogs pretreated with Antabuse caused the blood acetaldehyde to rise to about 0.11 mg%.

Forster (F9) studied the effect of alcohol ingestion on the blood acetaldehyde level of human subjects. He determined acetaldehyde by a modification of the method of Burbridge *et al.* (B23), and reported normal acetaldehyde levels of 0.04–0.13 mg%. After his subjects had ingested alcohol to give blood alcohol levels of 100–160 mg%, the blood acetaldehyde level rose to 1.1–3.0 mg%.

An enzyme method for blood acetaldehyde, using ADH, was developed by Brahm-Vogelsanger and Wagner (B18). They employed ADH plus $DPNH_2$ and no semicarbazide. The acetaldehyde goes to ethanol, with corresponding conversion of $DPNH_2$ to DPN, and the decrease of $DPNH_2$ is read at 366 m$\mu$. The method is said to determine blood acetaldehyde levels as low as 0.1 mg%. Using this method, Wagner (W1) reported the normal blood acetaldehyde level of rats to be 0–0.09 mg%, which was not elevated by administering alcohol to give a blood alcohol level up to 150 mg%. When alcohol was given after Antabuse medication, the blood acetaldehyde level rose to 0.1–0.3 mg%. Several other drugs, administered prior to alcohol, also caused the blood acetaldehyde to rise to levels not far from those resulting from Antabuse-alcohol. Wagner felt that the much higher blood acetaldehyde levels reported by earlier workers are due to lack of specificity in the analytical methods employed.

Janitzki (J1) stated that using this modified ADH method she found the normal blood acetaldehyde level to be around 0.03 mg%, which may rise tenfold after Antabuse plus alcohol.

## 3. LIVER

Mallov and Bloch (M3) gave rats 6.2 gm/kg of alcohol and sacrificed them 15–18 hours later. Liver lipid was much increased over that of controls. DiLuzio (D2) repeated this type of experiment with rats and found that the lipid increase was mostly in the triglyceride fraction.

Eger and Ottensmeier (E1) reported that administration of 4 gm/kg of alcohol to rats and guinea pigs caused, within 8 hours, a decrease in the liver glycogen of the rats but not in the guinea pigs.

Polyakova (P10) conducted a galactose liver tolerance test with thirty-three subjects with and without the additional ingestion of 100 ml of 40% alcohol. He reported that alcohol lowered carbohydrate metabolic function of the liver.

During a 14-day period, Clark *et al.* (C10) gave three fasting dogs a daily dose of 4 gm/kg of alcohol, gave four fasting dogs only water, and used four fed dogs as controls. At the end of the period, the livers were analyzed for total lipid and glycogen. The averaged analytical results for the fed controls, fasting controls, and fasting controls receiving alcohol were, respectively: liver lipid, 2.6, 5.3, and 20.5; liver glycogen, 4.9, 1.9, and 0.23 (expressed as per cent of fresh liver).

### 4. Adrenal Hormones

Perman (P4) measured the output of adrenaline and noradrenaline from one adrenal gland of cats by analyzing the venous return from the gland. When alcohol (0.6–1.0 gm/kg) was administered intravenously the output of both amines was increased.

That the urinary excretion of adrenaline and noradrenaline is increased by administration of alcohol was reported by Klingman and Goodall (K11), Perman (P4), and Abelin *et al.* (A6). However, Goddard (G9) found that, while the urinary excretion of noradrenaline of glider students was increased during flight, this increase was prevented by the ingestion of alcohol prior to the flight.

### 5. Brain

Hakkinen (H4) gave rats, by stomach tube, 0.43 gm/kg of alcohol. One hour later, the $\gamma$-aminobutyric acid (GABA) content of the brain was elevated to a maximum of 34% over that of controls without alcohol. Alcohol plus glutamine, or glutamine alone, elevated the brain GABA 18 and 20%, respectively.

### B. Changes in Body Functions

### 1. Gastric Secretion

It has long been known that a small oral dose of alcohol will temporarily increase the production of HCl by the glands of the stomach. To test where this effect is produced, Woodward *et al.* (W17) formed Heidenhain pouches in the fundus area of dogs' stomachs. Weak alcohol solutions placed in such a pouch did not stimulate formation of HCl, but when alcohol solutions were placed in the antrum of the stomach HCl was produced copiously, both in the stomach and in the pouch, indicating that the stomach area affected by alcohol is the portion near the pylorus. Intravenous administration of alcohol stimulated some gastric production of HCl, so part of the alcohol effect may be of central nervous system origin.

## 2. Brain Metabolism

Sutherland *et al.* (S24) incubated brain tissue slices with and without 0.056 *M* alcohol in the medium. The alcohol caused no increase in the uptake of oxygen or glucose in slices of human brain from lobotomized patients or in rat brain slices.

Continuing the earlier studies of Quastel, Beer and Quastel (B6) determined the consumption of oxygen by incubated slices of rat brain cortex. Using a medium containing 0.1 *M* KCl, they added alcohol to give concentrations of 0.4–0.8 *M* ethanol. At 0.4, 0.6, and 0.8 *M* alcohol the oxygen uptake was reduced 52%, 68%, and 90%, respectively.

The concentration of alcohol used by Sutherland *et al.* was 258 mg%, which is considerably below the fatal level. However, the alcohol concentrations employed by Beer and Ouastel, 0.4–0.8 *M* or 1840–3680 mg%, are about three and six times the fatal concentration. Such concentrations can shed little light on the brain effects of alcohol in living subjects.

## 3. Thymus Contraction

Santisteban (S4) reported that subcutaneous administration of alcohol to mice caused a shrinkage of the thymus. Groups of mice receiving 3, 5, or 7 gm/kg of alcohol, and sacrified 48 hours later, showed an average decrease in thymus weight of 42 and 63%, respectively. With adrenalectomized mice, the administration of hydrocortisone caused the same type of shrinkage of the thymus, indicating that shrinkage of the thymus by administration of alcohol may be due to overproduction of corticosteroids.

## 4. Physical Efficiency after Moderate Doses of Alcohol

Garlind *et al.* (G1) conducted a battery of tests, including heart rate, $O_2$ uptake, R.Q., blood lactate, work capacity, and mechanical efficiency, on nine healthy subjects, with and without the ingestion of 0.32 or 0.64 gm/kg of alcohol. The alcohol caused more sweating, but no change in any of the test results. After 0.64 gm/kg of alcohol the blood alcohol level rose to 50–70 mg% in 1 hour.

## 5. Blood Sedimentation Rate

Pilotti and Pisani (P8) reported that human subjects with blood alcohol levels above 200 mg% had abnormally high erythrocyte sedimentation rates.

6. NYSTAGMUS

This term comes from a Greek word meaning *drowsiness*. Medically, nystagmus signifies an involuntary rhythmic oscillation of the eyeballs. The movements are commonly horizontal, but they may be vertical. The speed of movement is quite rapid in one direction, with a much slower return movement. The type of nystagmus movement is designated as *right* or *left*, indicating the direction of the rapid portion of the oscillation. Closing or opening the eyelids does not affect the nystagmus, except that it is somewhat more regular with the eyelids closed. Nystagmus is produced by various physical means. Among these are: stimulation of the inner ear by heat, cold, pressure, or electric impulses; rotation of the body; and fixation of vision on an intermittent light beam. Certain drugs, including alcohol, will induce nystagmus.[3]

A number of investigators have recently studied the relationship between blood alcohol level and three types of nystagmus:

*a. Rotation Nystagmus.* Rotation nystagmus was used by Taschen (T2) as a measure of impairment from alcohol. His procedure is quite simple. The subject is rotated five times around the vertical axis during 10 seconds, the movement is quickly stopped, and the subject's gaze is directed toward a point about 10 inches away. With nonalcoholic subjects, there is a mild nystagmus lasting 4–8 seconds. Various levels of body alcohol prolonged the duration of nystagmus to a maximum of 20 seconds, or more, and increased the frequency and amplitude of the oscillations of the eyeball.

Schulte and Roth (S12) used Taschen's rotation nystagmus test with 240 subjects. The duration of nystagmus, with increasing blood alcohol level, which they found was: no blood alcohol, 0–13 seconds; 10–68 mg% blood alcohol, up to 29 seconds; and 70–150 mg% blood alcohol, more than 29 seconds.

Lommer (L9) studied the correlation between blood alcohol level and results of the Taschen rotation nystagmus test in 1723 observations. He reported a statistical relationship between the two, and proposed a formula for calculating blood alcohol level from the duration of the nystagmus.

*b. Spontaneous Positional Nystagmus.* Alcohol-induced nystagmus was extensively studied by Aschan *et al.* (A14). Their subjects were tested lying down, either in the right lateral or the left lateral position, and with the eyes closed. To record frequency and amplitude of the nystagmus, electrodes were attached to the outside margins of the eyelids and connected to an electrocardiograph apparatus. The experimental results

[3] For literature, prior to 1954, on alcohol-induced nystagmus see reviews by Elbel and Schleyer (E4) and Aschan *et al.* (A14).

covered twenty-one tests with seventeen subjects who ingested 0.23–0.97 gm/kg of alcohol, as brandy, in 1–2 minutes and were studied during a period of 2½ to 13 hours. The resulting nystagmus was in two phases, the average duration of which, expressed as time following the drinking, was: phase I, from ½ to 3.3 hours; phase II, from 4.7 to 6.5 hours; with a period without nystagmus between phase I and phase II lasting an average of 1.4 hours. During phase I, the direction of nystagmus was right in the right lateral position and left in the left lateral position. These directions were reversed in phase II. The amplitude and frequency of the nystagmus were much increased in phase II. Figure 5 shows the average

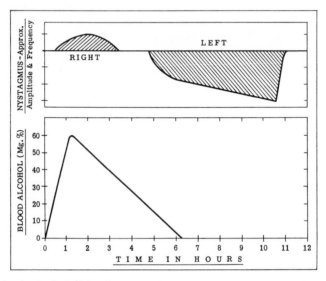

Fig. 5. Blood alcohol level and resulting positional nystagmus. Alcohol dosage 0.23–0.97 gm/kg, ingested within 2 minutes. Graphs give average data from twenty-one experiments with seventeen subjects. Condensed from data reported by Aschan, Bergstedt, Goldberg, and Laurell (A14).

data for these twenty-one experiments. It will be observed that phase II began during the descending phase of blood alcohol and at a rather low alcohol level, and continued long after the subject was alcohol-free. The blood alcohol level at which phase I began varied from 15 to 45 mg% and ranged from 70 mg% to zero when this phase ended.

   *c. Optokinetic Nystagmus.* Krauland *et al.* (K18) produced nystagmus by having the subject fix his gaze on an intermittent beam of light. The oscillation frequency of the resulting nystagmus was recorded with an electrocardiograph apparatus, the leads of which were attached to electrodes at the temporal margins of the eyelids. Ingestion of alcohol was found to reduce, or abolish, this type of nystagmus. Krauland *et al.* reported a fairly good correlation between decrease in nystagmus frequency and increase in blood alcohol level, in the range of blood alcohol of 50–280 mg%.

Rauschke (R4) conducted rotation nystagmus tests with twenty drinking subjects and measured positional nystagmus values with twenty-seven persons. He reported that the correlation between degree of nystagmus and impairment and blood alcohol level was much better with the positional nystagmus than with nystagmus produced by rotation.

Since nystagmus is associated with many types of body pathology, including brain damage, multiple sclerosis, etc., this test is no more specific for alcohol than the other physical tests commonly used.

### 7. Pupillary Width and Reaction to Light

Schleyer and Wichmann (S8) have made a statistical study of the records of about 2000 examinations of subjects where blood alcohol level, pupil width, and pupillary reaction to light were determined. For presenting the eye data, the subjects were grouped according to blood alcohol level. The results for the groups with the highest and lowest blood alcohol are given in Table VII.

TABLE VII

Pupillary Findings of Subjects in Two Blood Alcohol Zones[a,b]

| Blood alcohol (mg%) | Reaction to light | | Pupil width | | |
|---|---|---|---|---|---|
| | Prompt | Sluggish | Medium | Wide | Narrow |
| 0–50 | 90% | 10% | 72% | 24% | 4% |
| 220–240 | 30% | 70% | 56% | 33% | 11% |

[a] Percentage distribution of subjects.
[b] Condensed from data presented by Schleyer and Wichmann (S8).

For intermediate blood alcohol levels the results were between those given in Table VII. It will be noted that elevation of blood alcohol level increased the percentage of subjects with sluggish reaction to light, but even at 240 mg% blood alcohol almost one third of the subjects still exhibited normal pupillary reaction to light. While the incidence of dilated pupils rose somewhat with increase of blood alcohol level, the incidence of contracted pupils rose even more. Schleyer and Wichmann stated: "In individual cases the pupil width gives no conclusive evidence regarding blood alcohol level."

## C. Rising versus Falling Alcohol Level; Adaptation; Tolerance

### 1. IMPAIRMENT AND RISING OR FALLING ALCOHOL LEVEL

Some of the earlier studies purport to show that at a given blood alcohol level during the rising phase there is more impairment than at the same level during the falling phase; these studies really prove very little because the alcohol analyses were made on cubital vein blood (H8). As mentioned in Section IV,A, during active absorption of alcohol the level in cubital vein blood may lag far behind that in arterial blood and brain.

However, fingertip blood was used in the studies by Goldberg (G11) and Eggleton (E2). With three of Goldberg's test methods he reported no difference between rising and falling phases as regards impairment from a given level of blood alcohol. With his other four test procedures, the impairment threshold was somewhat higher during the decreasing phase of blood alcohol.

Eggleton's paper presents very limited data from three experiments with two subjects. In two of these experiments the first blood sample taken was at the peak of the blood alcohol curve, probably because of a very rapid rate of absorption with this subject. During the falling phase the impairment curve dropped more rapidly than the blood alcohol curve.

In a recent study by Rauschke (R2), nineteen subjects ingested 1 gm/kg of alcohol in 15 minutes and were given four tests of impairment at frequent intervals during the period of alcoholemia. Rauschke estimated the blood alcohol level by breath analysis, which would be analogous to the use of arterial or fingertip blood. His four tests of impairment were: reaction time to light and to sound; choice and reaction time to light or sound stimulus, altered at random; and the Elbel ring test.[4] The last two tests involve not only manual dexterity but also some elements of attention and judgment. The average data for Rauschke's nineteen subjects are shown in Fig. 6. These results certainly do not indicate any lessened impairment during the phase of falling blood alcohol level, but, if anything, somewhat greater impairment during this phase.

With the alcohol-induced nystagmus studied by Aschan *et al.* (A14; see Fig. 5), phase I usually began while the blood alcohol level was rising, but the greatest degree of phase I nystagmus occurred while the blood alcohol level was falling. Phase II of the nystagmus did not start until the alcohol level was approaching zero and continued long after the person was alcohol-free. Likewise, alcohol-induced hypoglycemia first appeared

---

[4] In the Elbel ring test the subject must thread ten curtain rings on a wooden rod in the least possible time. Record is kept of time and also of certain errors: missing the end of the rod, dropping the rings, or failure to pick up rings.

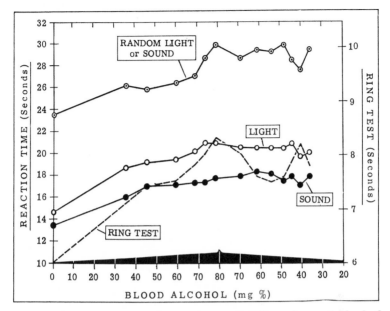

Fig. 6. Relative impairment during rising and falling phases of blood alcohol level, as shown by four tests. Alcohol dosage, 1 gm/kg, ingested within 15 minutes. Abscissa scale is not proportional to time intervals. Redrawn from Rauschke (R2).

while the blood alcohol level was falling and continued during the "hangover" (see Section VI,A,1).

2. ADAPTATION

This term was proposed by Mirsky *et al.* (M14) to designate a reported lessening of impairment from alcohol when a given level of blood alcohol was kept approximately constant for several hours. However, they analyzed cubital vein blood[5] and their reported blood alcohol levels prior to the maximum are probably far below the corresponding arterial levels during this period. A recent study of this problem by Loomis and West (L10), using much more quantitative measurements of impairment, showed no evidence of "adaptation" in any of ten subjects whose blood alcohol was maintained at an almost constant level for a period of 5 hours.

3. TOLERANCE

Further evidence that prolonged administration of alcohol to animals results in less impairment from a given level of blood alcohol have been reported by Kinard and Hay (K7) and Troshina (T5), both using rats

[5] Personal communication from Dr. Mirsky. Also, from the dosages of alcohol administered, the maximum blood alcohols reported seem unbelievably high.

(see Section V,B,7). From the data for humans reported by Goldberg (G11) and Loomis and West (L10) (see Fig. 7 for the latter), Harger

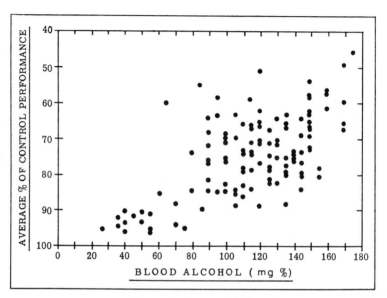

Fig. 7. Blood alcohol level and individual performance scores for 120 simulated driving tests, employing ten subjects. Each point represents the average deterioration for reaction to two light signals and time off the road. From data in Table I of Loomis and West (L10).

(H9) has estimated that for a large group of human subjects the range of blood alcohol level required to produce a given degree of impairment may vary ±30 or 40% from the mean. Thus, the maximum degree of tolerance for alcohol is quite small when compared with the tolerance which some people develop for morphine.

## D. Fatal Acute Alcoholism

### 1. HUMAN CASES

Kaye and Haag (K4) conducted alcohol analyses on post-mortem blood samples from ninety-four cases of fatal acute alcohol intoxication which were not complicated by aspiration pneumonia, other drugs, etc. Terminal blood alcohol levels ranged from 180 to about 600 mg%. From these results, and the duration of coma, Kaye and Haag estimated that the maximum blood alcohol of all of the victims was 500–600 mg%, which level may kill in a short time, or may produce sufficient brain damage to cause death after some hours, during which period the blood alcohol falls considerably.

Fazekas (F1) reported four fatalities which occurred 4–12 hours following the ingestion of 1.4–2.0 gm/kg of alcohol. At autopsy, Fazekas found that the adrenals of three of the victims weighed much less than the average for the victim's age, while the thymus weight was two or three times the normal value. He ascribed these deaths to hypersensitivity to alcohol caused by endocrine imbalance. However, the heart blood of one victim contained 568 mg% alcohol, so the alcohol intake of this victim must have exceeded the amount reported.

Koppanyi (K16) has published a good review of suggested procedures for treating acute alcoholic intoxication. He concluded:

> It is unfortunate that no reliable treatment for severe alcoholic coma is available. The best remedy is probably the symptomatic treatment by good and continuous nursing care for at least 12 hours to keep the respiratory passages free, to keep the patient warm, to turn the patient frequently, administer antibiotics to prevent pneumonia and, if necessary, to employ artificial respiration and/or transfusions of whole blood or plasma expanders. Insulin and glucose or fructose may be employed to accelerate the combustion of alcohol.

Koppanyi also suggested that massive infusion of saline may help to remove alcohol from the body by urinary excretion.

## 2. ANIMAL STUDIES

Klingman and Haag (K12) and Klingman *et al.* (K13) have made extensive studies of blood and urinary changes during lethal alcohol intoxication in dogs. An alcohol dose of 9.0–9.5 gm/kg, given orally in divided doses during 4 hours, killed about two thirds of the dogs within 24 hours. Continuous intravenous infusion of alcohol at a rate of 1.9 gm/kg/hour killed most of the dogs within 5 hours. The chief blood abnormalities produced by either method of alcohol administration were: increase, up to threefold, in blood sugar; drop of about 30% in serum potassium during the initial coma; rise in hematocrit of 30–60%; and decrease in blood pH from about 7.4 to 7.1, which means a doubling of hydrogen ion concentration. The increase in hematocrit was accompanied by a contraction of the spleen, but after splenectomy alcohol still caused some increase in the hematocrit value as compared with controls receiving the same volume of water without alcohol. Administration of a ganglion-blocking agent, hexamethonium chloride, lessened the alcohol-induced hyperglycemia and hypokalemia, but did not abolish the rise in hematocrit. With the urine, the minute volume was markedly decreased within 6 hours, and anuria occurred within 9 hours, the excretion of Na,

K, and urea being decreased proportionally. If the dog lived less than 12 hours after alcohol administration was started, death was usually due to respiratory failure. However, where the fatal period was 12–24 hours after the experiment began, the blood pressure had dropped to shock levels shortly prior to death.

Estable and Grezzi (E7) determined the fatal blood alcohol level for dogs, guinea pigs, and mice from the intraperitoneal administration of 40% alcohol from pure alcohol or from four types of alcoholic beverage. The average fatal blood level was 980 mg%, with a range of 850 to 1450. The average and range were essentially the same for pure alcohol and for the four alcoholic beverages, indicating no effect from the congeners.

## E. Harmful, or Beneficial, Effects of Other Drugs

### 1. CNS (Central Nervous System) Stimulants

*a. Caffeine.* Newman and Newman (N7) gave seven subjects 0.08 gm/kg of alcohol at 20-minute intervals for 2 hours and determined blood alcohol level and reaction to four impairment tests: balance while standing on one foot, hand steadiness, vision, and electroencephalogram. Later, the procedure was repeated, 45 minutes after administering 300 mg of caffeine. The blood alcohol level at which definite impairment in each of the tests began was essentially the same without and with caffeine.

Rutenfranz and Jensen (R9) tested two subjects on the Graf driving machine before and after the ingestion of 0.5 gm/kg of alcohol. Impairment from alcohol was not diminished by giving 200 mg of caffeine.

Hughes and Forney (H26) trained rats to respond to a light stimulus followed by an electric shock, and then gave them 1 gm/kg of alcohol, or the same dose plus 50–150 mg/kg of caffeine. This dose of alcohol alone, or 50 or 100 mg/kg of caffeine alone, produced little blocking of the response to the light or shock stimulus, but alcohol plus caffeine greatly increased the blocking effect. This blocking effect persisted an hour or more after the rats became alcohol-free. On escaping from the shock chamber the rats had a choice of a lighted chamber with a charged floor or a dark chamber with insulated floor. After training, and without alcohol or caffeine, they always chose the latter chamber. Alcohol or caffeine alone caused some errors in this choice, and alcohol plus caffeine greatly increased the number of errors of choice. This effect, too, persisted after the alcohol was gone. Caffeine alone in a dose of 150 mg/kg greatly impaired choice and reaction. The dosages of caffeine used would be very high for a human.

Promill-Ex, an alleged "sobering" agent containing caffeine, was tried on twelve drinking subjects by Mallach (M2). He observed no beneficial effect from it.

*b. Dexedrine and Methamphetamine.* In connection with their studies with caffeine, Newman and Newman also tested their subjects after administering 15 mg of dexedrine. As with caffeine, there was no definite beneficial effect from dexedrine. Rutenfranz and Jensen (R9) reported that administration of 9 mg of methamphetamine (Pervitin) to subjects with a blood alcohol level of 50 mg% caused certain functions, but not all, to return to normal.

## 2. CNS DEPRESSANTS

*a. Morphine.* Eerola *et al.* (E6) used mice to study the toxic effects of various doses of alcohol (4–8 gm/kg) plus morphine (0.05–0.8 gm/kg). They reported, "the joint effect of ethyl alcohol and morphine is not the sum of the effects of these drugs when administered separately but a potentiatative type of synergism."

*b. Dolophine (Polamidone).* Wagner (W2) reported a case of a Dolophine addict who had apparently given himself an intravenous injection of 33 mg of Dolophine while drinking, and was found dead. The blood contained 126 mg% of alcohol. Dolophine was isolated from the liver. The death was attributed to the combined effects of alcohol and Dolophine.

*c. Barbiturates.* Aston and Cullumbine (A15) used mice to test the combined toxic effects of alcohol plus seconal or phenobarbital. They concluded that the combined effect was additive, but that there was no potentiation. Weinig and Schwerd (W7) reviewed the literature on this matter and came to the same conclusion.

Graham (G15) studied the degree and length of coma in patients with barbiturate poisoning, half of whom had also ingested alcohol. In each of eleven pairs of such patients the barbiturate level was about the same, but one member of the pair had also consumed 4–5 fl oz of whisky or gin. With nine of the eleven pairs the member who had taken alcohol exhibited deeper and more lasting coma. Graham also gave mice 25%, 50%, or 75% of the $LD_{50}$ of alcohol, plus 100 minus this per cent of the $LD_{50}$ of pentobarbital. All of these mixtures killed about half of the mice, indicating a simple additive effect. He found that administration of alcohol had no effect on the blood barbiturate level of rats which received a given dose of pentobarbital, showing no change in the rate of absorption of the barbiturate.

*d. Paraldehyde.* Weatherby and Clements (W5) used mice to study the effect of paraldehyde on the toxicity of alcohol. The $LD_{50}$ of the two compounds, given intraperitoneally, was found to be: alcohol, 7 gm/kg; and paraldehyde, 1.77 gm/kg. Simultaneous administration of various fractions of these two doses showed that each compound increased the toxicity of the other, but the fraction of the animals killed was less than the calculated fraction, assuming full additive effect of the two compounds. When the paraldehyde was administered 1–5 hours after the alcohol, the increase in toxicity due to the paraldehyde became progressively less.

3. TRANQUILIZERS

*a. Chlorpromazine (Thorazine).* Kopf (K15) reported that pretreatment with chlorpromazine increased the hypnosis of mice caused by alcohol, but that the potentiation greatly decreased after successive doses of the chlorpromazine.

Zirkle *et al.* (Z1) gave twenty-four subjects a daily dose of 200 mg of chlorpromazine for 1 week and then sufficient alcohol to produce a blood alcohol level of about 50 mg%, after which the subjects were given eight tests of impairment. They reported somewhat greater impairment after alcohol plus chlorpromazine than from alcohol alone. However, the average scores with and without chlorpromazine did not differ greatly.

Hughes and Rountree (H27) gave rats 1 mg/kg of chlorpromazine with, or without, 0.5 gm/kg of alcohol, and tested the rats during a 4-hour period with the electric shock device mentioned in Section VI,E,1 above. Chlorpromazine alone caused some blocking of response to the light stimulus, particularly during the first hour, and some errors in choice of the chamber with insulated floor; alcohol alone caused less impairment of these two functions; while alcohol plus chlorpromazine considerably increased the blocking of the light stimulus and the errors in choice. These impairments continued after the animals became alcohol-free.

Sutherland *et al.* (S23) gave nine subjects 1 gm/kg of alcohol and determined the arterial blood alcohol level and degree of impairment at intervals during the following hour. During the next week the subjects received daily doses of chlorpromazine, starting with 25 mg and ending with 400 mg, and the alcohol tests were then repeated. After chlorpromazine the blood alcohol levels were 10–40% higher than from alcohol alone, and the degree of impairment was greater. With some of the patients, this increased impairment lasted up to 3 hours after the 60-minute test period.

*b. Meprobamate.* Zirkle *et al.* (Z2) tested the effect of meprobamate (400 mg), plus alcohol to give a blood level of 50 mg%, on twenty-two subjects, who were then given the eight impairment tests mentioned in

Subsection VI,E,3,*a* above. Meprobamate added to the impairment from alcohol in about the same amount as that from chlorpromazine.

Hughes and Rountree (H27) also tested the combined effects of meprobamate and alcohol with rats, in the procedure they used for chlorpromazine. Meprobamate added somewhat to the impairment caused by alcohol alone.

### 4. Brain Amines

While these amines are found in some other parts of the body, they seem to be concentrated in certain areas of the brain and may be involved in neurochemical changes associated with cerebration. Rosenfeld (R8) gave mice 4.5 gm/kg of alcohol, intraperitoneally. This caused no deaths, and an average hypnosis period[6] of 74 minutes. Administration, $\frac{1}{2}$ hour after the alcohol, of 35–80 mg/kg of serotonin (5-hydroxytryptamine), tryptamine, and dopamine (3-hydroxytyramine) killed 10–30% of the animals and increased the hypnosis period three- to six-fold. When these doses of the amines were given without alcohol there were no deaths or hypnosis. Tyramine, 125 mg/kg, caused a slight increase in the toxicity of ethanol, and GABA ($\gamma$-aminobutyric acid), 188 mg/kg, had no effect. If 180 or 125 mg/kg, respectively, of serotonin or tryptamine were administered when the mice had just recovered from the hypnosis caused by 4.5 gm/kg of alcohol alone, part of the animals soon fell asleep again. None of the amines caused any increase of $\beta_{60}$.

### 5. Triiodothyronine

As mentioned in Section V,B,5, Goldberg *et al.* (G13) reported that this hormone greatly increased $\beta_{60}$ in deeply intoxicated humans. They also reported a marked "sobering up" effect of the hormone with these patients. Since separate subjects were used as controls, this work should be repeated, using the same experimental subjects as the controls.

### 6. Corticosteroids

Hofle *et al.* (H23) administered 50 mg of Prednisolone (Solu-Decortin-H) to a deeply intoxicated patient with rectal temperature of 34.3°C. Rapid recovery was observed.

### 7. Antabuse and Related Polysulfides

Alha *et al.* (A10) investigated five deaths which they attributed to the combined effect of alcohol plus Antabuse. The blood alcohol levels ranged from 1 to 189 mg%. A similar fatality was reported by Jones (J4).

[6] Interval during which the animal could not right itself when lying on its back.

Korabley (K17) used mice to study the potentiating effect of disulfiram (Antabuse), tetramethylthiuram disulfide, sodium diethyldithiocarbamate, and sodium dimethyldithiocarbamate on the toxicity of alcohol. The dosage of the sulfur compounds was 200 mg/kg for 4 days prior to the alcohol. The thio compounds prolonged and intensified the alcohol effects and lowered the $LD_{50}$.

8. FRUCTOSE

While some workers have reported that intravenous fructose hastens the recovery in severe alcoholic intoxication in humans, tests with rabbits by Avery (A18) led him to conclude that "neither fructose nor glucose was found to have sufficient effect to warrant its use in the treatment of alcohol poisoning."

9. CARBON MONOXIDE

Pecora (P3) exposed dogs to 100 ppm of CO, 6 hours per day, 5 days per week, for 21 weeks. Part of the dogs received alcohol to maintain the blood alcohol at 150 mg% during these periods of exposure to CO. Neither the control dogs exposed to CO alone nor the dogs exposed to CO plus alcohol showed any abnormalities in hemoglobin values, liver function, or electrocardiogram, and none exhibited any neurologic abnormalities.

F. Alcohol Level and Impairment

Earlier investigations on the range of blood alcohol level causing beginning impairment and the range producing frank intoxication have been reviewed by Harger and Hulpieu (H13). Thirteen further studies published since 1953, using more revealing tests than those employed in part of the earlier studies, are summarized in Table VIII.

In the extensive driving tests conducted by Abele (A2), he recorded abnormal speeding and steering and erratic steering wheel movements. These results he presented statistically, giving only the means and deviation ranges, but not the individual scores. The maximum blood alcohol level was about 150 mg%, but he reported marked impairment during the rising phase of blood alcohol, and also during the falling phase even when the blood alcohol had fallen to a low level. In the study by Coldwell et al., all but six of the fifty subjects exhibited impairment before their blood alcohol level reached 100 mg%. With the forty subjects employed by Drew et al., the maximum blood alcohol levels from the largest dose given (0.65 gm/kg) ranged from 55 to 93 mg%, but some of the ten subjects who did not show impairment from this dose had blood alcohol levels much below 93 mg%. The individual results of the study by Loomis and West are

## TABLE VIII
STUDIES CORRELATING BLOOD ALCOHOL LEVEL AND IMPAIRMENT

| Investigator(s) | Date | Number of subjects | Type of impairment test | Level impairing all subjects (mg%) |
|---|---|---|---|---|
| Abele (A2) | 1958 | 33 | Automobile driving | See text |
| Aksenes (A8) | 1954 | 14 | Aviation link trainer | 80 |
| Bohne *et al.* (B11) | 1957 | 15 | Neurophysical measurements | 100 |
| Brecher *et al.* (B19) | 1955 | 14 | Duration of induced double vision | 100 |
| Chardon *et al.* (C5) | 1959 | 25 | Electroencephalo-graph | 40 |
| Chastain (C7) | 1961 | 6 | Automobile driving | 100 |
| Cohen *et al.* (C11) | 1958 | Not given | Automobile driving | 50 |
| Coldwell *et al.* (C13) | 1958 | 50 | Automobile driving | 138 |
| Drew *et al.* (D5) | 1958 | 40 | Simulated driving | 93 (for thirty subjects) |
| Forster and Starck (F12) | 1959 | 6 | Light and dark adaptation | 150 |
| Hoppe and Bachmann (H25) | 1960 | 15 | Verbal-motor measurements | 25 |
| Loomis and West (L10) | 1958 | 10 | Simulated driving | 75 (see Fig. 7) |
| Martin *et al.* (M6) | 1958 | 4 | Simulated driving | 100 |

given in Fig. 7. (Section VI,C,3) As shown by this figure, some subjects were definitely impaired with a blood alcohol level as low as 35 mg%.

# VII. Abnormal Changes in Alcohol Level

## A. Stability of Alcohol in Stored Blood

Krauland and colleagues (K19, K20) stored 684 samples of blood, collected i sterile veules adn analyzed for alcohol, in a refrigerator and performed a second analysis after storage for periods ranging from 90 to 686 days. Of these 684 samples, 130 were preserved with fluoride. Whether the remaining samples contained any anticoagulant is not stated. Analyses of serum or plasma were made by the Widmark and ADH methods. There was a very gradual drop in alcohol level, amounting to 3–4 mg% per 100 days in the samples without fluoride and 1 mg% per 100 days in the samples containing fluoride. After being stored 934 days, about 70% of the fluoride-containing samples were found to be sterile. The remaining 30% contained a few organisms, but the drop in alcohol content was about the same as with the sterile samples. Long storage resulted in much hemolysis, with decrease in hematocrit and increase in specific gravity of the serum. On adjusting the factor of 1.2 originally used to calculate the whole blood alcohol level from that of the serum or plasma to one corresponding to the final water distribution between serum or plasma and clot, the calculated whole blood alcohol level was found to have undergone practically no change during storage. Factors for various time intervals are given. Thus, with blood samples stored in sterile venules, the results of the original analysis may be reliably checked at any time up to almost 3 years.

Karger and Sachs (K3) discussed a common claim that blood samples stored in a stoppered bottle, which is only partly filled with the blood, will lose a substantial fraction of alcohol by vaporization into the air above it in the bottle. They questioned this claim because of the very high blood/air alcohol distribution ratio, which is about 10,000/1 at 10°C and about 5,000/1 at 20°C. This means that if the volume of air in the bottle is ten times the volume of blood, the blood will lose only 1/1000 of its alcohol to the air at 10°C (see Harger *et al.*, H17). Subsequently, Sachs (S1) collected five samples of blood from alcoholic subjects, placed them in rubber-stoppered bottles having a volume five to seven times that of the blood sample, added fluoride, and stored the bottles in a refrigerator. Repeated analyses over a period of 23 days showed no demonstrable drop in the blood alcohol content of the samples.

## B. Possible Post-mortem Changes

### 1. DIFFUSION OF ALCOHOL FROM STOMACH

Publications on this subject prior to 1958 have been reviewed by Elbel and Schleyer (E4) and Harger (H9).

Further evidence that an artificially high level and volume of alcohol in the stomach may cause diffusion of alcohol from stomach contents to pericardial fluid, and sometimes to heart blood, has been published by Hebold (H19). He introduced 250 ml of 15% alcohol solution into the stomachs of each of twelve alcohol-free cadavers, which were then stored, refrigerated, for 1½–24 hours. At the end of the storage period, the bodies were autopsied and certain samples analyzed by the ADH method. No alcohol was found in the femoral vein blood or spinal fluid. The pericardial fluid contained 50–724 mg% alcohol. With four of the cadavers, the heart blood contained no alcohol while with the other eight the heart blood contained 11–149 mg% of alcohol. There was a heart infarct with pericardial obliteration in one cadaver, and a stomach ulcer in another.

Abele and Scholtz (A5) relate the case of a man who died shortly after a traffic accident. Heart blood taken 1½ hours after death showed 19 mg% alcohol. Sixty hours after death the alcohol level in heart blood was 79 mg% and the level in femoral vein blood was 14 mg%. The chest and abdomen were not opened and there was no analysis of stomach contents. If this body was not refrigerated during the 60 hours of storage there is a possibility of neoformation of alcohol in the heart blood. This phenomenon is discussed in the following section. This case emphasizes the need of further, extensive studies in which samples of heart blood, femoral vein blood, and stomach contents are taken shortly after death, and again following refrigeration storage for 12–24 hours.

Two recent studies of post-mortem distribution of alcohol in routine human autopsy cases were reported by Sunshine (S22) and Freireich (F14).[7] Both investigators concluded that their findings showed no evidence of significant post-mortem migration of alcohol from stomach contents to heart blood.

In Sunshine's series of seventy-six cases, the level of alcohol in stomach contents was above 0.5% in twenty-five cases and exceeded 1.0% in only fifteen cases, the maximum being 5.3%. These results indicate that persons do not die with their stomachs full of strong liquor, because of the speed with which ingested alcohol is absorbed. The data from Sunshine's cases where the concentration of alcohol in stomach contents exceeded 0.5% are given in Table IX. In his remaining fifty-one cases, the small gradient between the alcohol levels in stomach contents and heart blood would seem to preclude any significant diffusion.

In sixteen of the twenty-five cases listed in Table IX, the alcohol levels in heart blood and venous blood agreed within ±7%, in two the heart level was below the venous level by 9–15%, and in seven the heart level exceeded the venous level by 8–25%. In three of the last seven cases the venous blood alcohol level exceeded the urine level, showing that death occurred during active absorption, at which time there is a normal lag in the alcohol level of peripheral venous blood. In cases 10 and 25, the urine/heart blood alcohol ratio was within normal limits indicating no abnormal rise in the heart blood level.

Freireich (F14) determined alcohol levels in brain, heart blood, and femoral vein blood in forty-two autopsy cases involving alcohol. The period between death and autopsy ranged from 2 to 22 hours. In twenty-nine of these forty-two cases the heart and femoral vein blood alcohol levels agreed within ±7%, in five cases the level in the heart was 11–28% below that in the femoral vein, and in eight cases the heart level exceeded that of the femoral vein by 9–28%. With five of these last eight cases the

[7] We are indebted to Drs. Sunshine and Freireich for supplying us with prepublication copies of their manuscripts.

TABLE IX
ALCOHOL LEVELS IN ROUTINE HUMAN AUTOPSY CASES[a,b]

| Case no. | Death to autopsy (hr) | Alcohol in stomach contents (%) | Alcohol level in: | | | Ratio of heart blood/ venous blood |
|---|---|---|---|---|---|---|
| | | | Urine (mg%) | Heart blood[c] (mg%) | Venous blood[d] (mg%) | |
| 1 | 14 | 5.3 | 170 | 220 | 180 | 1.22[e] |
| 2 | 8 | 3.2 | 80 | 210 | 180 | 1.17[e] |
| 3 | 12 | 2.5 | — | 190 | 180 | 1.06 |
| 4 | — | 2.4 | — | 20 | 20 | 1.00 |
| 5 | — | 2.0 | — | 220 | 210 | 1.05 |
| 6 | — | 2.0 | — | 250 | 220 | 1.14 |
| 7 | 13 | 1.8 | 360 | 330 | 320 | 1.06 |
| 8 | 13 | 1.6 | 320 | 220 | 220 | 1.00 |
| 9 | 14 | 1.6 | 590 | 490 | 470 | 1.04 |
| 10 | — | 1.6 | 280 | 250 | 200 | 1.25 |
| 11 | 8 | 1.4 | 450 | 340 | 330 | 1.03 |
| 12 | 27 | 1.3 | 210 | 170 | 170 | 1.00 |
| 13 | — | 1.3 | 230 | 160 | 160 | 1.00 |
| 14 | 8 | 1.2 | 260 | 230 | 210 | 1.09 |
| 15 | — | 1.2 | — | 90 | 90 | 1.00 |
| 16 | 13 | 0.8 | 480 | 450 | 440 | 1.02 |
| 17 | — | 0.8 | 330 | 310 | 290 | 1.07 |
| 18 | 1 | 0.8 | 140 | 630 | 580 | 1.08[e] |
| 19 | 2 | 0.7 | — | 200 | 190 | 1.05 |
| 20 | 7 | 0.7 | 210 | 170 | 200 | 0.85 |
| 21 | — | 0.7 | — | 200 | 210 | 0.95 |
| 22 | 10 | 0.6 | — | 300 | 330 | 0.91 |
| 23 | 18 | 0.6 | — | 60 | 60 | 1.00 |
| 24 | — | 0.6 | — | 270 | 290 | 0.93 |
| 25 | — | 0.6 | 110 | 80 | 70 | 1.14 |

[a] Cases with over 0.5% alcohol in stomach contents.
[b] Condensed from data reported by Sunshine (S22).
[c] Blood from right heart.
[d] Blood from right femoral vein or inferior vena cava.
[e] Urine alcohol below venous blood alcohol, indicating active absorption with probable lag in alcohol level of venous blood.

femoral vein blood/brain alcohol ratio ranged from 0.79 to 1.00, which low ratio would occur during active absorption where the femoral vein blood level lags behind that of heart blood. In none of Freireich's forty-two cases was the heart blood/brain alcohol ratio abnormally high, which should have been the case if post-mortem alcohol diffusion from stomach to heart blood had occurred.

## 2. PUTREFACTION OR FERMENTATION

Redetzki *et al.* (R6) placed nine cadavers in a refrigerated room about 12 hours after death. During the next 3 days blood samples were collected in sterile venules and analyzed immediately by the Widmark and ADH methods. The results of the two methods agreed quite well in four cases, but in four others the Widmark result exceeded the ADH result by 27–350%. After storing the venules at 37° for 24 days, the blood samples were again analyzed. The results by both methods showed an increase in alcohol in some samples, no change in a few, and a decrease in others. With three putrid cadavers, two of which had been in cold water for about 40 days and one under a feather mattress for 2 days, femoral vein blood contained 0–15 mg% alcohol (40 mg% by Widmark in one case), while blood from the right heart and thoracic cavity showed 80–263 mg% alcohol by the Widmark method and 40–56 mg% by the ADH method. Fresh blood collected in sterile venules containing fluoride and stored 4 weeks at room temperature changed only slightly in alcohol content. Redetzki *et al.* concluded that post-mortem putrefaction or fermentation can cause destruction, or neoformation, of alcohol.

Bonnichsen *et al.* (B13) analyzed blood, urine, stomach contents, and certain tissues taken from four cadavers about 24 hours after death. Although recent ingestion of alcohol was excluded, the Zeisel alkoxy and ADH methods agreed in indicating 0–390 mg% alcohol varying greatly in different parts of the same cadaver. In two cadavers the blood alcohol was 0 and 19–23 mg%, while the stomach contents and pleural fluid levels were over 300 mg% and 200 mg%, respectively in one, and the kidney and brain 79 mg% and 31 mg% in the other. With the other two cadavers the blood levels were 164 and 237 mg%, while the levels in stomach contents were 12–23 mg%. They also reported analyses by the Widmark and alkoxy methods of blood and urine from thirty-four other cadavers. Where the period between death and autopsy was not over 2 days, the results by the two methods agreed within 20 mg%. Where this period was 3–15 days, the results by the Widmark method were much higher than those by the ADH method, the difference ranging from 22 to 230 mg% for blood, but much less for urine.

Abele and Scholz (A5) analyzed blood and/or urine from 227 cadavers by the Widmark and ADH methods. The data are presented statistically, with average deviations from the mean, but individual data are not given. The results by the two methods agreed quite well and do not appear to indicate any post-mortem changes in alcohol level. However, the period between death and autopsy is not given.

Paulus and Janitzki (P1) collected bloods from nonalcoholic subjects in sterile venules. After being kept at room temperature up to 14 days, analyses by the ADH method showed no alcohol. Similar samples, placed in cork-stoppered tubes, showed 10 mg% alcohol after 3 days and up to 16 mg% after 14 days. They also used the Widmark and ADH methods to analyze samples of blood from 200 cadavers. In 121 samples, where the ADH reading was zero, the Widmark results were zero in seventy-five samples and ranged from 10 to 70 mg% in the remaining forty-six samples. In twenty-four cases, with no history of drinking, where the period between death and autopsy was 1–14 days, the ADH results ranged from 10 to 20 mg% alcohol and the Widmark results showed 0–52 mg% alcohol. With the remaining twelve cadavers, which represented drinking subjects, the blood alcohol level by the Widmark method generally exceeded that by the ADH method, being greater by 50% or more in two thirds of the samples. The time between death and autopsy for these 124 cadavers is not given.

Weinig and Schwerd (W8) reported that putrefaction or fermentation of blood within a cadaver can rather rapidly form some ethanol, higher alcohols, and even traces of methanol. They warn against the forensic use of alcohol analyses made on blood from a putrefied body.

3. DROWNING

Schweitzer (S14) administered by stomach tube about 2.6 gm/kg of alcohol, as 20% solution, to fifteen rabbits. After 1½ hours blood samples were drawn from an ear vein for alcohol analysis, and the animals were then killed by immersion in water for about 10 minutes until the heart ceased to beat. Femoral vein blood was taken immediately afterward. In one animal the alcohol level was the same as that in the ear vein before death, with eleven there was a drop of 3–12% (average, 7%), and with three there was a rise of 2–20% (average, 9%). Schweitzer ascribes the fall in blood alcohol to blood dilution from inhaled water.

4. BURNING

Vidoni and Redenti (V5) subjected rabbits under Evipan narcosis to fatal burning and found no reducing substance in heart blood or thoracic cavity fluid. Alcohol was administered to a second group of rabbits, and blood samples were taken 1 hour later and then immediately following fatal burning, as with the first group. The burning caused no change in the alcohol level of heart blood. The alcohol experiment was repeated, with the second blood sample taken 6–7 hours after death, and the result was the same.

## VIII. Medicolegal Interpretation of Blood Alcohol Level

### A. Legislation

1. EARLY MEASURES

In 1926, Norway passed a law providing that if a motor vehicle operator's blood contains over 50 mg% of alcohol "it shall be presumed that he was under the influence of intoxicating liquor" (I2). This law is still in effect (W16). The next such legislation was enacted in Sweden in 1934. It stipulated that if a driver's blood alcohol level was 150 mg%, or above, "he shall be considered to have been under the influence . . ." and be given a heavy fine or jail sentence. The Swedish law also provided a lesser penalty for driving with blood alcohol level between 80 and 150 mg%, but did not label the particular offense. In 1957, this zone was lowered to 50 mg%.

2. LATER LEGISLATION

Between 1939 and 1960, thirty-four states of the U.S.A. and the District of Columbia enacted legislation providing for chemical tests for intoxication in traffic cases and specifying the presumptive medicolegal interpretation for three zones of blood alcohol level (N3). All of these jurisdictions, except North Dakota, have followed a model act recommended in 1938–39 by the National Safety Council and American Medical Association (A12), which divided drinking drivers into three zones, to be interpreted as follows:

*Zone I.* Blood alcohol below 50 mg%, *no one* under influence.

*Zone II.* Blood alcohol 50–150 mg%, some people, but not all, under the influence.

*Zone III.* Blood alcohol 150 mg%, or above, *all* persons under the influence.

North Dakota's recently enacted law changes the boundary between Zone II and Zone III to 100 mg%, which follows present day views that the 150 mg% limit, suggested over 20 years ago, is too high. Variations in certain details of the chemical test laws in the U.S.A. have been reviewed by Donigan (D3, A12).

In 1954, New York State added a section to their chemical test law providing for revocation of license of a driver who, after arrest, refuses to submit to a chemical test for intoxication. This type of *implied consent* law was subsequently enacted in seven other states of the U.S.A., and in Saskatchewan Province of Canada and in the Province of Queensland, Australia.

As with poison analyses, the results of chemical tests for intoxication are usually admissible evidence in jurisdictions not having laws specifying the medicolegal interpretation of the level of blood alcohol, and this is true in all other states of the U.S.A., in Canada, and in many countries of Europe and other parts of the world. In these jurisdictions the chemical test results must be supported by expert testimony, or by judicial decree. The Dominion of Canada 1951 law provides for chemical test evidence, but stipulates no presumptive limits of blood alcohol. A 1956 paper by Wolff (W16) stated, "in Denmark and Finland there is no statutory limit but it is generally assumed that a person is intoxicated at a concentration of 1.0 per mil (100 mg%)."

In most jurisdictions having chemical test legislation the law permits calculation of the blood alcohol level from analysis of urine, saliva, or breath.

### B. Recommendations of Scientific Bodies

In 1954, the West German Government appointed a committee of medicolegal experts to consider the matter of chemical tests for intoxication and the blood alcohol level at which all drivers are under the influence. The committee endorsed the 0.15% (1.5 per mil) blood alcohol limit (W9) in the following language:

> The motor vehicle operator requires a sensitive perception-and-judgment ability for every unusual and unexpected moving change of the traffic situation within his sphere, he must literally anticipate the future traffic situation. Especially this ability to feel one's way in the traffic events is adversely affected with certainty at a blood alcohol concentration of 1.5 pro mille even in alcohol-habituated motor vehicle operators. Because of all this, no scientifically established facts are known which permit assuming that driving fitness still exists above a blood alcohol concentration of 1.5 pro mille. [1.5 pro mille equals 0.15%.] (Translation by Dr. Kurt M. Dubowski.)

At a symposium on alcohol and road traffic held at Indiana University in 1958 a special technical committee issued the following report (P12):

> As a result of the material presented at this Symposium, it is the opinion of this Committee that a blood alcohol concentration of 0.05% will definitely impair the driving ability of some individuals and, as the blood alcohol concentration increases, a progressively higher proportion of such individuals are so affected, until at a blood alcohol concentration of 0.10%, all individuals are definitely impaired.

The members of this committee who voted unamiously for this recommendation were: Rolla N. Harger, Indiana; Leonard Goldberg, Sweden; Herman A. Heise, Milwaukee (Chairman, A.M.A. Committee on Medicolegal Problems); Ted A. Loomis, Seattle; Henry W. Newman, San

Francisco; D. W. Penner, Manitoba, Canada; and H. Ward Smith, Toronto, Canada.

A British Medical Association Special Committee reported in 1959 as follows (B21):

> The committee considers that a concentration of 50 mg of alcohol in 100 ml of blood while driving a motor vehicle is the highest that can be accepted as entirely consistent with the safety of other road users. While there may be circumstances in which individual driving ability will not depreciate significantly by the time this level is reached, the committee is impressed by the rapidity with which deterioration occurs at blood levels in excess of 100 mg./100 ml. This is true even in the case of hardened drinkers and experienced drivers. he committee cannot conceive of any circumstances in which it could be considered safe for a person to drive a motor vehicle on the public roads with an amount of alcohol in the blood greater than 150 mg./100 ml.

In 1960, the U.S. National Safety Council's Committee on Alcohol and Drugs unanimously approved the following statement (N3):

> That the Committee on Alcohol and Drugs of the National Safety Council urges the State Legislatures when amending or enacting chemical test laws to establish the three blood alcohol levels at 0 to 0.05 per cent, 0.05 per cent to 0.10 per cent, 0.10 per cent and above.

On the recommendation of the American Medical Association's Committee on Medicolegal Problems, the A.M.A. Board of Trustees and House of Delegates recommended in 1960 that (A12, 1960 Addendum):

> Blood alcohol of 0.10% be accepted as *prima facie* evidence of alcoholic intoxication, recognizing that many individuals are under the influence in the 0.05% to 0.10% range.

## IX. Analytical Methods for Body Alcohol

A large number of analytical methods for alcohol published prior to 1954 have been reviewed by Friedemann and Dubowski (F15) and by Harger (H9).

### A. Modified Dichromate Methods

#### 1. WIDMARK DIFFUSION PROCEDURES

Weinig (W6) has modified the Widmark method, particularly for cadaver blood. The blood is diluted, treated with $HgSO_4$, tungstate, and 1.7 $N$ $H_2SO_4$, and distilled. An aliquot of the distillate is placed in the Widmark cup, one drop of $HgSO_4$ solution and one drop of 10% NaOH are added, and the remaining Widmark procedure is carried out. Weinig claims much less interference from nonalcohol substances in cadaver blood.

To determine the end point in the Widmark titration of excess dichromate, Schmidt *et al.* (S11) have replaced the starch indicator by measurement of change in potential. They reported an accuracy of 0.1–0.3%.

Kael and Bina (K1) enlarged the Widmark flask from 50 ml to 118 ml and widened the neck of the flask. They claim these changes facilitate dilution of the reaction fluid prior to the titration and help to avoid wetting the flask neck with the standard thiosulfate solution.

Kent-Jones and Taylor (K5) proposed a slightly altered Cavett (C4) method by conducting the diffusion for 4 hours at 37° instead of 2 hours at 70°. (The original Cavett method is essentially the Widmark method with the dichromate reaction fluid 18 $N$ instead of 36 $N$ (conc.) $H_2SO_4$, and the excess dichromate titrated with the $FeSO_4$–methyl orange reagent of Harger (H9).

Nickolls (N10) has described a "modified Cavett method," although it is more nearly a macro Widmark method, employing 2 ml of blood or urine. The diffusion chamber is a 16-oz, wide mouth, screw-capped bottle, with the top of the neck ground plane to effect closure with a circular glass plate inside the cap. The jar contains 10 ml of $N/10$ $K_2Cr_2O_7$ in 18 $N$ $H_2SO_4$. The sample of blood or urine is placed in a 2-inch Petri dish which is supported on a glass tripod inside the jar. After diffusion has proceeded for 8 hours at 37° the reaction fluid is diluted to 12 fl oz, KI and starch are added, and the fluid is titrated with 0.1 $N/10$ thiosulfate.

## 2. CONWAY CELL METHODS

Williams *et al.* (W12) place dichromate in 18 $N$ $H_2SO_4$ in the center compartment and 0.1 ml of blood plus 1 ml of 20% $Na_2CO_3$ in the outer portion. Diffusion proceeds for 1 hour at 55–60°. The center compartment fluid is transferred to a 25-ml volumetric flask, diluted somewhat, and 3 ml of a 1% brucine solution in 10% $H_2SO_4$ are added. The fluid is made up to 25 ml and the blue color read at 425 m$\mu$. The authors claim an average accuracy of ±2.0%.

Boiteau (B12) uses 0.03 $N$ dichromate in 10 $N$ $H_2SO_4$ in the center compartment with the blood sample plus $Na_2CO_3$ in the outer chamber and diffuses 2 hours at room temperature. Excess dichromate is titrated with $FeSO_4$, using diphenylamine-$p$-sulfonate as indicator. Excess dichromate is also determined by spectrophotometer at 349 m$\mu$. Accuracy claimed, ±1% by the titration method and ±2% by spectrophotometry.

## 3. OTHER DICHROMATE METHODS

The method of Cordebard (C16), which is official in France, uses concentrated HNO$_3$ instead of H$_2$SO$_4$, and the conversion of alcohol to acetic acid is said to be complete in 1 minute at 20–25°. Ten milliliters of urine plus 2 ml of 20% NaPO$_3$ are distilled into a tube containing 5 ml of 0.1 N dichromate in concentrated HNO$_3$, until the volume in the receiving tube reaches 10 ml. This fluid is then diluted ten-fold, KI and starch are added, and the liberated iodine titrated with thiosulfate. Griffon and LeBreton (G16) reported that the accuracy of this method is within ±8%.

Kirk *et al.* (K9) have developed a variant of the Kozelka–Hine dichromate method, employing a complicated glass unit which serves as steam generator, distillation chamber, and alkaline mercury scrubber. This unit consists of a 1-inch all glass scrubber tube entirely surrounded by a 2-inch glass shell. A short length of ⅝-inch tubing, sealed to the top of the scrubber inlet, is for holding a roll of filter paper on which the blood sample is absorbed. The scrubber tube outlet passes through the jacket wall and connects with a delivery tube extending to the bottom of a narrow receiving tube. The mouth of the shell is closed with a glass stopper and a glass inlet tube enters near the bottom of the shell. The scrubber tube contains alkaline HgSO$_4$, and about 15 ml of water are placed in the bottom of the shell. The receiving tube contains 5 ml of 0.1 N dichromate plus 5 ml of concentrated H$_2$SO$_4$, which, on being mixed, reach an initial temperature of about 110°. A roll of dry filter paper, impregnated with NaH$_2$PO$_4$ and MgCl$_2$, is inserted into the top of the scrubber inlet and 1 ml of blood is absorbed in this paper. Air is drawn through the glass unit and receiver at a rate of 200–300 ml/minute and the water in the glass shell is kept gently boiling over a small flame. Distillation and oxidation of the alcohol are completed in about ½ hour. The contents of the receiving tube, now measuring 15 ml, are diluted to 50 ml and the excess dichromate is determined by the usual KI-thiosulfate titration, or read with a spectrophotometer. Results with bloods deviated 1–9% from the correct values, so this method seems to offer little improvement over those using inexpensive, conventional apparatus.

## B. Acid Permanganate Methods

For determining very low concentrations of alcohol in breath, Harger and colleagues (H10, P6) have decreased the volume of 0.05 N KMnO$_4$ per 10 ml of 16 N H$_2$SO$_4$ to 0.2 ml, instead of 1.0 ml. This modified reagent was subsequently employed by Goldbaum (G10) to analyze air equilibrated with alcoholic blood in a glass syringe. Lester and Greenberg (L5) have reported an acid permanganate micro method for determining alcohol in biological fluids. The sample of fluid, containing not over 35 μg of alcohol, and a volume of 0.2 ml or less, is spread on a 2-cm square of filter paper within a 30-ml flask. The flask is heated to 100° and a current of nitrogen, 100 ml/minute, is passed for 10–15 minutes through the flask and into a receiving tube containing 10 ml of 16 $N$ $H_2SO_4$. The tube connecting flask and receiver is heated to prevent moisture condensation. One milliliter of 0.01 $N$ $KMnO_4$ is now added to the 10 ml of fluid in the receiver and at the end of 5 minutes the color of the remaining permanganate is read at 520 m$\mu$ with a spectrophotometer. The standard deviation is said to be ±1%.

## C. Alcohol Dehydrogenase Methods

Brink *et al.* (B20) have modified the original Bonnichsen and Theorell method (B15), chiefly by greatly increasing the concentration of ADH, so that the reaction to DPN-$H_2$ goes to completion, as in the method of Bucher and Redetzki (B22).

A concise and clear review by Redetzki and Johannsmeier (R5) compares the two ADH methods of the Swedish group with the method developed by the German investigators, and discusses the application of the Michaelis constant to the reactions involved. They state that the presence of fluoride in amounts usually added to blood does not inhibit the reaction.

Lundquist and Wolthers (L14) have modified the ADH method to determine very low serum alcohol concentrations. For serum alcohol concentrations of 20–50 mg% the final dilution of the serum was 300:1; for 2–20 mg% alcohol it was 60:1; and for concentrations below 2 mg% the final dilution was 15:1.

Machata (M0) has studied the various steps in the ADH method of Bucher and Redetzki and gives suggestions for attaining maximum accuracy. To obtain a standard solution of alcohol containing 1% ethanol, he dissolves 303 mg of glycine ethyl ester hydrochloride in 10 ml of 2 $N$ NaOH and allows the solution to stand for 35 minutes at room temperature.

Kirk *et al.* (K9) have described an ADH method using a 0.1-ml sample of blood placed on a small filter paper roll inside a 30-ml diffusion flask containing the ADH-DPN-semicarbazide-buffer reagent. At room temperature they found that diffusion of alcohol into, and reaction with, the reagent was complete in 90 minutes. Their diffusion device is much like those used by Abels and Sheftel for their respective dichromate methods (A7, S15).

Kaplan and Ciotti (K2) substituted the acetylpyridine derivative of DPN (APDPN) in the ADH method for ethanol. They reported that reduced APDPN has a maximum light absorption at 365 m$\mu$, as compared with 340 m$\mu$ for reduced DPN.

Brahm-Vogelsanger and Wagner (B18) have developed an ADH method for acetaldehyde. Instead of DPN, they use DPN-$H_2$, and measure the decrease in reduced DPN photometrically at 366 m$\mu$, acetaldehyde being converted to ethanol.

## D. Alcohol Dehydrogenase Plus Diaphorase

In 1958, Teller (T3) reported a modification of the ADH method yielding a visible color change.[8] To the ADH-DPN-semicarbazide reagent he added the flavoprotein enzyme, *diaphorase,* and 2,6-sodium dichlorophenolindophenol. The last is the blue dye long used in the determination of ascorbic acid. Under the influence of diaphorase, the DPN-H$_2$ initially formed in the oxidation of alcohol to acetaldehyde reacts with the dye, decreasing the depth of blue color. This color change is read at 600 m$\mu$, which eliminates the use of ultraviolet spectrophotometry. The maximum color change is reached in about 2 minutes, so serial readings must be made. He reported that 1 $\mu$g of ethanol causes a decrease of about 0.09 in optical density. To analyze blood, the serum or plasma is diluted 1:100 with saline or water and 0.1 ml of the diluted solution is employed. The accuracy with known solutions of alcohol was said to be ±6%.

Subsequently, Machata (M1) investigated this method, using enzymes made in Germany. In his hands, the accuracy of the method was unsatisfactory, due to variable oxidation of the reduced dye by air.

## E. Gas Chromatography

This analytical method employs the principles of chromatography commonly used to separate liquid or solid compounds, but the compounds to be separated enter and leave the column as gases. On entering the column, the gas dissolves in a high boiling liquid which coats the inert, solid granules of the column, or is adsorbed on the column, if the latter is of the adsorptive type. This segment of dissolved, or adsorbed, gas is caused to travel along the column by means of a *carrier gas,* which flows through the column at a constant rate. The compounds present in the gas travel at different speeds and, using the proper column ingredients, each compound in the gas mixture should leave the column as a separate fraction. The moving carrier gas really distills the compound from the back to the front of its particular dissolved segment.

In 1958, Cadman and Johns (C1) described a method for determining ethanol in blood employing the Beckman Model GC-2 gas chromatograph. The coiled ¼-inch column is filled with 42- to 60-mesh firebrick, impregnated with 28% of a 15:10:3 mixture of Flexol, diisodecylphthalate, and polyethylene glycol 600. One milliliter of the blood plus 1 gm of

---

[8] Dr. Teller kindly furnished us with a copy of his paper, which has not yet been published.

$K_2CO_3$ is extracted with 1 ml of *n*-propylacetate which removes about 77% of the alcohol. An aliquot of the extract (0.020–0.035 ml) is introduced into the vaporizing chamber connected to the column. This chamber, the column, and thermal conductivity detector at the end of the column are heated to 120°C, which vaporizes the ethanol and its solvent. The thermal conductivity changes of the detector are recorded on a moving strip chart. Helium is the carrier gas, the flow rate being 60 ml/minute. With the 6-ft column the ethanol appears in the conductivity detector during an interval of about 1 minute, beginning around 3 minutes after the sample enters the vaporizing chamber. The *n*-propylacetate appears about 4 minutes later. With the 12-ft column the ethanol response begins about 7 minutes after the start. The quantity of ethanol is proportional to the area under the peak on the moving strip chart. The satisfactory working range is 5–60 $\mu$g of ethanol. For complete separation of ethyl ether, methanol, acetone, and ethanol, which appear in this order, the 12-ft column was needed. The authors reported an accuracy of ±3 mg% ethanol, but their results with sixteen samples of alcoholic blood showed deviations of 1–17 mg% (average, 6 mg%) between their gas chromatography results and those by the Kozelka–Hine method. A later paper by Cadman and Johns (C2) gives further information on the use of gas chromatography for determining ethanol and other volatile compounds.

Fox (F13) used distillates of blood or urine and placed 0.05–0.10 ml of the distillate directly into the column of the Perkin–Elmer gas chromatograph. He reported an accuracy of about ±5%.

Chundela and Janak (C8) conducted blood ethanol analyses with a British gas chromatograph employing thermal conductivity and an apparatus made in Prague which used flame ionization detection. In part of their analyses they introduced 0.1 ml of the blood directly into the instrument, but had to refill the column after about fifteen analyses. With the first procedure, the results were 8–15% below those by the Widmark method, and the column did not separate ethanol and methanol. The second instrument gave good separation of these two alcohols, but some of the duplicate analyses for ethanol did not agree too well.

Janitzki (J2) reported a preliminary study with the Beckman GC-2 gas chromatograph in which he experimented with various materials for the column, stationary phase, and carrier gas. He used a large number of volatile substances which might be present in blood.

We are told that the properties of a given chromatograph column change with use, so that it is necessary to routinely use a standard alcoholic blood to check the results.

## F. Other Blood Alcohol Methods

### 1. VANADATE METHOD

Vidic (V3, V4) employs the Widmark desiccation flask but substitutes for the $H_2SO_4$-$K_2Cr_2O_7$ reagent a reagent made by dissolving 4.3 gm of $NaVO_3$ in 100 ml of concentrated $H_2SO_4$ plus 13 ml of $H_2O$. Three milliliters of this latter reagent are placed in the flask and 0.5 ml of blood or urine in the cup. After 3 hours at 85°, 20 ml of water are added to the fluid in the flask, and the resulting blue color is read photometrically, using a standard made by adding blue $VOSO_4$ to the diluted reagent.

### 2. ACETALDEHYDE-THIOSEMICARBAZONE METHOD

This method, developed by Schmidt and Manz (S9), oxidizes the alcohol to acetaldehyde in a diffusion cell containing 0.5 N $H_2SO_4$, 5% $K_2Cr_2O_7$, and 0.5% $CrCl_2$. The resulting, volatilized acetaldehyde reacts with a solution of thiosemicarbazide in a separate chamber, and the thiosemicarbazone formed is determined spectrophotometrically at 260 m$\mu$.

## G. Breath Alcohol Procedures

### 1. PLASTIC BREATH CONTAINERS

Salem *et al.* (S3) reported that plastic bags made of *Saran*, which is a polymer of vinylidine chloride and vinyl chloride, serve excellently for storing breath samples containing alcohol vapor. Air equilibrated with a water solution of alcohol, and placed in bags made of Saran with a wall thickness of about 0.001 inch, had lost only 3–6% of its alcohol after 24 hours storage. A 1956 paper by Harger *et al.* (H10) also presents data on the migration of alcohol vapor through certain bag materials.

### 2. BREATHALYZER

This instrument was announced by Borkenstein in 1954 (B16) and was later described in detail by Borkenstein and Smith (B17). It employs a 52.5-ml sample of alveolar air collected in a metal cylinder, which is then passed through 3 ml of 18 N $H_2SO_4$ containing 0.25 mg of $K_2Cr_2O_7$ per ml. The decrease in yellow color is measured by means of an ingenous photometer. The light source is moved between the test ampule and a standard ampule until the light passing through the two ampules causes equal response in identical photocells placed back of the ampules, as shown by a null-point ammeter. The instrument dial indicates this movement of the light source, and the weight of alcohol oxidized is directly proportional to the dial reading. This is because both light intensity/distance and transmittance/concentration are logarithmic functions, making the ratio between the two functions linear. With other photoelectric instruments, the scale is logarithmic. This linearity of the Breathalyzer scale eliminates errors due to small variations in the dichromate concentration of the ampule fluid, or changes in line voltage. It also permits successive analyses with the same ampule, until practically all of the dichromate is reduced. The weight of alcohol oxidized in the test is multiplied by 40 to give the weight of alcohol in 2100 ml of alveolar air, which is the weight of alcohol in 1 ml of the subject's blood (N2).

### 3. Intoximeter, Photoelectric Type

Forrester's previous Intoximeter absorbed the alcohol and carbon dioxide from a sample of ordinary breath and the weights of alcohol and $CO_2$ caught were later determined by a chemist. The blood alcohol level was calculated from the alcohol:$CO_2$ ratio. A rough quantitative test, using permanganate in 10 $N$ $H_2SO_4$, was performed at the time of collecting the breath. A photoelectric instrument employing alveolar air was recently developed by Forrester (F7). Alveolar air is collected in two 105-ml metal cylinders. One of the alveolar air samples is passed through 4 ml of approximately 18 $N$ $H_2SO_4$ containing 0.21 mg of $K_2Cr_2O_7$ per ml and the decrease in yellow color is measured photoelectrically with a modified Klett null-point instrument. The weight of alcohol oxidized times 20 equals milligrams alcohol per 2100 ml alveolar air, or milligrams alcohol per milliliter blood. The second sample of alveolar air is passed through a tube containing solid magnesium perchlorate, to be used for later check analysis.

### 4. Drunkometer, Using Rebreathed Air

This modification, which eliminates the $CO_2$ determination used in the former Drunkometer, was reported by Harger *et al.* in 1956 (H10). The subject exhales into a warm 2-qt polyethylene bag and rebreathes this air four times. The rebreathed air is then passed through the usual reagent (10 ml of 16 $N$ $H_2SO_4$ plus 1 ml of 0.05 $N$ $KMnO_4$) until the end point is reached. The weight of alcohol caught (0.169 mg) times 2100/ volume of rebreathed air used equals weight of alcohol per 2100 ml of rebreathed air, or weight of alcohol per milliliter of blood. Rebreathed air and alveolar air contain the same concentration of alcohol. The volume of rebreathed air used in the test is measured by means of a compact, dry, glass metering suction pump.

5. Gas Chromatography

The Beckman instrument used by Cadman and Johns for analyzing blood for alcohol was also used by them for determining the alcohol content in 10 ml of alveolar air (C2). Analyses of blood and alveolar air from a subject indicated that the blood alcohol level could be calculated from the alcohol level in alveolar air, employing the commonly accepted 2100:1 ratio.

The Beckman instrument was used by Lins and Randonat (L7) to determine how long the breath contained alcohol after a nondrinker rinsed his mouth with a strong solution of alcohol.[9]

A compact, portable gas chromatograph for determining the alcohol level of alveolar air has been announced by Wilson (W14) of the Aerojet-General Corporation of California.

In 1962, Lester (L3) reported the use of an Aerograph Model A-600-B gas chromatograph, equipped with a hydrogen flame ionization detector, to study the problem of the "endogenous" alcohol (see Section II). He reported that this apparatus will detect as little as 0.002 μg of ethanol in a 7-ml sample of alveolar air.

6. Alcotest Modification

This device, originated by Grosskopf (G17), has been widely used in continental Europe as a preliminary test for breath alcohol. It is a small sealed glass tube about 3 cm in length filled with silica gel, a section of which is impregnated with concentrated $H_2SO_4$ containing dissolved $K_2Cr_2O_7$. To perform the test, the ends of the tube are opened, a 1-liter plastic bag is attached to the distal end, and the subject blows 1 liter of breath through the tube. The length of the impregnated part which changes from yellow to green is a rough measure of the weight of alcohol in the liter of breath used. Pfeil and Goldbach (P5) place 0.2–0.3 gm of "Blaugel" (a moisture indicator) just ahead of the impregnated section. They stated that this gel will lose all of its blue color with the passage of approximately 1 liter of breath, making the plastic bag unnecessary.

H. Specificity of Methods

1. Garlic Odor of Breath

Fazekas and Deak (F2) had human subjects consume large amounts

[9] Lins and Randonat discarded the first 200 ml of exhaled breath and then used the next 10 ml for the analysis. The alcohol levels they found are probably much higher than if they had used alveolar air, rebreathed air, or a 2-liter sample of mixed expired air. Even so, all alcohol had disappeared in 15 minutes.

of garlic and analyzed their blood by the Widmark method and their breath by the Harger permanganate method. No reducing substance was found. Prolonged administration of garlic extract to rabbits gave the same negative result on testing the blood by the Widmark method.

## 2. CANDLE WAX

Audrlicky and Beran (A16) received test tube samples of blood where melted candle material had been dropped on top of the blood to eliminate the air space above it. Melted candle wax was added to water containing 60 mg% of alcohol. Analyses of the water solution 24–96 hours later showed no increase in alcohol content.

## 3. SKULL TRAUMA

Wagner and Wagner (W3) performed alcohol analyses by the Widmark and ADH methods on blood samples from 551 cases of skull injury. Agreement of the two methods indicated no formation of an alcohol-like substance which would alter the Widmark results.

## 4. DIABETES

Paulus and Mallach (P2) used the Widmark and ADH methods to analyze blood and urine samples from twenty-six diabetics, some of whom had pronounced acetonuria. The "alcohol" levels in the blood, expressed as mg%, were: Widmark: 10–49, average, 14; ADH: for nineteen diabetics, 0, and for seven, 1–6. The corresponding results for eleven urines containing much acetone were: Widmark: 9–55, average, 34; ADH: for nine, 0, for one, 1, and for one, 2.

Blotner (B9) has reported that diabetics, who had taken no alcohol, sometimes showed "alcohol" in the blood and urine, the highest reading observed by him being 78 mg% for blood and 149 mg% for urine.

Coldwell and Grant (C12), using the Breathalyzer, found no "alcohol" in the breath of diabetics who were receiving insulin.

The reaction of acetone in the dichromate alcohol methods depends on the concentration of sulfuric acid used, the temperature employed for the reaction, and the time of heating. The results reported by Paulus and Mallach and by Blotner suggest the need for further study of the blood, urine, and breath of severe diabetics with acetonemia, using various analytical procedures.

## 5. CHLORINATED HYDROCARBONS

Schleyer (S7) exposed a subject to a high concentration of tetrachlorethylene vapor for 130 minutes. At the end of the period the blood showed no alcohol by the Widmark method, and Breathalyzer analyses indicated 10–20 mg% "alcohol" in the blood. Schleyer stated that the low Breathalyzer readings are within the usual variation of results with this instrument. Lob (L8) added trichlorethylene to blood, but analysis by the ADH method gave a reading of zero. However, on adding 600 mg% of trichlorethylene to blood, the Nicloux method gave a reading of 100 mg% "alcohol."

### 6. ETHER

Alha and Karlsson (A11) tested blood samples from twenty-six physicians present during open ether anesthesia administration, using the Widmark method. The average result was 0.7 mg%, the highest being 4.6 mg%, expressed as ethanol.

### 7. ALIPHATIC ESTERS

Klein (K10) obtained high blood alcohol values by the ADH method in a subject who had inhaled the vapor of ethyl acetate. Weyrich and Hauck (W10) killed guinea pigs by exposure to the vapors of a cement solvent containing methyl and ethyl acetate. With two of the animals, the blood "alcohol" figures were: Widmark method, 71 and 92 mg%; ADH method, 51 and 54 mg%. Weyrich and Hauck also studied the case of a workman at the end of a day during which he was exposed to the vapors from this cement and had consumed about 1 liter of beer. His blood alcohol at the end of the day, by the Widmark and ADH methods, was no higher than could be accounted for from the beer ingested.

## X. Investigations of the Accuracy of Analytical Methods

The accuracy to be expected from a given method for determining body alcohol is usually estimated from a statistical study of many analyses. On a probability basis, the results may be expressed in three ways:
(1) *Standard Deviation, Probable Error or Sigma.* If this is expressed as $x$, two thirds of an infinite number of analyses will give results within $\pm x$ from the correct figure.
(2) *Confidence Limit of 95% (3 Sigma).* Ninety-five of 100 analytical results will be within $\pm 3 x$ from the correct figure.
(3) *Maximum Error.* This is the greatest deviation encountered in a given series of analyses. It should be known, because defense attorneys may overemphasize it.
*Units for Sigma and Maximum Error.* Two types of unit are employed:
(1) *Arithmetical Deviation.* The magnitude of the deviation is presumed to be independent of the particular level. For a blood alcohol method with a probable error (sigma) of $\pm 10$ mg%, this

is supposed to hold regardless of whether the blood alcohol level is 50 mg% or 250 mg%.

(2) *Relative Deviation.* This is expressed on a percentage basis. Thus, a probable error of 10 mg% in blood alcohol level would be a relative error of 20% for a blood alcohol of 50 mg%, but a relative error of only 4% for a blood alcohol of 250 mg%.

With most analytical methods for alcohol it is customary to choose an aliquot where the actual weight of alcohol analyzed is within the optimal range for the method used, and where the degree (percentage) error, but not the arithmetical deviation, for the alcohol level reported would be about constant. It would therefore seem that the relative deviation is the fairer criterion of the accuracy of most analytical methods for alcohol.

In the recent studies reviewed below, some investigators have reported sigma or maximum error in arithmetical units and some in relative (percentage) units. The reader should bear this in mind.

### A. Widmark Method

Bonnichsen and Lundgren (B14), from almost 900 analyses of blood by the Widmark method, calculated that the standard deviation of a single analysis was ±4–6 mg%. The difference encountered, when analyzing three samples taken simultaneously from fifty subjects, ranged from 0 to 23 mg%, averaging 9 mg%.

Schmidt and Manz (S10) made an extensive study of the errors which may occur in each step of the Widmark procedure and recommended certain precautions for eliminating them. Using their modifications, they reported that the deviation with 95% of their results was within ±0.6% to 1.4% of the correct figure, depending on the blood alcohol level.

Nagel (N1) reported a study where, for 1 year, monthly samples of serum of known alcohol content were analyzed independently by six German laboratories, using the Widmark method. The maximum error was within ±6%.

### B. ADH (Alcohol Dehydrogenase) Method

Bonnichsen and Lundgren (B14), on the basis of almost 900 ADH analyses, reported the standard deviation for a single analysis to be 5–6 mg%.

Dotzauer *et al.* (D4) stated that the probable error of a single analysis of deproteinized blood by the ADH method is ±0.8%.

Michon and Michon (M13) studied the accuracy of the ADH method using water and blood solutions of alcohol and found a probable error of ±1.5%, with a maximum error of ±4%.

## C. Other Blood Alcohol Methods

Michon and Michon (M13) reported that with water solutions of alcohol the probable error by the Kozelka–Hine method was 2–6%, and the maximum error observed was 28%. They also studied the Nicloux method. It gave an average error of —4% to +18%, with a maximum error of 36%.

Dettling (D1) reported a cooperative study in Switzerland in which seven laboratories participated. Variations from the mean of the extreme values reported ranged from 4 to 9%, with a deviation of 24% for one analysis. He felt that the blood alcohol analyses in his country were usually accurate within ±5%, which he considered ample for practical purposes.

Kent-Jones and Taylor (K5) published the results of an investigation where nine British laboratories made repeated analyses of a sample of blood and a sample of urine, taken from master samples of known alcohol content. The analysts employed a modified Cavett method and the Kozelka–Hine method. Each result submitted was the average of duplicate analyses. With the Cavett method the probable error (sigma) was +1.6% for urine and —1.4% for blood; the maximum error ranged from —0.7% to +11.5% for urine, and from —9% to +9.8% for blood; and the greatest difference between the results from two analysts was ±24% for blood. Deviations with the Kozelka–Hine method were: probable error, —0.6% for urine and —3.3% for blood; maximum error, —3.7% to +1.2% for urine and —7.7% to +1.5% for blood; greatest difference between two analysts, ±14%. The authors stated: "If each analyst makes two analyses of a sample, the distribution of the mean results will have a standard error of about 14 (Cavett) or 8 (K–H) mg. per 100 ml."

Coldwell and Grant (C12)[10] made duplicate analyses on thirty-six samples of blood and thirty-five samples of urine, using the gas chromatographic method of Cadman and Johns (C1) and the desiccation method of Smith (S17). The alcohol levels ranged from 1 to 81 mg%, averaging about 40 mg%. With the gas chromatograph, the mean difference between duplicate analyses was 2.5 mg% for blood and 1.1 mg% for urine; and the standard error was 2.05 mg% for blood and 1.32 mg% for urine. With the Smith method the mean difference between duplicate analyses was 3.1 mg% for blood and 3.9 mg% for urine; and the standard error was 2.12 mg% for blood and 1.48 mg% for urine. For a given sample of blood, the maximum deviation between the results of the two methods ranged from +12.4 to —12.4 mg%.

[10] We are indebted to Dr. Coldwell for furnishing us with a prepublication copy of this paper by himself and Grant.

## D. Breath Alcohol Methods

Since breath alcohol results are used for estimating the alcohol level of the subject's blood, studies of the accuracy of breath methods usually correlate the results of direct analysis of blood with the blood level calculated from analysis of a sample of breath, taken simultaneously. It should be pointed out that errors inherent to all blood alcohol methods may contribute to some of the apparent deviations between the blood findings and those calculated from breath analyses. Also, most of the published blood-breath studies have employed cubital vein blood, which, during an hour after the end of drinking, may have a significantly lower alcohol level than that of arterial blood (H8, H9), although the latter controls the levels of alcohol in brain and breath.

A number of investigators have made extensive studies comparing the results of direct analysis of blood with the calculated level obtained from a particular breath alcohol method. The results of eleven of these studies are summarized in Table X. The first three studies listed were made by a technical subcommittee of the U.S. National Safety Council, headed by Dr. C. W. Muehlberger, Michigan State Toxicologist (N2).

In the study by Harger *et al.* using the rebreathed air–Drunkometer procedure (H10), almost all blood samples taken within 2 hours after the end of drinking were from the finger tip.

With the four investigations of the Breathalyzer, most of the results which differed from those obtained by direct analysis of blood were too low. Thus, the fraction of the total tests where the breath result deviated from the blood result by more than +15% was, respectively: Chastain, 0; Fennell, 0; Caldwell and Smith, 11%; and Bayly *et al.*, 3%.

Burger (B24) and Vamosi (V0) have reported that the Breathalyzer results agree with those from the Widmark blood method within ±10%.

A blood-breath study with the Drunkometer, using mixed expired air and comprising twelve tests with three subjects, was reported by Sillery *et al.* (S16). A few of the low breath results considerably exceeded the blood results, but cubital vein blood was used and the subjects continued to drink during most of the 2½-hour period employed.

To ascertain how well the Grosskopf *Alcotest* breath alcohol tube will indicate whether the blood alcohol level is below or above about 80 mg%, several investigators have checked the results against direct blood analysis. Abele (A3) reported that the length of green color is often not proportional to the blood alcohol content. He recommended taking a sample of blood whenever the Alcotest result is positive for alcohol. The same conclusions were reached by Leithoff and Weyrich (L1) from com-

TABLE X

ACCURACY OF ESTIMATING BLOOD ALCOHOL LEVEL FROM ANALYSIS OF BREATH

| Investigator(s) | Instrument | Breath type | Estimation from | Subjects | Total tests | Blood-breath correlation[a] | | | |
|---|---|---|---|---|---|---|---|---|---|
| | | | | | | Fraction within | | | Fraction beyond |
| | | | | | | ±5% (%) | ±10% (%) | ±15% (%) | ±15% (%) |
| Muehlberger et al. (N2) | Alcometer | Alveolar air | 2100 ml | 38 | 38 | 32 | 76 | 92 | 8 |
| Muehlberger et al. (N2) | Intoximeter | Mixed expired air | 200 mg $CO_2$ | 44 | 44 | 45 | 77 | 86 | 14 |
| Muehlberger et al. (N2) | Drunkometer | Mixed expired air | 190 mg $CO_2$ | 48 | 48 | 23 | 65 | 79 | 21 |
| Harger et al. (H11) | Drunkometer | Mixed expired air | 190 mg $CO_2$ | 33 | 100 | 34 | 63 | 80 | 20 |
| Harger et al. (H11) | Drunkometer | Mixed expired air | 3200 ml[b] | 33 | 90 | 38 | 58 | 81 | 19 |
| Harger et al. (H10) | Drunkometer | Rebreathed air | 2100 ml | 31 | 93 | 54 | 87 | 98 | 2 |
| Chastain (C6) | Breathalyzer | Alveolar air | 2100 ml | 34 | 34 | 38 | 62 | 91 | 9 |
| Fennell (F3) | Breathalyzer | Alveolar air | 2100 ml | 116 | 116 | 40 | 68 | 84 | 16 |
| Coldwell and Smith (C14) | Breathalyzer | Alevolar air | 2100 ml | 77 | 251 | 30 | 51 | 68 | 32 |
| Bayly et al. (B4) | Breathalyzer | Alveolar air | 2100 ml | 101 | 122 | 26 | 52 | 72 | 28 |
| Lereboullet et al. (L1a) | Breathalyzer | Aleovlar air | 2100 ml | — | 52[c] | 56 | 77 | 85 | 15 |

[a] The figures in the four columns under *Blood-breath correlation* represent per cent of total tests in the four categories.

[b] The volume of mixed expired air used in the test is measured at 25°C after removal of $CO_2$.

[c] Pairs with blood alcohol above 0.30 mg/ml. This paper contains data from 128 pairs of blood and breath, but in 76 of the pairs the blood alcohol was below 0.30 mg/ml (51 bloods were exactly 0.17 mg/ml). In the zone below 0.30 mg/ml blood alcohol the average percentage deviation between blood and breath was much greater than where the blood alcohol level was above 0.30 mg/ml.

parative tests with 141 alcoholic subjects. Misleading results with the Alcotest occurred in only 3–5% of 812 tests according to Hallermann and Sachs (H6), and in 2–9% of the subjects studied by Tara (T1).

## XI. Other Aliphatic Alcohols

### A. Methanol

A 1956 monograph by Koivusalo of Helsinki (K14) contains a comprehensive review of previously published studies on the metabolism of methanol and formaldehyde, and presents extensive *in vivo* and *in vitro* experimental work on this subject by the author. The blood methanol curves of rabbits, given methanol in doses of 0.8–3.8 gm/kg orally, or 0.8 gm/kg intravenously, showed an almost linear drop in methanol level, with a $\beta_{60}$ of about 2.4. (The ethanol $\beta_{60}$ for rabbits averages around 30.) With doses of 0.8–1.6 gm/kg, about 8% of the administered methanol was excreted unchanged in the urine during the disappearance period for the methanol. Since excretion in breath does not greatly exceed that in the urine, these findings do not support earlier claims that administered methanol is mostly lost by these two routes. In these *in vivo* experiments no formaldehyde could be detected in the blood of the rabbits, and there was no increase in their normal urinary output of formic acid. Simultaneous administration of ethanol in a dosage one to two times that of the methanol caused a marked slowing of the utilization of methanol, during the period when ethanol was being metabolized. Disulfiram, administered orally in a dose of 0.7–1.0 gm/kg 12 hours prior to the methanol, caused some slowing of the disappearance of methanol from the rabbits' blood.

With Koivusalo's *in vitro* experiments he used homogenized, or sliced, tissues from guinea pigs or rats. The tissues were incubated aerobically at the optimum pH of 7.4, with 15–36 mg% of methanol in the incubation fluid. Using liver tissue and an incubation period of $1\frac{1}{2}$ hours, the methanol concentration dropped to half, or less, of the original level and the incubation fluid contained formaldehyde in a concentration representing 5–10% of the utilized methanol. Kidney and spleen tissue were about half as active as liver; lung, testis, and heart tissues showed lesser activity; and skeletal muscle and brain, none. Ethanol, in a concentration of 19–95 mg%, inhibited the liver homogenate utilization of methanol by 13–79% and decreased the accumulation of formaldehyde by 5–66%. Other substances which were found to inhibit, or suppress, the utilization of methanol and the accumulation of formaldehyde were iodoacetate, malonate, cyanide, and disulfiram. When the concentration of cyanide was $10^{-4.3}$ to $10^{-3.3}$ $M$, methanol utilization had dropped about 85% and no formaldehyde could be detected in the incubation fluid. A 2-hour incubation of the liver tissue homogenate with formaldehyde only in a concentration of 3.6 mg% caused a disappearance of about half of the formaldehyde. Control experiments with boiled homogenate showed no drop in formaldehyde.

Copeman and Venter (C15) have published analyses of liver, kidney, stomach, and intestine in five cases of fatal methanol poisoning. The methanol levels in liver, expressed as mg%, were: 449, 368, 220, 69, and 65. Levels in the other organs were about the same. With cases three and four, ethanol was also present, in concentrations of 70 and 15 mg%, respectively. Blood methanol levels in ten cases of poisoning reported earlier by Hulpieu and Harger (H30) show similar results, the high levels being where the fatal period was only a few hours.

Eulner (E8) reported a case of illness and partial blindness in a woman whose skin was exposed to compresses soaked, by mistake, with methanol. Eulner and Gedicke (E9) shaved a 12-sq cm area on the backs of rats, applied an absorbent pad to this area, covered the pad with part of a rubber glove to prevent evaporation and inhalation, and injected methanol into the pad. Within 30 minutes, all animals showed ataxia, with later narcosis. Some of the rats died within 12 to 14 hours. The fatal dose, calculated from the loss of methanol from the pad, was about 5.2 ml for a 100–120 gm rat. The oral fatal dose was 1.75 ml. To further test skin absorption, they used a device consisting of a small glass cylinder ending a narrow tube, with the small cylinder surrounded by a somewhat larger cylinder, leaving an annual air space between the two. The open end of the two cylinders was applied to a shaved area of the skin of rabbits or dogs, and a slight vacuum applied to a side arm of the larger cylinder to maintain a tight fit with the skin. The small cylinder and attached narrow tube were then filled with methanol. The absorption of methanol, estimated from the fall of liquid in the narrow tube, was found to average 0.013 ml/sq cm/hour. This would represent absorption of 2.2 ml of methanol from a 12-sq cm area in 14 hours. Since the apparatus somewhat restricted the blood flow to this skin area, they felt that skin absorption from a compress would be greater. They also confirmed earlier reports that inhalation of methanol vapor in concentrations of 50–120 mg/liter can kill rats after 3–25 hours of exposure.

Battey *et al.* (B2) determined cerebral blood flow and oxygen consumption in five cases of methanol poisoning. During the intoxication the blood flow averaged 28% below normal and the brain oxygen uptake was about 30% low, as compared with normal controls.

Aurele and Schreener (A17) recommended body dialysance in the treatment of methanol and ethanol poisoning.

## B. Propyl and Butyl Alcohols

Durwald and Degen (D6) described the case of a woman who was found unconscious and died 4½ hours later, where post-mortem analysis showed 100 ml of n-propanol in the gastrointestinal tract. They estimated that the deceased took 400–500 ml of this alcohol.

Wallgren (W4) tested the intoxicating effects of certain aliphatic alcohols on rats, using the tilting plane technique to estimate degree of impairment. On the basis of mols per kilogram the relative intoxicating effects were: ethanol, 1.0; n-propanol, 2.5; isopropanol, 2.7; n-butanol, 6.3; isobutanol, 3.6; sec-butanol, 4.4; and tert-butanol, 4.8. With the propanols, the duration of impairment was longer than that from ethanol.

Ginther and Finch (G8) have described a method for determining isopropanol and acetone in distillates from body materials. The free acetone is determined by the usual salicylaldehyde-NaOH procedure. A second aliquot of the distillate is reacted with persulfate at 80° to convert the isopropanol to acetone, $NaHSO_3$ is then added to reduce excess persulfate, and the total acetone determined as before. Isopropanol is calculated from the increase in acetone.

## C. Congeners of Whisky

Haag et al. (H1) have studied the acute toxicity and irritating properties of certain substances present in, or related to, the congeners of whisky. They found that the $LD_{50}$ for rats, expressed as grams per kilogram, for the following substances was: furfural, 0.14; aldehyde, 1.0; fusel oil, 1.9; acids, 2.8; and esters, 3.2–3.5. With pure ethanol, the $LD_{50}$ was 10.4. The authors speculated on the possible ill effects from drinking whisky containing these congeners. However, they should have mentioned the extensive analyses of raw and aged whisky published by Liebmann and Scherl (L6) and later work by Snell (S20), both of which show the extremely small concentration of these substances in whisky. Thus, the number of fatal doses of ethanol found in the volume of whisky furnishing a fatal dose of the three most toxic congener constituents would be, respectively: aldehyde, 520; furfural, 270; and fusel oil, 30. The irritation studies employed the rabbit's eye and showed that the concentrations required to produce definite irritation were: ethanol, 18.3%; acids, 1.2%; and aldehydes, fusel oil, esters, and furfural, 5–6%.

Mecke and deVries (M10) extracted certain congeners from alcoholic beverages with a pentane-ether mixture, evaporated the extract from 300 ml of beverage to 0.2 ml, and passed this residue through a Perkin–Elmer gas chromatograph. This resulted in a good separation of the various compounds present. To successively remove certain compounds from the concentrated extract, they saponified the esters, combined the aldehyde with 2-phenylacetyl-1,3-indandione-1-hydrazine, and converted the alcohols to the 3,5-dinitrobenzoates.

REFERENCES

(A1) Abele, G. *Deut. Z. Ges. Gerichtl. Med.* **44**, 374 (1955).
(A2) Abele, G. *Deut. Z. Ges. Gerichtl. Med.* **47**, 447 (1958); **48**, 58 (1958).
(A3) Abele, G. *Zent. Verkehrs-Med.* **4**, 212 (1958); Abstr. in *Deut. Z. Ges. Gerichtl. Med.* **49**, 332 (1960).
(A4) Abele, G., and Kropp, R. *Deut. Z. Ges. Gerichtl. Med.* **48**, 68 (1958).
(A5) Abele, G., and Scholtz, R. *Deut. Z. Ges. Gerichtl. Med.* **48**, 393 (1959).
(A6) Abelin, I., Herren, C., and Berli, W. *Helv. Med. Acta* **25**, 591 (1958).
(A7) Abels, J. *Proc. Soc. Exptl. Biol. Med.* **34**, 346 (1936).
(A8) Aksenes, E. G. *J. Aviation Med.* **25**, 680 (1954).
(A9) Alha, A. R. *Ann. Med. Exptl. Biol. Fenniae* (*Helsinki*) **29**, 125 (1951); *Chem. Abstr.* **46**, 2686g (1952).
(A10) Alha, A. R., Hjeldt, E., and Tamminen, V. *Acta Pharmacol. Toxicol.* **13**, 277 (1957).
(A11) Alha, A. R., and Karlsson, K. *Ann. Med. Exptl. Biol. Fenniae* (*Helsinki*) **33**, 56 (1955); Abstr. in *Quart. J. Studies Alc.* **17**, 520 (1956).
(A12) Am. Med. Assoc., Comm. on Medicolegal Problems, "Manual on Chemical Tests for Intoxication." Am. Med. Assoc., Chicago, Illinois, 1959; also, see 1960 Addendum. Am. Med. Assoc., Chicago.
(A13) Apel, G. *Deut. Z. Ges. Gerichtl. Med.* **49**, 388 (1960).
(A14) Aschan, G., Bergstedt, M., Goldberg, L., and Laurell, L. *Quart. J. Studies Alc.* **17**, 381 (1956).
(A15) Aston, R., and Cullumbine, H. *Toxicol. Appl. Pharmacol.* **1**, 65 (1959).
(A16) Audrlicky, I., and Beran, J. *J. Soudni Lek.* **3**, 161 (1958); Abstr. in *Deut. Z. Ges. Gerichtl. Med.* **49**, 329 (1959).
(A17) Aurele, J. M., and Schreener, G. *J. Clin. Invest.* **39**, 882 (1960).
(A18) Avery, M. A. *Bull. Georgetown Univ. Med. Center* **11**, 79 (1958).
(B1) Bartlett, G. R., and Barnet, H. N. *Quart. J. Studies Alc.* **10**, 381 (1949).
(B2) Battey, L. L., Patterson, L. L., and Heyman, A. *A.M.A. Arch. Neurol. Psychiat.* **76**, 252 (1958).
(B3) Bayly, R. C., and McCallum, N. E. W. *Med. J. Australia* **II**, 173 (1959).
(B4) Bayly, R. C., McCallum, N. E. W., and Preston, W. L. K. *Proc. Roy. Australian Chem. Inst.* **27**, 157 (1960).
(B5) Beck, W. *Muench. Med. Wochschr.* **103**, 200 (1961); Abstr. in *Deut. Z. Ges. Gerichtl. Med.* **51**, 705 (1961).
(B6) Beer, C. T., and Quastel, J. H. *Can. J. Biochem.* **36**, 543 (1958).
(B7) Bernstein, A., Pletscher, A., and Renschler, H. *Klin. Wochschr.* **33**, 488 (1955).
(B8) Bernstein, A., and Staub, H. A. *Helv. Med. Acta* **15**, 494 (1948).
(B9) Blotner, H. *J. Am. Med. Assoc.* **175**, 542 (1961).
(B10) Bogen, E. Personal communication.
(B11) Bohne, G., Luff, K., and Trautmann, H. *Deut. Z. Ges. Gerichtl. Med.* **46**, 226 (1957).
(B12) Boiteau, H. *Ann. Med. Legale Criminol. Police Sci. Toxicol.* **39**, 449 (1959).
(B13) Bonnichsen, R., Halstrom, F., Moller, K. O., and Theorell, H. *Acta Pharmacol. Toxicol.* **10**, 101 (1954).

(B14) Bonnichsen, R., and Lundgren, G. *Acta Pharmacol. Toxicol.* **13,** 256 (1957).
(B15) Bonnichsen, R. F., and Theorell, H. *Scand. J. Clin. Lab. Invest.* **3,** 58 (1951).
(B16) Borkenstein, R. F. "Breath Tests to Determine Alcoholic Influence," 2nd ed. Indiana State Police, Indianapolis, Indiana, 1957.
(B17) Borkenstein, R. F., and Smith, H. W. *Med. Sci. Law* **1,** 13 (1961).
(B18) Brahm-Vogelsanger, A., and Wagner, H.-J. *Deut. Z. Ges. Gerichtl. Med.* **46,** 66 (1957).
(B19) Brecher, G. A., Hartman, A. R., and Leonard, D. D. *Am. J. Ophthalmol.* **39,** 44 (1955).
(B20) Brink, N. G., Bonnichsen, R., and Theorell, H. *Acta Pharmacol. Toxicol.* **10,** 223 (1954).
(B21) British Med. Assoc., Special Comm. Report: "Relation of Alcohol to Road Accidents." *Brit. Med. J.* **I,** 269 (1960).
(B22) Bucher, T., and Redetzki, H. *Klin. Wochschr.* **29,** 615 (1951).
(B23) Burbridge, T. N., Hine, C. H., and Schick, A. F. *J. Lab. Clin. Med.* **35,** 983 (1950).
(B24) Burger, E. *Zentr. Verkehrs-Med.* **5,** 23 (1959); Abstr. in *Deut. Z. Ges. Gerichtl. Med.* **49,** 506 (1959).
(B25) Burger, E. *Zentr. Verkehrs-Med.* **5,** 28 (1959); Abstr. in *Deut. Z. Ges. Gerichtl. Med.* **49,** 502 (1960).
(C1) Cadman, W. J., and Johns, T. "Gas Chromatographic Determination of Ethanol and Other Volatiles from Blood." Paper presented at Pittsburgh Conference on Anal. Chem. and Appl. Spectroscopy (1958).
(C2) Cadman, W. J., and Johns, T. *J. Forensic Sci.* **5,** 369 (1960).
(C3) Casier, H., Polet, H., and Bruyneel, N. *Arch. Intern. Pharmacodyn.* **120,** 498 (1959).
(C4) Cavett, J. W. *J. Lab. Clin. Med.* **23,** 543 (1938).
(C5) Chardon, G., Boiteau, H., and Bogaert, E. *Ann. Med. Legale Criminol. Police Sci. Toxicol.* **39,** 462 (1959).
(C6) Chastain, J. D. "Correlation of Blood Alcohol Levels as Determined by Alcometer, Breathalyzer and Direct Blood Analysis." Texas Dept. of Public Safety, Austin, Texas, 1957.
(C7) Chastain, J. D. "Effects of 0.10 Per Cent Blood Alcohol on Driving Ability." Texas Dept. of Public Safety, Austin, Texas, 1961.
(C8) Chundela, B., and Janak, J. *J. Forensic Med.* **7,** 153 (1960).
(C9) Clark, W. C., and Hulpieu, H. R. *Quart. J. Studies Alc.* **19,** 47 (1958).
(C10) Clark, W. C., Wilson, J. E., and Hulpieu, H. R. *Quart. J. Studies Alc.* **22,** 365 (1961).
(C11) Cohen, J., Dearnaley, E. J., and Hansel, C. E. M. *Brit. Med. J.* **I,** 1438 (1958).
(C12) Coldwell, B. B., and Grant, G. L. *J. Forensic Sci.* **8,** 220 (1963).
(C13) Coldwell, B. B., Penner, D. W., Smith, H. W., Lucas, G. W. H., Rodgers, R. F., and Darroch, F. *Quart. J. Studies Alc.* **19,** 590 (1958).
(C14) Coldwell, B. B., and Smith, H. W. *Can. J. Biochem. Physiol.* **37,** 43 (1959).
(C15) Copeman, P. R., and Venter, J. A. *J. Forensic Med.* **3,** 131 (1956).
(C16) Cordebard, H. *Bull. Soc. Chim. Biol.* **41,** 133 (1959).
(C17) Coulthard, A. J. *J. Forensic Med.* **5,** 185 (1958).
(D1) Dettling, J. *Schweiz. Med. Wochschr.* **88,** 151 (1958).
(D2) DiLuzio, N. R. *Am. J. Physiol.* **194,** 453 (1958).
(D3) Donigan, R. L. "Chemical Tests and the Law." Northwestern Univ. Traffic Institute, Evanston, Illinois, 1957.

(D4) Dotzauer, G., Redetzki, H., Johannsmeier, K., and Bucher, T. *Deut. Z. Ges. Gerichtl. Med.* **41**, 15 (1952).
(D5) Drew, C. G., Colquhoun, W. P., and Long, H. A. *Medico-Legal J.* **26**, 94 (1958).
(D6) Durwald, W., and Degen, W. *Arch. Toxicol.* **16**, 84 (1956).
(E1) Eger, W., and Ottensmeier, H. *Med. Monatsschr.* **8**, 85 (1954); *Chem. Abstr.* **48**, 7195 i (1954).
(E2) Eggleton, M. G. *Brit. J. Psychol.* **32**, 5261 (1941).
(E3) Elbel, H. *Experientia* **14**, 255 (1958); *Chem. Abstr.* **53**, 4551b (1959).
(E4) Elbel, H., and Schleyer, F. "Blutalkohol," 2nd ed. Thieme, Stuttgart, Germany, 1956.
(E5) Ellerbrook, L. D., and VanGassbeek, C. B. *J. Am. Med. Assoc.* **122**, 996 (1943).
(E6) Eerola, R., Venho, I., Vartiaianen, O., and Venho, E. V. *Ann. Med. Exptl. Biol. Fenniae (Helsinki)* **33**, 353 (1955); Abstr. in *Quart. J. Studies Alc.* **17**, 518 (1956).
(E7) Estable, J. J., and Grezzi, J. W. *Arch. Soc. Biol. Montevideo* **21**, 47 (1954); Abstr. in *Quart. J. Studies Alc.* **17**, 680 (1956).
(E8) Eulner, H-H. *Arch. Toxicol.* **15**, 73 (1954).
(E9) Eulner, H-H., and Gedicke, K-H. *Arch. Toxicol.* **15**, 409 (1955).
(F1) Fazekas, I. G. *Arch. Toxicol.* **17**, 183 (1958); *ibid.* **18**, 205 (1960).
(F2) Fazekas, I. G., and Deak, S. *Zacchia* **33**, 455 (1958); Abstr. in *Deut. Z. Ges. Gerichtl. Med.* **49**, 502 (1960).
(F3) Fennell, E. J. Proceedings of the Conference on Alcohol and Road Traffic, Indiana University, Bloomington, 1958, pp. 88–109.
(F4) Ford, W. H. *J. Elliott Soc. Nat. Hist. Charleston, South Carolina,* (1859); *J. Physiol. (London)* **34**, 430 (1906).
(F5) Forney, R. B., and Hulpieu, H. R. *Diabetes* **6**, 28 (1957).
(F6) Forney, R. B., Hulpieu, H. R., and Harger, R. N. *J. Pharmacol. Exptl. Therap.* **98**, 8 (1950).
(F7) Forrester, G. C. "Alcohol, Traffic Accidents and Chemical Test Evidence; The Photo-Electric Intoximeter." Intoximeter Assoc., Niagara Falls, New York, 1960.
(F8) Forsander, O., Vartia, O. K., and Krusius, F-E. *Ann. Med. Exptl. Biol. Fenniae (Helsinki)* **36**, 416 (1958); Abstr. in *Quart. J. Studies Alc.* **22**, 489 (1961); *Chem. Abstr.* **53**, 14326b (1959).
(F9) Forster, B. *Deut. Z. Ges. Gerichtl. Med.* **45**, 221 (1956).
(F10) Forster, B. *Deut. Z. Ges. Gerichtl. Med.* **47**, 599 (1958).
(F11) Forster, B., Schulz, G., and Starck, H-J. *Blutalkohol* **1**, 2 (1961); Abstr. in *Deut. Z. Ges. Gerichtl. Med.* **52**, 145 (1961).
(F12) Forster, B., and Starck, H-J. *Deut. Z. Ges. Gerichtl. Med.* **49**, 66 (1959).
(F13) Fox, J. K. *Proc. Soc. Exptl. Biol. Med.* **97**, 236 (1958).
(F14) Freireich, A. W. "Second International Meeting on Forensic Pathol. Med.," p. 49, Abstr. 10-1. New York Univ. Med. Center, New York, 1960.
(F15) Friedemann, T. E., and Dubowski, K. *In* "Manual of Chemical Tests for Intoxication" (Am. Med. Assoc., Comm. on Medicolegal Problems, ed.), Chapter V. Am. Med. Assoc., Chicago, Illinois, 1959.
(G1) Garlind, T., Goldberg, L., Graf, K., Perman, S., Strandell, T., and Strom, G. *Acta Pharmacol. Toxicol.* **17**, 106 (1960).
(G2) Gettler, A. O., and Freireich, A. W. *J. Biol. Chem.* **92**, 199 (1931).
(G3) Gettler, A. O., and Freireich, A. W. *Am. J. Surg.* **27**, 328 (1935).

(G4) Gettler, A. O., Freireich, A. W., and Schwartz, H. *Am. J. Clin. Pathol.* **14,** 366 (1944).

(G5) Gettler, A. O., Niederl, J. B., and Benedetti-Pilcher, A. A. *J. Am. Chem. Soc.* **54,** 1476 (1932).

(G6) Gerchow, J., and Sachs, V. Private Publication, Kiel, 1959; Abstr. in *Deut. Z. Ges. Gerichtl. Med.* **49,** 318 (1959).

(G7) Gerchow, J., and Steigleder, E. *Blutalkohol* **1,** 43 (1961).

(G8) Ginther, G. B., and Finch, R. C. *Anal. Chem.* **32,** 1894 (1960).

(G9) Goddard, P. J. *J. Appl. Physiol.* **13,** 118 (1958).

(G10) Goldbaum, L. "Second International Meeting on Forensic Pathol. Med.," p. 49, Abstr. 10-2. New York Univ. Med. Center, New York, 1960.

(G11) Goldberg, L. *Acta Physiol. Scand.* **5,** (Suppl.) No. 16 (1943).

(G12) Goldberg, L. "Proceedings, First International Conference on Alcohol and Road Traffic," p. 90. Kugelsbergs, Stockholm, 1953.

(G13) Goldberg, M., Hehir, R., and Hurowitz, M. *New Engl. J. Med.* **263,** 1336 (1960).

(G14) Gonzales, T. A., Vance, M., Helpern, M., and Umberger, C. J. "Legal Medicine, Pathology and Toxicology," 2nd ed., p. 1112. Appleton, New York, (1954).

(G15) Graham, J. D. P. *Toxicol. Appl. Pharmacol.* **2,** 14 (1960).

(G16) Griffon, H., and LeBreton, R. *Ann. Med. Legale Criminol. Police Sci. Toxicol.* **37,** 237 (1957).

(G17) Grosskopf, K. *Angew. Chem.* **66,** 10 (1954).

(G18) Gruner, O. *Deut. Z. Ges. Gerichtl. Med.* **46,** 10 (1957).

(G19) Gruner, O. *Deut. Z. Ges. Gerichtl. Med.* **46,** 744 (1958).

(G20) Gruner, O. *Deut. Z. Ges. Gerichtl. Med.* **48,** 4 (1958).

(G21) Gruner, O. *Deut. Z. Ges. Gerichtl. Med.* **46,** 53 (1957).

(G22) Gruner, O. *Deut. Z. Ges. Gerichtl. Med.* **49,** 234 (1959).

(G23) Gruner, O., Luff, K., and Weiss, K. *Zentr. Verkehrs-Med.* **5,** 89 (1959); Abstr. in *Deut. Z. Ges. Gerichtl. Med.* **49,** 506 (1959).

(G24) Gruner, O., and Sattler, H. *Deut. Z. Ges. Gerichtl. Med.* **47,** 276 (1958).

(G25) Gumbel, B. *Muench. Med. Wochschr.* **98,** 337 (1956); Abstr. in *Quart. J. Studies Alc.* **19,** 337 (1958).

(G26) Gumbel, B. *Deut. Med. Wochschr.* **81,** 1850 (1956); Abstr. in *Quart. J. Studies Alc.* **19,** 337 (1958).

(H1) Haag, H. B., Finnegan, J. K., Larson, P. S., and Smith, R. B. *Toxicol. Appl. Pharmacol.* **1,** 618 (1959).

(H2) Haggard, H. W., and Greenberg, L. *J. Pharmacol. Exptl. Therap.* **52,** 157 (1934).

(H3) Haggard, H. W., Greenberg, L., and Cohen, L. H. *New Engl. J. Med.* **219,** 466 (1938).

(H4) Hakkinen, H. M., and Kulonen, E. *Nature* **184,** 726 (1959).

(H5) Hald, J., Jacobsen, E., and Larsen, V. *Acta Pharmacol. Toxicol.* **5,** 179 (1949).

(H6) Hallermann, W., and Sachs, V. *Zentr. Verkehrs-Med.* **6,** 81 (1960); Abstr. in *Deut. Z. Ges. Gerichtl. Med.* **51,** 262 (1961).

(H7) Hallermann, W., Sachs, V., and Steigleder, E., *Deut. Z. Ges. Gerichtl. Med.* **49,** 431 (1960).

(H8) Harger, R. N. *J. Forensic Sci.* **1,** 27 (1956).

(H9) Harger, R. N. *In* "Toxicology: Mechanisms and Analytical Methods" (C. P. Stewart and A. Stolman, eds.), Vol. II, Chapter 4. Academic Press, New York, 1961.

(H10) Harger, R. N., Forney, R. B., and Baker, R. S. *Quart. J. Studies Alc.* 17, 1 (1956).
(H11) Harger, R. N., Forney, R. B., and Barnes, H. B. *J. Lab. Clin. Med.* 36, 306 (1950).
(H12) Harger, R. N., and Goss, A. L. *Am. J. Physiol.* 112, 374 (1935).
(H13) Harger, R. N., and Hulpieu, H. R. *In* "Alcoholism" (G. N. Thompson, ed.), Chapter 2. Thomas, Springfield, Illinois, 1956.
(H14) Harger, R. N., Hulpieu, H. R., and Cole, V. V. *Federation Proc.* 4, 123 (1945).
(H15) Harger, R. N., Hulpieu, H. R., and Lamb, E. B. *J. Biol. Chem.* 120, 689 (1937).
(H16) Harger, R. N., Lamb, E. B., and Hulpieu, H. R. *J. Am. Med. Assoc.* 110, 779 (1938).
(H17) Harger, R. N., Raney, B. B., Bridwell, E. G., and Kitchel, M. F. *J. Biol. Chem.* 183, 197 (1950).
(H18) Hebbelinck, M. *Arch. Intern. Pharmacodyn.* 119, 521 (1959); *ibid.* 120, 402 (1959).
(H19) Hebold, G. *Deut. Z. Ges. Gerichtl. Med.* 47, 619 (1958).
(H20) Hebold, G. *Deut. Z. Ges. Gerichtl. Med.* 48, 257 (1959).
(H21) Herold, H., and Prokop, O. *Deut. Z. Ges. Gerichtl. Med.* 50, 1 (1960).
(H22) Hine, C. H. *Proc. Am. Acad. Forensic Sci.* 1, 161 (1951).
(H23) Hofle, K. H., Linheimer, W., and Marx, H. *Medizinische* 47, 2280 (1959).
(H24) Hogberg, H. *Nord. Kriminaltekn.* 30, 61 (1960); Abstr. in *Deut. Z. Ges. Gerichtl. Med.* 51, 98 (1961).
(H25) Hoppe, C., and Bachmann, H. *Wiss. Z. Karl-Marx-Univ. Leipzig Math-Naturw. Reihe* 9, 535 (1960); Abstr, in *Deut. Z. Ges. Gerichtl. Med.* 52, 144 (1961).
(H26) Hughes, F. W., and Forney, R. B. *Proc. Soc. Exptl. Biol. Med.* 108, 157 (1961).
(H27) Hughes, F. W., and Rountree, C. B. *Arch. Intern. Pharmacodyn.* 133, 418 (1961).
(H28) Hulpieu, H. R., Clark, W. C., and Onyett, H. P. *Quart. J. Studies Alc.* 15, 189 (1954).
(H29) Hulpieu, H. R., and Cole, V. V. *Quart. J. Studies Alc.* 7, 89 (1946).
(H30) Hulpieu, H. R., and Harger, R. N. *In* "Pharmacology in Medicine" (V. A. Drill, ed.), 2nd ed., Chapter 16. McGraw-Hill, New York, 1958.
(I1) Illchmann-Christ, A. *Deut. Z. Ges. Gerichtl. Med.* 49, 113 (1959).
(I2) "Proceedings, First International Conference on Alcohol and Road Traffic," pp. 1–82. Kugelsbergs, Stockholm, 1953.
(J1) Janitzki, U. *Deut. Z. Ges. Gerichtl. Med.* 49, 183 (1959).
(J2) Janitzki, U. *Deut. Z. Ges. Gerichtl. Med.* 52, 22 (1961).
(J3) Johannsmeier, K., Redetzki, H., and Pfleiderer, G. *Klin. Wochschr.* 32, 560 (1954).
(J4) Jones, R. O. *Can. Med. Assoc. J.* 60, 609 (1949).
(K1) Kael, K., and Bina, K. *Soudni Lek.* 3, 150 (1958); Abstr. in *Deut. Z. Ges. Gerichtl. Med.* 49, 330 (1960).
(K2) Kaplan, N. O., and Ciotti, M. M. *J. Biol. Chem.* 221, 823 (1956); *ibid.* 221, 833 (1956).
(K3) Karger, J. V., and Sachs, V. *Deut. Z. Ges. Gerichtl. Med.* 47, 614 (1958).
(K4) Kaye, S., and Haag, H. B. *J. Am. Med. Assoc.* 165, 451 (1957).
(K5) Kent-Jones, D. W., and Taylor, G. *Analyst* 79, 121 (1954).

(K6) Kinard, F. W., and Cox, E. C. *Quart. J. Studies Alc.* **19**, 375 (1958).
(K7) Kinard, F. W., and Hay, M. G. *Am. J. Physiol.* **198**, 657 (1960).
(K8) Kinard, F. W., Hay, M. G., and Kinard, F. W., Jr. *Federation Proc.* **21**, 214 (1962).
(K9) Kirk, P. L., Gibor, A., and Parker, K. P. *Anal. Chem.* **30**, 1418 (1958).
(K10) Klein, H. *Klin. Wochschr.* **33**, 590 (1955); *Chem. Abstr.* **49**, 13347b (1955).
(K11) Klingman, G. I., and Goodall, M. J. *J. Pharmacol. Exptl. Therap.* **121**, 313 (1957).
(K12) Klingman, G. I., and Haag, H. B. *Quart. J. Studies Alc.* **19**, 203 (1958).
(K13) Klingman, G. I., Haag, H. B., and Bane, R. *Quart. J. Studies Alc.* **19**, 543 (1958).
(K14) Koivusalo, M. *Acta Physiol. Scand.* **39**, Suppl. No. 131, 103 pp. (1956).
(K15) Kopf, R. *Arch. Intern. Pharmacodyn.* **110**, 56 (1957).
(K16) Koppanyi, T. *J. Forensic Med.* **4**, 132 (1957).
(K17) Korabley, M. V. *Farm. Toksikol.* **22**, 259 (1959); Abstr. in *Quart. J. Studies Alc.* **22**, 149 (1961).
(K18) Krauland, W., Schuster, R., and Klein, R. *Deut. Z. Ges. Gerichtl. Med.* **51**, 429 (1961).
(K19) Krauland, W., Vidic, E., Freudenberg, K., Schmidt, B., and Lenk, V. *Deut. Z. Ges. Gerichtl. Med.* **50**, 34 (1960).
(K20) Krauland, W., Vidic, E., and Freudenberg, K. *Deut. Z. Ges. Gerichtl. Med.* **52**, 76 (1961).
(K21) Kulonen, E., and Forsander, O. *Arch. Intern. Pharmacodyn.* **123**, 1 (1959); **123**, 8, 21 (1959).
(K22) Kulpe, W., and Mallach, H. J. *Med. Sachverstandige* **56**, 270 (1960); Abstr. in *Deut. Z. Ges. Gerichtl. Med.* **52**, 145 (1961).
(K23) Kulpe, W., and Mallach, H. J. *Z. Klin. Med.* **156**, 432 (1961); *Chem. Abstr.* **55**, 20065h (1961).
(L1) Leithoff, H., and Weyrich, G. *Arch. Kriminol.* **123**, 133 (1959); Abstr. in *Deut. Z. Ges. Gerichtl. Med.* **50**, 124 (1960).
(L1a) Lereboullet, J., Amstutz, Cl., Leluc, R., and Biraben, J.-N. *Rev. Alcoolisme* **7**, 87 (1961).
(L2) Lester, D. *Quart. J. Studies Alc.* **22**, 554 (1961).
(L3) Lester, D. *Quart. J. Studies Alc.* **23**, 17 (1962).
(L4) Lester, D., and Greenberg, L. A. *Quart. J. Studies Alc.* **12**, 167 (1951).
(L5) Lester, D., and Greenberg, L. A. *Quart. J. Studies Alc.* **19**, 331 (1958).
(L6) Liebmann, A. J., and Scherl, B. *Ind. Eng. Chem.* **41**, 534 (1949).
(L7) Lins, G., and Randonat, H. W. *Deut. Z. Ges. Gerichtl. Med.* **52**, 242 (1962).
(L8) Lob, M. *Med. Lavoro* **51**, 587 (1960); Abstr. in *Deut. Z. Ges. Gerichtl. Med.* **51**, 692 (1961).
(L9) Lommer, E. *Deut. Z. Ges. Gerichtl. Med.* **49**, 281 (1959).
(L10) Loomis, T. A., and West, T. C. *Quart. J. Studies Alc.* **19**, 30 (1958).
(L11) Lowenstein, J., Morgan, T. E., Jr., and Newman, H. W. *Stanford Med. Bull.* **15**, 14 (1957).
(L12) Ludin, M. *Deut. Z. Ges. Gerichtl. Med.* **45**, 530 (1956).
(L13) Lundquist, F. *Acta Pharmacol. Toxicol.* **18**, 231 (1961).
(L14) Lundquist, F., and Wolthers, J. *Acta Pharmacol. Toxicol.* **14**, 265 (1958).
(L15) Lundquist, F., and Wolthers, H. *Acta Pharmacol. Toxicol.* **14**, 290 (1958).
(L16) Lundsgaard, E. *Bull. Johns Hopkins Hosp.* **63**, 15 (1938).
(M0) Machata, G. *Deut. Z. Ges. Gerichtl. Med.* **51**, 447 (1961).
(M1) Machata, G. *Deut. Z. Ges. Gerichtl. Med.* **48**, 26 (1958).

(M2) Mallach, H. *Arzneimittel-Forsch.* 9, 389 (1959); Abstr. in *Quart. J. Studies Alc.* 22, 147 (1961).

(M3) Mallov, S., and Bloch, J. L. *Am. J. Physiol.* 184, 29 (1956).

(M4) Marcellini, D. *Neuropsichiatria (Genoa)* 13, 325 (1957); Abstr. in *Quart. J. Studies Alc.* 22, 145 (1961).

(M5) Marshall, E. K., and Fritz, W. F. *J. Pharmacol. Exptl. Therap.* 109, 431 (1953).

(M6) Martin, R., LeBreton, R., and Roche, M. *Ann. Med. Legale Criminol. Police Sci. Toxicol.* 37, 56 (1957).

(M7) Matsumoto, Y. *Folia Pharmacol. Japon.* 51, 376 (1955); *Chem. Abstr.* 50, 15920e (1956).

(M8) McCallum, N. E. W., and Scroggie, J. G. *Med. J. Australia* II, 1031 (1960).

(M9) McManus, I. R., Contag, A. O., and Olson, R. E. *Science* 131, 102 (1960).

(M10) Mecke, R., and deVries, M. Z. *Anal. Chem.* 170, 326 (1959).

(M11) Mehrtens, H. G., and Newman, H. W. *A.M.A. Arch. Neurol. Psychiat.* 30, 1092 (1933).

(M12) Meyer, K-H. Doctoral Dissertation University of Bonn, Germany, 1957; Abstr. in *Quart. J. Studies Alc.* 20, 785 (1959).

(M13) Michon, R., and Michon, P. *Ann. Med. Legale Criminol. Police Sci. Toxicol.* 37, 136 (1957).

(M14) Mirsky, A., Piker, P., Rosenbaum, M., and Lederer, H. *Quart. J. Studies Alc.* 2, 35 (1941).

(M15) Muehlberger, C. W. *In* "Legal Medicine" (R. B. H. Gradwohl, ed.), Chapter 26. Mosby, St. Louis, Missouri, 1954.

(N1) Nagel, G. *Lebensmittelchem. Gerichtl. Chem.* 15, 27 (1961); Abstr. in *Deut. Z. Ges. Gerichtl. Med.* 52, 143 (1961).

(N2) National Safety Council, Committee on Tests for Intoxication. "Evaluating Chemical Tests for Intoxication." National Safety Council, Chicago, Illinois, 1953.

(N3) National Safety Council, Committee on Alcohol and Drugs, Report. National Safety Council, Chicago, Illinois, 1961.

(N4) Nelson, D., and Jensen, C. E. *Federation Proc.* 20, 189 (1961).

(N5) Nelson, G. H., and Kinard, F. W. *Quart. J. Studies Alc.* 20, 1 (1959).

(N6) Newman, H. W. *A.M.A. Arch. Internal Med.* 94, 417 (1954)

(N7) Newman, H. W., and Newman, E. J. *Quart. J. Studies Alc.* 17, 406 (1956).

(N8) Newman, H. W., and Smith, M. E. *Nature* 183, 689 (1959).

(N9) Newman, H. W., Smith, M. E., and Newman, E. J. *Quart. J. Studies Alc.* 20, 213 (1959).

(N10) Nickolls, L. C. *Analyst* 85, 840 (1960).

(P1) Paulus, W., and Janitzki, U. *Deut. Z. Ges. Gerichtl. Med.* 48, 403 (1959).

(P2) Paulus, W., and Mallach, H. J. *Deut. Med. Wochschr.* 79, 1045 (1954); Abstr. in *Quart. J. Studies Alc.* 16, 753 (1955).

(P3) Pecora, L. J. *Am. Ind. Hyg. Assoc. J.* 20, 235 (1959).

(P4) Perman, E. S. *Acta Physiol. Scand.* 48, 323 (1960).

(P5) Pfeil, E., and Goldbach, H-J. *Polizei-Praxis* 48, 92 (1957); Abstr. in *Deut. Z. Ges. Gerichtl. Med.* 46, 656 (1957).

(P6) Pietz, D. G., Rosenak, B. D., and Harger, R. N. *Am. J. Gastroenterol.* 34, 140 (1960).

(P7) Pihkanen, T. A. *Quart. J. Studies Alc.* 18, 183 (1957); *Ann. Med. Exptl. Biol. Fenniae (Helsinki)* 35, Suppl. No. 9, 152 pp. (1957); Abstr. in *Quart. J. Studies Alc.* 20, 131 (1959).

(P8) Pilotti, G., and Pisani, G. *Minerva Med.* I, 1823 (1954); *Chem. Abstr.* 51, 20466f (1959).

(P9) Plesso, G. I., and Fuskov, V. S. *Sb. Nauch.* No. 13, 254 (1957); *Chem. Abstr.* 53, 20466f (1959).

(P10) Polyakova, V. I. *Terapevt. Arkh.* 31, 67 (1959); *Chem. Abstr.* 53, 22543g (1959).

(P11) Ponsold, A., and Heite, H-J. *Deut. Z. Ges. Gerichtl. Med.* 50, 228 (1960).

(P12) Proceedings of the Conference on Alcohol and Road Traffic, Indiana University, Bloomington, 1958.

(R1) Raby, K. *Quart. J. Studies Alc.* 15, 21 (1954).

(R2) Rauschke, J. *Deut. Z. Ges. Gerichtl. Med.* 43, 27 (1954).

(R3) Rauschke, J. *Muench. Med. Wochschr.* 96, 1446 (1954); Abstr. in *Quart. J. Studies Alc.* 17, 145 (1956).

(R4) Rauschke, J. *Medizinische* 12, 460 (1958); Abstr. in *Quart. J. Studies Alc.* 21, 143 (1960).

(R5) Redetzki, H., and Johannsmeier, K. *Arch. Toxicol.* 16, 73 (1956).

(R6) Redetzki, H., Johannsmeier, K., and Dotzauer, G. *Deut. Z. Ges. Gerichtl. Med.* 41, 424 (1952).

(R7) Robljek-Priversek, T. *Deut. Z. Ges. Gerichtl. Med.* 46, 740 (1958).

(R8) Rosenfeld, G. *Quart. J. Studies Alc.* 21, 584 (1960).

(R9) Rutenfranz, J., and Jensen, G. *Intern. Z. Angew. Physiol.* 18, 62 (1959); Abstr. in *Deut. Z. Ges. Gerichtl. Med.* 50, 345 (1960).

(S1) Sachs, V. *Deut. Z. Ges. Gerichtl. Med.* 48, 400 (1959).

(S2) Sachs, V. *Deut. Z. Ges. Gerichtl. Med.* 50, 246 (1960).

(S3) Salem, H., Lucas, G. W. H., and Lucas, D. M. *Can. Med. Assoc. J.* 82, 682 (1960).

(S4) Santisteban, G. A. *Quart. J. Studies Alc.* 22, 1 (1961).

(S5) Schiller, J., Peck, R. E., and Goldberg, M. A. *A.M.A. Arch. Neurol.* 1, 129 (1959).

(S6) Schleyer, F. *Med. Sachverstandige* 55, 151 (1959); Abstr. in *Deut. Z. Ges. Gerichtl. Med.* 50, 124 (1960).

(S7) Schleyer, F. *Arch. Toxicol.* 18, 187 (1960).

(S8) Schleyer, F., and Wichmann, D. *Blutalkohol* 1, 58 (1961).

(S9) Schmidt, O., and Manz, R. *Klin. Wochschr.* 33, 82 (1955); Abstr. in *Quart. J. Studies Alc.* 17, 329 (1956).

(S10) Schmidt, O., and Manz, R. *Deut. Z. Ges. Gerichtl. Med.* 47, 309 (1958).

(S11) Schmidt, O., Starck, H. J., and Forster, B. *Deut. Z. Ges. Gerichtl. Med.* 49, 649 (1960).

(S12) Schulte, K., and Roth, H. *Zentr. Verkehrs-Med.* 3, 144 (1957); Abstr. in *Quart. J. Studies Alc.* 20, 784 (1959).

(S13) Schweitzer, H. *Deut. Z. Ges. Gerichtl. Med.* 43, 18 (1954).

(S14) Schweitzer, H. *Deut. Z. Ges. Gerichtl. Med.* 49, 699 (1960).

(S15) Sheftel, A. G. *J. Lab. Clin. Med.* 23, 534 (1937).

(S16) Sillery, R. J., Williams, R. J., and Langtry, A. C. *J. Lab. Clin. Med.* 54, 613 (1959).

(S17) Smith, H. W. *J. Lab. Clin. Med.* 38, 762 (1951).

(S18) Smith, M. E., and Newman, H. W. *Proc. Soc. Exptl. Biol. Med.* 104, 282 (1960).

(S19) Smith, M. E., Newman, E. J., and Newman, H. W. *Proc. Soc. Exptl. Biol. Med.* 95, 541 (1957).

(S20) Snell, C. A. *Quart. J. Studies Alc.* 19, 69 (1958).
(S21) Stotz, E. A. *J. Biol. Chem.* 148, 585 (1943).
(S22) Sunshine, I. "Post-Mortem Distribution of Ethyl Alcohol." Presented at the 1957 Meeting of the Am. Acad. Forensic Sci. and distributed in mimeographed form.
(S23) Sutherland, V. C., Burbridge, T. N., and Simon, A. *J. Appl. Physiol.* 15, 189 (1960).
(S24) Sutherland, V. C., Hine, C. H., and Burbridge, T. N. *J. Pharmacol. Exptl. Therap.* 116, 469 (1956).
(T1) Tara, S. *Rev. Alc.* 6, 392 (1960); Abstr. in *Deut. Z. Ges. Gerichtl. Med.* 51, 262 (1961).
(T2) Taschen, B. *Med. Monatsschr.* 9, 25 (1955); Abstr. in *Quart. J. Studies Alc.* 16, 745 (1955).
(T3) Teller, J. D. "Colorimetric Determination of Ethyl Alcohol." Paper presented at the Am. Chem. Society Meeting, September, 1958. Unpublished.
(T4) Tipton, D. L., Jr., Sutherland, V. C., Burbridge, T. N., and Simon, A. *Am. J. Physiol.* 200, 1007 (1961).
(T5) Troshina, A. E. *Sb. Tr. Ryazansk. Med. Inst.* 4, 1 (1957); Abstr. in *Quart. J. Studies Alc.* 20, 783 (1959).
(T6) Tuovinen, P. I. *Skand. Arch. Physiol.* 60, 1 (1930).
(U1) Umberger, C. J. "A Study of the Ethyl Alcohol Normally Present in Blood." Ph.D. Thesis, New York University, New York, 1939.
(V0) Vamosi, M. *Soudni Lek.* 4, 42 (1959); Abstr. in *Deut. Z. Ges. Gerichtl. Med.* 50, 343 (1960).
(V1) VanHecke, W., Handovsky, H., and Thomas, F. *Ann. Med. Legale Criminol. Police Sci. Toxicol.* 31, 291 (1957).
(V2) Vartia, O. K., Forsander, O. A., and Krusius, F-E. *Quart. J. Studies Alc.* 21, 597 (1960).
(V3) Vidic, E. *Deut. Z. Ges. Gerichtl. Med.* 43, 88 (1954).
(V4) Vidic, E. *Arzneimittel-Forsch.* 4, 506 (1954); Abstr. in *Deut. Z. Ges. Gerichtl. Med.* 44, 649 (1956).
(V5) Vidoni, G., and Redenti, L. *Minerva Medicolegale* 80, 132 (1960); Abstr. in *Deut. Z. Ges. Gerichtl. Med.* 51, 262 (1961).
(W1) Wagner, H-J. *Deut. Z. Ges. Gerichtl. Med.* 46, 70 (1957).
(W2) Wagner, H-J. *Arch. Toxicol.* 17, 159 (1958).
(W3) Wagner, K., and Wagner, H-J. *Deut. Med. Wochschr.* 81, 869 (1956); Abstr. in *Quart. J. Studies Alc.* 18, 306 (1957).
(W4) Wallgren, H. *Acta Pharmacol. Toxicol.* 16, 217 (1960).
(W5) Weatherby, J. H., and Clements, E. L. *Quart. J. Studies Alc.* 21, 394 (1960).
(W6) Weinig, E. *Deut. Z. Ges. Gerichtl. Med.* 40, 318 (1951).
(W7) Weinig, E., and Schwerd, W. *Fortschr. Med.* 74, 497 (1956); Abstr. in *Deut. Z. Ges. Gerichtl. Med.* 46, 803 (1958).
(W8) Weinig, E., and Schwerd, W. *Beitr. Gerichtl. Med.* 21, 114 (1961); Abstr. in *Deut. Z. Ges. Gerichtl. Med.* 51, 705 (1961).
(W9) West German Government, Health Office Commission. "Blood Alcohol and Traffic Offenses," p. 46. Borgman, Bielefeld, Kirschbaum, Bonn, 1955.
(W10) Weyrich, G., and Hauck, G. *Arch. Toxicol.* 18, 120 (1960).
(W11) Widmark, E. M. P. "Die theoretischen Grundlagen und die praktische Verwendbarkeit der gerichtlich-medizinischen Alkoholbestimmung," 140 pp. Urban & Schwartzenberg, Munich, Germany, 1932.

134         *Rolla N. Harger and Robert B. Forney*

(W12) Williams, L. A., Linn, R. A., and Zak, B. *Clin. Chim. Acta* **3**, 169 (1958).
(W13) Willner, K. *Deut. Z. Ges. Gerichtl. Med.* **50**, 429 (1960).
(W14) Wilson, E. M. Aerojet-General Corp., Azusa, California. Personal communication.
(W15) Wilson, R. H. L., Newman, E. J., and Newman, H. W. *J. Appl. Physiol.* **8**, 556 (1956).
(W16) Wolff, E. *Acta Med. Lagale Soc.* **9**, 11 (1956); Abstr. in *Quart. J. Studies Alc.* **19**, 691 (1958).
(W17) Woodward, E. R., Slotter, D. S., and Tilmans, V. C. *Proc. Soc. Exptl. Biol. Med.* **89**, 428 (1955).
(W18) Wuermeling, H. B., Leithoff, H., and Weyrich, G. *Medizinische II*, 1935 (1959); Abstr. in *Quart. J. Studies Alc.* **22**, 658 (1961).
(Z1) Zirkle, G. A., King, P. D., McAtee, O. B., and VanDyke, R. *J. Am. Med. Assoc.* **171**, 1496 (1959).
(Z2) Zirkle, G. A., McAtee, O. B., King, P. D., and VanDyke, R. *J. Am. Med. Assoc.* **173**, 1823 (1960).

# Acidic and Neutral Poisons

## by A. S. CURRY

*Forensic Science Laboratory, Harrogate, Yorkshire, England*

## I. Introduction

From 1950 to 1955 great advances were made in toxicological analysis with the increasing use of such purification procedures as paper chromatography, electrophoresis, and countercurrent distribution and the ready availability of ultraviolet spectrophotometers for identification and quantitation.

In contrast, 1955–1959 were years of consolidation in which these techniques entered all branches of the science and are no better demonstrated than by considering the history of the analysis of the barbiturates.

In the years 1960–1961 there were other major advances in the analysis of the group of poisons considered here and it is probable that these will produce as important results as those of the previous decade. These advances are gas and thin layer chromatography for the purification stage and micro infrared spectroscopy for identification. All are now in widespread use and not only have enlarged the armory of the toxicologist but also have presented him with much more sensitive and specific methods of identification.

Gas chromatography, by measurement of retention volumes, gives valuable information without loss of material and pyrolysis and the formation of derivatives on the column provide even higher criteria of identification on a microgram scale. The realization that gas chromatography can be applied to solids on columns well below the melting points of the compounds under investigation has produced a tool of research whose first fruits are only beginning to appear in the literature. For toxicologists the separation of the barbiturates by Parker and Kirk (P2) has dramatically demonstrated the potential of the method following, as it does, closely on the separation of steroids and alkaloids (S27, V1) and the experiments on pyrolysis by Janak (J5).

The increasing use of such a valuable technique as infrared spectroscopy was to be expected but with it have come developments which have vastly increased its value to toxicologists; these are the availability of focusing lenses and micro disc and solution holders which enable excellent curves to be obtained with as little as 10 $\mu$g of material and the appearance on the market of relatively inexpensive machines with scan times of as low as 3 minutes.

The isolation of the poison on a microgram scale can now be followed by its purification by paper, thin layer, or gas chromatography and its absolute identification by infrared spectroscopy. The following sections in this chapter must be examined with this approach in mind.

## II. Isolation Procedures

This stage of the analysis is nearly always the most tedious and often the least investigated. There have been no obviously outstanding papers noted since the publication of *Toxicology: Mechanisms and Analytical Methods* (S19) in 1960, most authors preferring to improve existing techniques by modification.

Direct extraction by organic solvent is back in favor mainly because the increase in sensitivity of methods for detecting poisons has meant that smaller volumes of blood or tissue can be used. Emulsions, previously caused by too small volumes of organic solvent, can now be avoided.

Chloroform and ether continue to be the solvents used by the majority of workers although ethyl acetate is preferred for the extraction of hydrochlorthiazide (S7) and glutethimide (A3) and amyl acetate for carboxytolbutamide (N2). Zaar and Gronwall (Z1) adsorb 1 ml of serum on filter paper before extracting barbiturates with 10 ml of ether by inversion shaking.

Several new solvent combinations have been used including acetonitrile–ether $(1 + 2)$ (A1) and ethanol–hexane–acetone $(1:2:2)$ (P1). This latter mixture has theoretical advantages if a universal solvent is required. Butyl ether has been recommended by Stevenson who described its use in the determination of barbiturates (S17) and salicylate (S16). The use of alcohols for extraction has been extended by Rieders (R1) who claims excellent recoveries for a wide variety of poisons using *n*-butanol and ammonium sulfate. A device using ethanol for the continuous extraction of alkaloids from plant material has been described (M9) and Mannering (M5) has made a modification to the continuous extractor of Curry and Phang (C13). This consists of an extension to the head and socket through which the ethanol from the condenser is returned to the extraction flask: the solvent is delivered about 2 inches *under* the tissue instead of on top as in the original paper. A small hole in the extension above the tissue is necessary to equilibrate pressure. Reports of the efficiency of this apparatus continue to be most encouraging; saponins, glycosides, cantharidin, and chlorinated insecticides have all been extracted from tissue by its use (W1) in addition to the classes of poisons described before. The advantages of an efficient extraction of several hundred grams of tissue in a few hours using only about 1½ liters of ethanol at 30°C in a simple recirculating apparatus requiring little or no attention are manifest and, although originally designed for countries where ethanol must be used as a preservative, it is coming now into widespread use (C20).

Bonnichsen *et al.* (B8), in a most important paper concerning the barbiturates, have described complete recovery experiments involving direct chloroform extraction, fat rejection, and paper chromatography. Results for six representative barbiturates added in therapeutic concentrations to blood and liver ranged from 65–94% with the majority of results about 80%. Their method is to macerate 10–50 gm of tissue, a few milliliters of either 1 *M* tartaric acid or 0.1 *N* hydrochloric acid to give pH 3–4, and 200–400 ml of chloroform. After centrifuging, filtering, and separating, two more extractions with 100 ml chloroform follow; the combined extracts are then evaporated. The residue is treated with 30–40 ml of hot water and the pH brought to 3–4. The solution is kept at 0°C for 30 minutes and filtered in the cold. Insoluble residue is extracted twice with 10–20 ml hot 0.01 *N* hydrochloric acid followed by filtration in the cold. The combined filtrates of about 50–60 ml are shaken vigorously for 1 minute with three portions of 100 ml each of chloroform. If tartaric acid was used it is now removed by shaking the combined chloroform extracts with two 20 ml portions of 0.5 *M* phosphate buffer (pH 7.2). The two buffer portions are removed and extracted twice with the same volume of chloroform. All chloroform solutions are combined, dehydrated over Na$_2$SO$_4$, and evaporated to dryness for paper chromatographic examination and quantitative assay by ultraviolet spectrophotometry.

### III. Purification Procedures

#### A. Paper Chromatography

After the extraction of the tissue with organic solvent, division into strong acid, weak acid, and neutral fractions is usually made by washing out with sodium bicarbonate and sodium hydroxide solutions. If micrograms of poison are to be detected a further purification stage is probably essential. Paper chromatography continues to be extensively used for this purpose.

In the investigation of the strong acid fraction, Tompsett (T2, T3, T4) has separated the phenolic acids and methoxy compounds in urine including vanillic, homovanillic, *p*-hydroxybenzoic, *p*-hydroxyphenylacetic, and *o*-hydroxyphenylacetic acids.

In the weak acid fraction the barbiturates continue to hold attention. Hensel and Abernethy (H3), using 5% sodium silicate impregnated paper and the bottom layer of chloroform: 0.880 ammonia (2:1), successfully separate many of the clinically important barbiturates. Their system is one of the very few using highly volatile solvents that works well and, provided that there is a prior 45-minute equilibration with the water phase of the solvent, with excellent reproducibility with little or no trailing of the spots. The outstanding value of this system is the wide separation of butobarbitone and amylobarbitone and a new barbiturate nealbarbitone (5-allyl, 5-neopentyl barbiturate) from amylobarbitone and secobarbitone.

Swedish workers (B8) reporting on investigations in over 600 cases of barbiturate poisoning reach the conclusion with which this author is in full agreement that two solvent systems are necessary for complete resolution. They prefer sodium carbonate–impregnated paper (0.05 $M$) and solvents of water-saturated *n*-butyl ether, chloroform, or diethyl ether with descending travel after a 4–6 hours equilibration time. In the United Kingdom the alcohol-ammonia solvents continue to be favored although, as indicated above, the Hensel–Abernethy system is a necessary adjunct. These methods, coupled with the permanganate spray reaction and the sulfuric acid dealkylation at 100°C (C12) for 1 hour, serve to distinguish all combinations of the common barbiturates. Other workers have used reversed phase systems with formamide-impregnated paper being favored and chloroform (L2, M2) or ethylene glycol (D4) as the recommended solvents. Neil and Payton (N1) tried the well-known Bush steroid system and separated cyclobarbitone, butobarbitone, and secobarbitone but not amylobarbitone from pentobarbitone. Street and Niyogi (S20, S21) have used ion-exchange paper with aqueous solvents followed by ionophoresis at right angles to give a separation of phenobarbitone, salicylic acid, and phenacetin; using Whatman DE20 and 0.2 N ammonia, Street (S22, S24) has detected salicylic acid and phenobarbitone after direct application of whole blood to the paper. The same worker has recognized that the main problem associated with barbiturate analyses is no longer identification but the speed with which the result can be achieved and, in an effort to reduce the time for chromatographic separations, he (S23) recommends tributyrin-impregnated paper (10% v/v in acetone dip) in an oven at 86°C with $M/15$ phosphate buffer at pH 7.4 as solvent; under these conditions excellent separations are obtained in 15–60 minutes. Cation-exchange paper has been used for the separation of sulfanil, sulfaguanidine, and sulfacetamide (L4).

The detection of the barbiturates on paper chromatograms is usually accomplished by inspection in 254-m$\mu$ light after exposure to the alkaline vapors of ammonia or after spraying with weak sodium hydroxide. If alkaline-impregnated papers have been used the spots can be seen without treatment although in any case a significant improvement in sensitivity is obtained by incorporating a fluorescent indicator into the paper or the spray. 0.005% fluorescein is excellent and Fischl and Segal (F3), using a mixture of 1% sodium hydroxide and 1% salicylamide in ethanol as a spray, say that 0.3–4.0 $\mu$g can be detected, the sensitivity depending on the particular barbiturate.

In Ivor Smith's book, *Chromatography and Electrophoretic Techniques,* Jackson (J1) contributed a chapter on "The Barbiturates" and Jackson and Moss (J2), a chapter on "Glutarimides and Other Neutral Drugs."

Both these chapters report the great advantages of paper chromatography. The popularity of compound barbiturate preparations is stressed, seven popular medicaments containing up to four different barbiturates in a single tablet or capsule being noted. In the classic paper of Bonnichsen and associates (B8) more than one drug was involved in 42% of the total while six cases had four barbiturates and one had five.

The phenols in hashish have been examined by paper chromatography by several workers (F1, K1, R2); de Ropp uses dimethylformamide and cyclohexane, Korte and Sieper (K1) prefer Dowex 1107 paper saturated in benzene with a solvent of ligroin (60–95°C): benzene:chloroform:methanol:water (2:2:1:4:1). Farmilo and McConnel Davis (F1) also use a technique involving dimethylformamide and cyclohexane and like the other workers stress that the physiologically active tetrahydrocannabinol can be separated and identified using paper chromatography. de Ropp (R2) used a macro separation by partition chromatography on Celite followed by high vacuum distillation for further purification but did not succeed in obtaining crystals.

Moss and Jackson (M12) use a multiple spray involving the following sequence for the detection of acidic and neutral poisons: inspection in 254-m$\mu$ light, spray with cobalt chloride solution, followed by exposure to ammonia vapor. These detect the barbiturates and are followed by a spray with ferric chloride for salicylates and finally a spray with 10% furfuraldehyde in ethanol and exposure to hydrochloric acid fumes to detect carbamates. Solvent systems suggested include isoamyl alcohol: water (190:10) and methanol:water (180:20). A new departure is the use of 50% acetic acid on Whatman No. 1 paper that has been dipped in 20% olive oil in acetone and dried. A useful reaction for the detection of methylprylone, glutethimide, thalidomide, bemegride, Sedulon, and Persedon is to dip the paper in a mixture of equal volumes of 6.6% hydroxylamine hydrochloride and 3.5% sodium hydroxide; after 30 minutes the paper is dipped in 12.5% ferric chloride when spots appear as purple on a colorless background.

Improvements in the well-known starch-iodide method for detecting all the compounds having a reactive nitrogen atom in the molecule which include carbromal, bromvaletone, Sedormid, methyprylone, glutethimide, thalidomide, bemegride, Sedulon, Persedon, meprobamate, mephenesin carbamate, and ethinamate have been described (G7). Ethinamate has been studied separately (F4) and the ethylenic group forms a reactive group for the formation of a silver complex which can be detected with sodium rhodizonate; in methanol:0.1 $N$ hydrochloric acid (1:1) it has an $R_f$ of 0.75.

The paper chromatographic separation of saponins has been described by Pasich (P3) who uses butanol:acetic acid:water (6:1:3) spraying with 25% ethanolic phosphotungstic acid for detection. Bonnichsen, Maehly, and Norlander (B7) after isolating caffeine, phenacetin, and antipyrine separate them on a 0.05 $M$ sodium carbonate–buffered paper using ether or butyl ether as solvent.

A general review of the use of paper chromatography in toxicology was given at the American Academy of Forensic Sciences, Toxicology Section Meeting, 1961 (C16).

Electrophoresis has not figured in the literature to any great extent in the examination of the acidic poisons; the metabolites of salicylate have however been examined in phthalate buffer at pH 3.2 (F8).

## B. Thin Layer Chromatography

This method of separating compounds has been studied mainly in Germany although there is a review paper by Wollish *et al.* (W3) in Analytical Chemistry. A thin layer, usually about 250 $\mu$, of silicic acid–

calcium sulfate is layered on a glass plate and after drying serves as an open plate chromatogram. The spots are usually discrete and the flow rate very rapid, and claims for greatly increased sensitivity over paper chromatography are made. Some of the barbiturates, salicylic acid, theobromine, theophylline, phenacetin, pyramidon, and antipyrine have been examined by Machata (M3) who uses a solvent of chloroform plus 15% ether. Unfortunately the resolution obtained in the case of the barbiturates is not very good, but no doubt as the technique is developed further improvements can be expected. Caffeine, phenobarbitone, phenacetin, theophylline, butazolidine, and amidopyrine have also been separated and 2% Leuchtstoff ZS-Super in 2% strength is incorporated into the layer (G1); its green fluorescence in UV light provides a means of detection similar to that used in paper chromatography. The steroids have also been examined by thin layer (B1).

## C. Gas Chromatography

As was indicated above, there has been a powerful addition to paper and thin layer chromatography in the form of gas chromtography. Although in the minds of many analysts gas chromatography is associated mainly with volatile liquids, and the patterns from peppermint, coffee, whisky, brandy, onions, cigarette, and cigar smoke described by MacKay *et al.* (M4) serve as general interest, Parker and Kirk's (P2) separation of the barbiturates illustrates the very great use and potential of the technique applied to the separation of what are normally considered nonvolatile compounds. Twenty-three barbiturates can be separated on a 4-ft column at 180°C on SE 30, 5% by weight on 100- to 120-mesh firebrick, with retention times ranging from 3.2 to 24.8 minutes. The trend towards multiple barbiturate preparations has also been emphasized by these workers; the value of the technique in cases from Coroners is especially mentioned.

Many other most interesting separations have been reported of compounds that are to be found in the organic solvent extract from acidic aqueous solution, for example, phenols (P5), dichlorbenzenes (C11), chlorinated hydrocarbons (U2), and pesticide residues (C10). The work of Farmilo and his colleagues (M6) is of special interest for they have followed the discovery of eighteen peaks from the essential oils from cannabis on a 2.5-meter column of 20% Apiezon M on Chromosorb W at 220°C with an examination of the phenols using 3% SE 30 on the same solid at 174°C on a 30-inch column. They found retention times of 9.3 minutes for cannabidiol, 13.5 minutes for tetrahydrocannabinol, and 18.3 minutes for cannabinol (F1). The recognition of the $\alpha$- and $\beta$-caryophyllins as being responsible for the Duquenois test and the absence of a positive Beams test from any of the peaks from the essential oil are interesting.

Horning has reported the separation of steroids also on a SE 30 column (H5).

The use of nondestructive methods of detecting the fractions as they come off the column or fraction collectors in parallel with the detection device means that each fraction can be separated and examined by infrared spectroscopy thus enabling absolute identification to be achieved. Leggon (L3) and Chang *et al.* (C3) have described traps suitable for the purpose. Anderson (A7) and Haslam *et al.* (H2) have described particular aspects of this technique and, although not directly related to toxicology, these workers indicate the general approach. There is no doubt that gas chromatography is an essential tool in toxicological analysis.

A most important variation is pyrolysis whereby thermal decomposition by means of an electrically heated platinum spiral at the top of the column gives a pattern of products which is often as characteristic as an infrared curve. Janak (J5), using a 30% squalane on Celite 545 column with hydrogen gas and a flame ionization detector, identified the 800°C pyrolysis products from phenobarbitone, barbitone, mephobarbitone, Dial, and Kalypnon. In Powell's hands (P8) the closely related compounds amylobarbitone, butobarbitone, and pentobarbitone produce entirely different pyrolytic products and give a pattern much more distinctive than the corresponding infrared curves.

# IV. Identification

## A. Infrared Spectroscopy

The main principles of the method are well known and are fully discussed in relation to toxicology in recent books. As long ago as 1952 Umberger and Adams (U1) published curves for the barbiturates, but few laboratories have had the necessary facilities to use the technique routinely. The availability of less expensive machines in the last 2 or 3 years, however, has found them installed in most toxicologists' laboratories. As in the case of ultraviolet spectra, a standard collection of curves must be prepared from pure compounds. Cleverley (C7) has indicated that grinding and pressing techniques can alter the spectrum of some barbiturates and has published curves for twenty (C8). Different spectra from polymorphic forms do not usually present insurmountable difficulties.

Alha and Tamminen (A4) have published a paper on the use of infrared spectroscopy in forensic chemical identification showing the investigations of thirty-one fatal cases of suspected poisoning. The majority of poisons in this paper fall into the group under consideration here and include meprobamate, phenacetin, aminopyrine, Sedormid, carbromal, phenobarbitone, bemegride, amylobarbitone, mesantoin, ethinamate, and a suspected case of DDT poisoning. The same workers also identified the metabolites of carbromal (A5) and bromvaletone (A6) by comparison with synthetic compounds. The infrared spectrum of a metabolite of ethinamate has been published (L2a) and although the identity of this compound is not yet known the spectrum will serve to characterize it. Sublimation of evaporated chloroform extracts onto a potassium bromide disc was used by Bonnichsen and his colleagues (B7) to prepare samples on a 5- to 50-$\mu$g scale when identifying caffeine, phenacetin, antipyrine, and barbiturates from tissue extracts.

Tetrahydrocannabinol has been isolated in a noncrystalline form (R2) and its infrared curve published. The determination of aldrin and dieldrin in aldrin-treated soil has also been described (B5).

## B. Investigations on Metabolites

There is an increasing tendency to search in the viscera for metabolites of ingested poison or drug when death follows after several days illness.

In the strong acid fraction 3:4:5 trimethylphenylacetic acid has been found as a major metabolite of mescaline in the dog (S13) and 3-*o*-tolyloxylactic acid is known as a metabolite of mephenesin (M1).

The barbiturates continue to be extensively studied (B6, S12) and Jackson and Moss (J3) have isolated 3-hydroxy-3-methylbutyl-5-ethylbarbiturate from human urine following a case of Tuinal ingestion. Identification was by paper chromatography and by X-ray diffraction pattern comparisons with an authentic specimen. No unchanged amylobarbitone could be detected and the metabolite was isolated by salting out with ammonium sulfate into large volumes of ether.

Ether has been indicted by Frey (F9) as tending to desulfurize thiobarbiturates during extraction procedures. Although chloroform does not have this tendency it should be remembered that many polar metabolites are much more soluble in ether than chloroform.

Jerslev and Ravn-Jonsen (J6, J7) have differentiated amylobarbitone and pentobarbitone by X-ray diffraction studies.

The bromoureides have been found to undergo a very interesting metabolism; debromination of carbromal and bromvaletone to 2-ethylbutyrylurea and 3-ethylbutyrylurea, respectively, has been established (A5, A6, C14). The production of inorganic bromide as a metabolite of these sedatives and the high blood bromide levels in cases of chronic addiction can therefore be easily understood. Such ureides have recently been placed on restricted sale in the United Kingdom.

The success of tolbutamide as an oral hypoglycemic agent means that it will probably be found in extracts although Nelson and O'Reilly (N3) have found a metabolite which has a half-life of 5.7 hours to be 1-butyl-3-*p*-carboxyphenylsulfonylurea. Nelson and Chulski (N2) say that only metabolite and no unchanged tolbutamide is excreted in the urine. They add 1 ml 5 *N* hydrochloric acid to 3 ml of urine (diluted if necessary) together with 6 ml of amyl acetate. After shaking and centrifuging, 4 ml of the organic layer is taken and added to 1 ml of 0.1% dinitrofluorobenzene in amyl acetate. After heating at 150°C for exactly 5 minutes and cooling, the optical density is read at 380 m$\mu$. Levels of 8–25 mg/100 ml were obtained for therapeutic doses.

Seventy-five per cent of ingested glutethimide has been found to be excreted in the bile and Algeri *et al.* (A2) recommend a search for its urinary excretion product 2-phenylglutarimide.

Investigations in a death from ethinamate led Lee (L2a) to the isolation of a metabolite from tissues; this had a melting point of 142°C and an empirical formula of $C_{21}H_{16}O$ but is, as yet, unidentified.

The much used stimulant, bemegride, ($\beta$-methyl-$\beta$-ethylglutarimide) has been labeled with $C^{14}$ in the side chains and its metabolism followed in the rat. More water-soluble compounds were found and the analyses indicated an intact glutarimide ring (N5).

## V. Analyses for Specific Poisons

A rapid scheme of analysis has been proposed by Sobolewski and Nadeau (S10) for the clinical chemist. Benzene and butanol are used as the extracting solvents with spot tests of Millon's reagent for barbiturates, the hydroxylamine/ferric chloride reaction for glutethimide, and the hydroquinine reaction for meprobamate. The toxic effects of benzene when used by inexperienced laboratory workers must not be ignored. These tests are presumably acceptable for confirmation of identity in the circumstances appertaining in an emergency but there seems little justification for not performing a quick separation of the isolated barbiturates by paper chromatography so as to assist the clinician even further. As Curry pointed out (C15), the extraction of 5 ml of blood, a rough estimate of the amount, and separation into short- or long-acting barbiturate can be completed in about 1 hour. Although Whatman CRL1 papers were recommended with butanol–6 *N* ammonia (1:1), top layer, as the solvent, the present trend to even quicker resolutions using the Street system (S23) or thin layer chromatography means that there is little reason for clinical chemists not performing these simple additional tests. A simple method for estimating barbiturate concentrations when an ultraviolet spectrophometer is not available has been described (Z1). One milliliter of serum is placed on a rolled-up filter paper and shaken with two 10-ml portions of ether. The ether is combined and evaporated and the residue dissolved in 5.0 ml of chloroform with 0.5 ml of the following solution added: dissolve 0.5 gm $Hg(NO_3)_2$ in 50 ml distilled water with a few drops of concentrated nitric acid, dilute 1 ml with 0.1 $M$ sodium bicarbonate to 50 ml, and filter. The chloroform layer, after shaking, is separated and filtered through Munktell 00 paper. Four milliliters are taken and shaken with 1 ml of 3.2 mg/100 ml of dithizone in chloroform. In the presence of barbiturate the green color is changed to orange and can be estimated at 605 m$\mu$ by measuring the optical density difference between the sample and a blank.

In the strong acid fraction Stevenson has described an assay for salicylate (S16) by extraction of 300 $\mu$l of serum or plasma with 3 ml of 0.4% malonic acid in butyl ether and measurement of the organic layer optical densities at 378, 314, 307, 300, and 280 m$\mu$. In a fatal case of ethyl-2,4-dichlorophenoxyacetate poisoning (C19) the corresponding acid levels in the tissues ranged from 4.5 to 40 mg%.

The weak acids continue to be a major source of poison with emphasis remaining on the barbiturates although glutethimide receives much attention. The fact that glutethimide is a weak acid seems to have been ignored by many workers and some extraction schemes even recommend washing the organic solvent with weak alkali to purify the sedative. Although in the conditions described in the published papers recovery experiments have been described there is a danger that the uninitiated will not recognize this and may assume that the cyclic imide structure is neutral; as was indicated in *Toxicology*, Volume II, this is not so (C17). The use of ultraviolet spectrophotometry to distinguish between barbiturates continues to attract attention: pentobarbitone and pentothal in blood and plasma for example (O3). These workers claim improvement in reliability and sensitivity for the quantitation by the use of Allen's correction factor. Stevenson (S17) makes use of consecutive extractions with borax and 1 N sodium hydroxide from butyl ether to distinguish the short- from the long-acting barbiturates; for example, under the described conditions extraction with 0.05 $M$ borax extracts 95% of phenobarbitone but only 22% of pentobarbitone. This paper, although suffering from a basic objection that it cannot adequately distinguish complex mixtures, is of great value because it reports comprehensively on the ultraviolet characteristics of twenty-one barbiturates and also on some partition coefficients. A comprehensive 57-page paper on barbiturates worthy of translation has been published by Schmidt (S4) and also a paper on a device for the extraction of barbiturates by Dressler and co-workers (D3).

As noted above, Bonnichsen et al. (B8) have reported on the chemical investigations in over 600 cases of barbiturate poisoning and this paper serves as an object lesson to be read in its entirety by all toxicologists. Few who read it will ever believe again a gravimetric barbiturate determination. The experience of these workers in Stockholm closely parallels those described in Volume II of Toxicology and when read together with the gas chromatographic work they represent the best up to the minute survey of barbiturates. The stability of barbiturates in exhumation cases has been discussed (W2) together with statistics for many other drugs; the probability that positive results will be obtained even after some years burial in temperate climates is suggested.

Glutethimide was discussed by Curry in relation to interference with barbiturate determinations (C17) and the rapid opening of the glutarimide ring by alkali with loss of the 235-m$\mu$ peak noted. Goldbaum and Williams (G2) used weak alcoholic potassium hydroxide (0.2 N potassium hydroxide in water, 1 part mixed with 3 parts absolute ethanol) and found that half the glutethimide was hydrolyzed about every 1000 seconds with a decrease of 200 seconds for every 6°C temperature rise. Extraction of 5 ml of blood, plasma, or urine is made with 25 ml of chloroform which after separating and filtering is washed with 5 ml 0.5 N sodium hydroxide and once with 5 ml 0.5 N hydrochloric acid. Twenty milliliters of the chloroform is carefully evaporated and the residue dissolved in 4 ml ethanol. A 3-ml aliquot is mixed with 1 ml of 0.2 N potassium hydroxide and measurements made at 280, 240, 235, and 225 m$\mu$ every 500 seconds. $E_{1cm}^{1\%}$ for glutethimide under these conditions at 235 m$\mu$ is given as 880. $\alpha$-Phenylglutarimide, the urinary metabolite, is hydrolyzed at twice the rate of glutethimide while bemegride, a possible source of interference, is not affected by this strength alkali. Phang et al. (P7) found difficulty in applying this method to fatty vomitus extracts and dissolved the residue in methanol. To a 1-ml portion containing less than 1 mg glutethimide they add 1 ml of 2 M hydroxylamine hydrochloride and 1 ml of 3.5 N sodium hydroxide. Thirty minutes later, 1.5 ml 3.5 N hydrochloric acid, 5 ml isobutanol, and 0.5 ml ferric chloride reagent (0.37 M FeCl$_3$ in 0.1 N HCl) are added. After shaking for 30 seconds the isobutanol layer is filtered through Whatman No. 1 paper and the purple color read at 510 m$\mu$. The toxicology of glutethimide has also been discussed by Schiebel (S3) together with that of Persedon and ethinamate.

The other cyclic imide, thalidomide, has been investigated simultaneously in England and Germany (B3, G5) and methods based on ultraviolet spectrophotometry after chloroform extraction recommended. The $E_{1cm}^{1\%}$ at the absorption maximum at 220 m$\mu$ in 0.1 N hydrochloric acid reaches the very high value of 1950.

Tolbutamide also appears in the weak acid fraction and Chulski (C5) published a spectrophotometric method for plasma determinations using Erhlich's reagent. One milliliter of oxalated plasma, 2 ml M/30 phosphoric acid, and 10 ml chloroform are shaken and after separation the chloroform layer is evaporated at room temperature. Two milliliters 0.4% p-dimethylaminobenzaldehyde in ethanol are added and controls of 2 ml of ethanol and 2 ml reagent are also prepared. After drying each at room temperature the tubes are heated at 70°C for 2½ hours. When cold, 10 ml of ethanol are added to each and readings at 395 m$\mu$ made within 8 minutes.

The ultraviolet spectra of cannabis extracts have been described by Scaringelli (S2) and de Ropp (R2). For tetrahydrocannabinol the latter worker gives absorption maxima at 275 and 282 m$\mu$ with log $\epsilon$ = 3.26 and 3.28, shifting in 0.1 N sodium hydroxide to 292 m$\mu$, log $\epsilon$ = 3.53, with a second peak at 325 m$\mu$.

In the neutral fraction the carbamates form the largest group; Harris and Reik (H1) hydrolyze urinary meprobamate extracts with 2 ml 1.0 N sodium hydroxide at 100°C for 10 minutes collecting any distillate in 4.0 ml of 0.75 N sulfuric acid. This acid is then added to the alkaline solution, when, after making up to 12.0 ml, a 2-ml aliquot is added to 1.0 ml of Nessler's reagent and a colorimetric assay made after 5 minutes. The basis of this method is the decomposition of the carbamate to free carbamic acid which spontaneously decomposes to give ammonia.

Ellis and Hetzel (E1), after ethereal extraction of meprobamate, take a 1-ml aqueous aliquot and add 1 ml of a chlorinating solution of 5.25% sodium hypochlorite diluted 1:30 with 0.05 M borate at pH 10.5. After shaking and 15 minutes at room temperature, 1 ml 0.5% phenol in 0.1 N hydrochloric acid is added and 5 minutes later 5 ml of 0.3% potassium iodide. Optical density measurements are taken 5 minutes later at 350 m$\mu$.

Rutter (R3) has found the absorption maximum at 245 m$\mu$ of the product of the concentrated sulfuric acid treatment at 100°C for 30 minutes of meprobamate described by Bedson (B4) to be preferable to the visible spectrum measurement. Lee's paper (L2a) on a fatality from ethinamate includes investigations into chemical tests for this acetylenic carbamate. Vidic also investigated this carbamate and meprobamate in relation to their reaction with p-dimethylaminobenzaldehyde and included in the enquiry Adalin, bromural, persedon, and Noludar (V2).

Mephenesin has been determined by ultraviolet spectrophotometry (M1). Sixty minutes after intravenous injection of 2 gm none was detectable in the blood although 0.5–0.6 mg/100 ml of 3-*o*-tolyloxylactic acid was present. Maximum blood levels of unchanged drug were in the range of 0.3–0.7 mg/100 ml. In this method 10 ml of plasma were extracted four times with 10–20 ml of ether which, after separating and concentrating to 10 ml, was read at 300 and 270 m$\mu$. The metabolite can then be isolated by adjusting the pH to 3 and repeating the ether extractions. It is assayed in 10 ml 0.1 N sodium hydroxide at the same wavelengths.

A three-sulfonamide mixture, sulfadiazine, sulfamerazine, and sulfathiazole, has been investigated by Marzys (M7) using ultraviolet spectrophotometry and reaction with 2-thiobarbituric acid.

For the determination of hydrochlorthiazide in urine Sheppard and co-workers (S7) extract 1 ml with 2 ml water and 18 ml ethyl acetate. After hydrolysis of the evaporated organic extract for 30 minutes at 100°C with 1 ml 5 N sodium hydroxide, and acidification with 1 ml concentrated hydrochloric acid, 1 ml 0.1% sodium nitrite is added and the solution stands for 4 minutes. One milliliter 0.5% ammonium sulfamate is then added and, after standing for 3 minutes, 1 ml 0.1% N-(1-naphthyl)-ethylenediamine dihydrochloride. Readings are taken in a colorimeter within 30 seconds to 1 minute. The same authors also distinguish hydrochlorthiazide from chlorthiazide by the chromotropic acid reaction for formaldehyde produced by hydrolysis of the former and not by the latter.

A useful color test for DDT and related compounds (I1) consists of heating the extract with a nitrating mixture of 1:1 nitric and sulfuric acids at 100°C for 1 hour. After cooling, dilute with 50–100 ml of ice-cold water and extract with 20 ml and then 10 ml of chloroform. Wash the combined chloroform extracts with 50 ml of 1% potassium hydroxide and then with three 50-ml portions of water. Dry the separated chloroform with anhydrous sodium sulfate and evaporate to dryness. Transfer the residue in chloroform to two separate spots on a white tile and evaporate off the solvent. To one spot add 1 drop of a 20% alcoholic potassium hydroxide (made by dissolving 5 gm potassium hydroxide in 2.5 ml water and diluting with 22.6 ml of ethanol). A positive reaction of colors going from rose to bright blue to green to yellow is obtained if DDT, DDE, DDA, DDD, DFDT, or methoxychlor is present in microgram quantities. To the other spot addition of 1 drop of alcoholic potassium hydroxide solution is followed by 1 to 2 drops of acetone. A positive result is bright blue changing to bright purple to grey to yellow.

Color tests for sulfonamides (S15), digoxin, digitoxin, and digitoxigenin (H4), and hydrochlorthiazide (Z3) have also been reported. Experiments in which colchicine was added to urine are most interesting (P6) and the fact that only 6–9% was recovered despite extensive investigations illustrates the difficulties that were met.

A very comprehensive paper (B9) giving Kofler melting points of over 300 compounds has been published and has fulfilled a long-felt want in this field.

## VI. General Toxicology

In the strong acid fraction salicylates are again predominant; the dangers of aspirin medication have been described (G6) and the relation of blood levels with effect discussed by Donne (D2). Reports of skin absorption with blood levels up to 40 mg/100 ml have been reported (S14). General opinion indicates that the probability of recovery with blood levels under 100 mg/100 ml, provided the clinician is experienced in the management of such cases, is high although death can occasionally occur with blood levels as low as 15 mg/100 ml. Death is probably inevitable if the level is over 100 mg/100 ml and certainly there is an increasing chance of a major metabolic upset at levels of 30 mg/100 ml and above. The artificial kidney has again been recommended in aspirin poisoning therapy if renal insufficiency developed (T1) and it is clear that there is a body of opinion in favor of this type of therapy in many types of poisoning: its use has been demonstrated not only with aspirin but also with some barbiturates (C6), glutethimide (S5), and ethinamate (D1). Bunker (B10) has put the case that portable artificial kidneys should be made available so that the seriously ill poisoned patient need not be moved. The response to dialysis in barbitone poisoning may be dramatic; in one case in my experience the blood level dropped from 29 mg/100 ml to 12 mg/100 ml in 6 hours and was certainly life-saving.

Clemmeson and Nilsonn (C6) have described the Scandinavian method for treating barbiturate poisoning and have achieved the remarkably low mortality of 1.5%. This is a statistically highly significant figure as the Copenhagen center alone treats 1500 cases a year. The combined effect of alcohol and barbiturate has again been studied (A8, G4) as has the combined effect of alcohol and meprobamate on coordination and judgment (Z2).

Bonnischen and his co-workers (B8) have found that in their extensive experience levels in the tissues with coincident alcohol were only about two-thirds those of cases without alcohol. Average levels in the blood at death of cases exclusively due to barbiturates were 2.7–2.8 mg/

100 ml for amylobarbitone and pentobarbitone while corresponding levels in the liver were 6.7 and 8.5 mg/100 ml. These are the most reliable yet reported being based on critically reported control recovery experiments fully described by the authors. These workers suggest that diffusion of barbiturate post mortem from the stomach into the liver may account for the high levels found in this organ. Sunshine and Curry (S25) have published figures showing a high liver to blood concentration ratio when there is a short time interval between ingestion and death. Further experiments are obviously necessary to show whether this finding is a real one or an artefact. The small amounts left in stomach contents, because of rapid absorption, initiated the combined English and American work and, although there may be a difference of opinion as to the cause of the high ratios, both sets of workers are agreed that heart blood is to be avoided.

The popularity of glutethimide as a mild sedative continues and the general consensus of opinion seems to be that blood levels of above 3 mg/100 ml are paralleled by a clinical state of deep coma. Several cases of poisoning have been reported and the suggestion made that in some cases of suicide the drug is used as an adjunct to more violent forms of death (C19).

Phenols in the form of sodium pentachlorophenol (L1) and an alkalanolamine salt of dinitro-*o-sec*-butylphenol have been reported (C2) as causing poisoning. In the latter case absorption from the skin of the right hand and from the gastrointestinal tract after the majority of a mouthful had been spat out led to a necrotizing renal tubule damage.

Blood levels of phenytoin, diphenylhydantoin, have been examined (S26) in epileptics during treatment and at doses of 14 mg/kg blood levels were stationary at about 4 mg/100 ml; in dose ranges of 3–8 mg/kg blood levels were about 2 mg/100 ml. A 30–55% loss per 24 hours after cessation of therapy was observed.

Thalidomide has been reported as causing peripheral neuritis (F7, F10, M10, S18) and has recently been withdrawn from sale because of the possibility of it being involved in cases in which abnormal fetuses have been noted. Before this occurred a case of poisoning followed by recovery after ingestion of 2.1 gm had been reported (S11).

In the chemically neutral fraction the carbamates, meprobamate, and ethinamate continue to be the subject of many papers describing their human toxicity and a new carbamate, 2-hydroxy-2-phenylethylcarbamate (C4, S1), has been described as muscle relaxant. An anaphylactic reaction to meprobamate (N4) was recorded which responded to hydrocortisone but hypotension seems to be the most serious effect of overdosage (F2). Combined with promazine, meprobamate gave rise to a suggestion of alarming side effects (Z4).

The bromoureides have been reported as causing poisoning in Australasia and Singapore (A9, F5, S8).

Two cases of hepatic failure involving peliosis hepatis and cholestasis associated with norethandrolone therapy have been reported (G3). Side effects from chlorthiazide have also been described (F6) and two cases of cantharidin poisoning with photographs of the eroded second degree burnt lips enlarge the list of cases since 1900 to twenty-six (O1).

Halogenated hydrocarbons such as dieldrin have caused poisoning in workers in spray teams engaged in malaria and filaria control and a case of acute poisoning in a child noted (C9). In the twenty cases reported by Patel and Rao (P4) the delayed effect of this poison (up to 15 days) is worthy of special attention. A case of chlordane poisoning following prolonged use for ant control in a private home has been described (S6). Perhaps the most striking report in this field has been the recognition of benzene hexachloride as the toxic agent of a porphyria outbreak in Turkey which was traced to the consumption of dressed wheat (M8, O2).

Other unusual cases of poisoning described in the literature include death after an intravenous injection of 3.2 gm of caffeine (J8), fresh cases of aminophylline poisoning in children (C19, J4), and a case of mephenesin poisoning characterized by a profound respiratory depression following ingestion of between 5.5 and 11 gm in a woman aged 43 (B2).

Self-administration of large doses of medicaments continue to cause trouble; phenacetin in particular has been noted as causing sulfhemoglobinemia which was only apparent during anesthesia (S9), and in another case of fatal nephritis (M11) a woman was subsequently found to have been taking ten to twenty-five compound aspirin, phenacetin, and codeine tablets a day for $5\frac{1}{2}$ years unknown to her medical attendants. As Hunter and Greenberg (H6) found in the case of barbiturate addiction, this medication can occur without the knowledge of close relatives, and such cases emphasize the need for toxicological investigations in routine clinical biochemistry.

## VII. Conclusions

The last 3 years have been dramatic years of development perhaps only paralleled by those of 1950–1952. The use of one or more chromatographic techniques followed by identification by spectroscopy is now the accepted approach and the detection and absolute identification of

152                                                                A. S. Curry

5–10 μg or the detection of one part of acidic or neutral poison or drug
in 50 million parts of tissue is to be considered not only possible but
routine.

(A1) Abernethy, R. F., Villaudy, J. A., and Thompson, E. R. Am. Acad. Forensic
     Sci., Chicago Meeting, 1959.
(A2) Algeri, E. J., Katsas, G. G., and McBay, A. J. *J. Forensic Sci.* 4, 111 (1959).
(A3) Algeri, E. J., and Katsas, G. G. *J. Forensic Sci.* 5, 217 (1960).
(A4) Alha, A. R., and Tamminen, V. *Ann. Med. Exptl. Biol Fenniae (Helsinki)*
     37, 157 (1959).
(A5) Alha, A. R., and Tamminen, V. *Suomen Kemistilehti B.* 32, 119 (1959).
(A6) Alha, A. R., and Tamminen, V. *Suomen Kemistilehti B.* 34, 9 (1961).
(A7) Anderson, D. M. W. *Analyst* 84, 50 (1959).
(A8) Aston, R., and Cullumbine, H. *Toxicol. Appl. Pharmacol.* 1, 65 (1959).
(A9) Atkinson, I. *Med. J. Australia* 2, 10 (1960).
(B1) Barbier, M., Jager, H., Tobias, H., and Wyss, E. *Helv. Chim. Acta* 42, 2440
     (1959).
(B2) Barron, D. W., and Milliken, T. G. *Lancet* i, 262 (1960).
(B3) Beckmann, R., and Kampf, H. H. *Arzneimittel-Forsch.* 11, 45 (1961).
(B4) Bedson, H. S. *Lancet* i, 268 (1959).
(B5) Blinn, R. C., Gunther, F. A., and Mulla, M. S. *J. Econ. Entomol.* 53, 1129
     (1960).
(B6) Block, W., and Ebight, I. *Arzneimittel-Forsch.* 10, 825 (1960).
(B7) Bonnichsen, R., Maehly, A. C., and Norlander, S. *J. Chromatog.* 3, 190 (1960).
(B8) Bonnichsen, R., Maehly, A. C., and Frank, A. *J. Forensic Sci.* 6, 411 (1961).
(B9) Brandstätter-Kuhnert, M., and Kuhnert, G. *Sci. Pharm.* 28, 287 (1960).
(B10) Bunker, N. V. D. *Brit. Med. J.* ii, 1402 (1959).
(C1) Cahiel, P. K. *Brit. Med. J.* ii, 1223 (1961).
(C2) Cann, H. M., and Verhulst, H. L. *Am. J. Diseases Children* 100, 947 (1960).
(C3) Chang, S. S., Ireland, C. E., and Tai, H. *Anal. Chem.* 33, 479 (1961).
(C4) Chesrow, E. J., Kaplitz, S. E., Musci, J. P., Breme, J. T., and Marquardt, G. H
     *J. Am. Geriat. Soc.* 8, 288 (1960).
(C5) Chulski, T. *J. Lab. Clin. Med.* 53, 490 (1959).
(C6) Clemmeson, C., and Nilsson, E. *Clin. Pharmacol. Therap.* 2, 220 (1961).
(C7) Cleverley, B., and Williams, P. P. *Chem. Ind. (London)* p. 49 (1959).
(C8) Cleverley, B. *Analyst* 85, 582 (1960).
(C9) Committee on Toxicology, *J. Am. Med. Assoc.* 172, 2077 (1960).
(C10) Coulson, D. M., Cavanagh, L. A., de Vries, J. E., and Walther, B. *J. Agr.
     Food Chem.* 8, 399 (1960).
(C11) Cowan, C. T., and Hartwell, J. M. *Nature* 190, 712 (1961).
(C12) Curry, A. S. *Nature* 183, 1052 (1959).
(C13) Curry, A. S., and Phang, S. E. *J. Pharm. Pharmacol.* 12, 437 (1960).
(C14) Curry, A. S. *Nature* 188, 58 (1960).
(C15) Curry, A. S. *Proc. Assoc. Clin. Biochem.* 1, 25 (1960).
(C16) Curry, A. S. *J. Forensic Sci.* 6, 373 (1961).
(C17) Curry, A. S. *In* "Toxicology: Mechanisms and Analytical Methods" (C. P.
     Stewart and A. Stolman, eds.), Vol. II, p. 179. Academic Press, New
     York, 1961.

(C18) Curry, A. S. *J. Pharm. Pharmacol.* **9**, 102 (1957).
(C19) Curry, A. S. *Brit. Med. J.* i, 687 (1962).
(C20) Curry, A. S. *In* "Poison Detection in Human Organs," p. 106. Charles C Thomas, Springfield, Illinois, 1963.
(D1) Davis, R. P., Blythe, W. B., Newton, M., and Welt, L. T. *Yale J. Biol. Med.* **32**, 192 (1959).
(D2) Donne, A. K. *Pediatrics* **26**, 800 (1960).
(D3) Dressler, A., Muller, M., and Schonfield, H. *Arch. Toxicol.* **17**, 286 (1958).
(D4) Dybing, F. *Scand. J. Clin. Lab. Invest.* **12**, 333 (1960).
(E1) Ellis, G. H., and Hetzel, C. A. *Anal. Chem.* **31**, 1091 (1959).
(F1) Farmilo, C. G., and McConnel Davis, T. W. *J. Pharm. Pharmacol.* **13**, 767 (1961).
(F2) Ferguson, M. J., Germanos, S., and Grace, W. J. *A.M.A. Arch. Internal Med.* **106**, 237 (1960).
(F3) Fischl, J., and Segal, S. *Clin. Chem.* **7**, 252 (1961).
(F4) Fisher, K., and Specht, W. *Arch. Toxicol.* **17**, 48 (1958).
(F5) Fischer, E. *Med. J. Australia* **2**, 13 (1960).
(F6) Fitzgerald, E. W. *J. A.M.A. Arch. Internal Med.* **105**, 305 (1960).
(F7) Florence, A. L. *Brit. Med. J.* ii, 1954 (1960).
(F8) Franz, J., Schotteluis, D., Arrendondo, E., Paul, W. D., and Routh, J. *Proc. Iowa Acad. Sci.* **69**, 205 (1959).
(F9) Frey, H. H. *Naturwissenschaften* **47**, 471 (1960).
(F10) Fullerton, P. M., and Kremer, M. *Brit. Med. J.* ii, 855 (1961).
(G1) Ganshurt, H., and Malzacher, A. *Arch. Pharm.* **293**, 925 (1960).
(G2) Goldbaum, L. R., and Williams, M. A. *Anal. Chem.* **32**, 82 (1960).
(G3) Gordon, B. S., Wolf, J., Krause, T., and Shai, F. *Am. J. Clin. Pathol.* **33**, 156 (1960).
(G4) Graham, J. D. P. *Toxicol. Appl. Pharmacol.* **2**, 14 (1960).
(G5) Green, J. N., and Benson, B. C. *J. Pharm. Pharmacol.* **13**. Suppl. 117T (1961).
(G6) Gregory, R. E. *J. S. Carolina Med. Assoc.* **66**, 258 (1960).
(G7) Greig, C. G., and Leaback, D. H. *Nature* **188**, 310 (1960).
(H1) Harris, E. S., and Reik, J. *J. Clin. Chem.* **4**, 241 (1958).
(H2) Haslam, J., Jeffs, A. R., and Willis, H. A. *Analyst* **86**, 44 (1961).
(H3) Hensel, E., and Abernethy, R. J. Personal communication.
(H4) Herrman, R. H. *Nature* **190**, 268 (1961).
(H5) Horning, E. C. *Clin. Chem.* **7**, 404 (1961).
(H6) Hunter, R. A., and Greenberg, H. P. *Lancet* ii, 58 (1954).
(I1) Irudayasamy, A., and Natarajon, A. R. *Anal. Chem.* **33**, 630 (1961).
(J1) Jackson, J. V. The barbiturates. *In* "Chromatography and Electrophoretic Techniques" (I. Smith, ed.), Vol. I, p. 379. Wiley (Interscience), New York, 1960.
(J2) Jackson, J. V., and Moss, M. S. Glutarimides and other neutral drugs. *In* "Chromatography and Electrophoretic Techniques" (I. Smith, ed.), Vol. I, p. 404. Wiley (Interscience), New York, 1960.
(J3) Jackson, J. V., and Moss, M. S. *Nature* **192**, 553 (1961).
(J4) Jadoul, R. *Rev. Med. Liege* **15**, 421 (1960).
(J5) Janak, J. *Nature* **185**, 685 (1960).
(J6) Jerslev, B., and Ravn-Jonsen, E. J. *Dansk. Tidsskr. Farm.* **34**, 153 (1960).
(J7) Jerslev, B., and Ravn-Jonsen, E. J. *Dansk. Tidsskr. Farm.* **34**, 186 (1960).

(J8) Jokela, S., and Vartisinan, A. *Acta Pharmacol. Toxicol.* **15**, 331 (1959).
(K1) Korte, F., and Sieper, H. *Tetrahedron* **10**, 153 (1960).
(L1) Lazarini, H. J., Dervillee, D., L'Epee, P., and Bossevain, L. *Arch. Maladies Profess. Méd. Travail et Sécurité Sociale* **22**, 71 (1961).
(L2) Ledvina, M. *Cesk. Farm.* **9**, 335 (1960).
(L2a) Lee, Kum-Tatt. *J. Pharm. Pharmacol.* **13**, 758 (1961).
(L3) Leggon, H. W. *Anal. Chem.* **33**, 1295 (1961).
(L4) Lewandowski, E. *Anal. Chim. Acta* **23**, 317 (1960).
(M1) Maas, A. R., Carey, P. J., and Heming, A. E. *Anal. Chem.* **31**, 1331 (1959).
(M2) Macek, A. *Arch. Pharm.* **293**, 545 (1960).
(M3) Machata, G. *Arch. Toxicol.* **18**, 338 (1960).
(M4) MacKay, D. A. M., Lang, D. A., and Berdick, M. *Anal. Chem.* **33**, 1369 (1961).
(M5) Mannering, G. Personal communication.
(M6) Martin, L., Morison Smith, D., and Farmilo, C. G. *Nature* **191**, 774 (1961).
(M7) Marzys, A. E. O. *Analyst* **86**, 460 (1961).
(M8) Matteis, de F., Prior, B. E., and Rimington, C. *Nature* **191**, 363 (1961) .
(M9) Mattocks, A. T. R. *Nature* **191**, 1281 (1961).
(M10) Mead, B. W., and Rosalki, S. B. *Brit. Med. J.* ii, 1223 (1961).
(M11) Moolten, S. E., and Smith, I. B. *Am. J. Med.* **28**, 127 (1960).
(M12) Moss, M. S., and Jackson, J. V. *J. Pharm. Pharmacol.* **13**, 361 (1961).
(N1) Neil, M. W., and Payton, J. E. *Med. Sci. Law* **2**, 4 (1961).
(N2) Nelson, O. R., and Chulski, T. *Clin. Chim. Acta* **5**, 774 (1960).
(N3) Nelson, E., and O'Reilly, I. *J. Pharmacol. Exptl. Therap.* **132**, 163 (1961).
(N4) Nevins, D. *Ann. Internal Med.* **53**, 192 (1960).
(N5) Nickolls, P. J. *Nature* **185**, 927 (1960).
(O1) Oaks, W. W., Dilunno, J. F., Magnani, T., Levy, J. A., and Mills, L. C. *A.M.A. Arch. Internal Med.* **105**, 574 (1960).
(O2) Ockner, R., and Schmid, R. *Nature* **189**, 499 (1961).
(O3) Oroszlau, S. I., and Maengwyn Davies, G. D. *J. Am. Pharm. Assoc. Sci. Ed.* **49**, 507 (1960).
(P1) Parker, B. "Group Isolation of Toxicological Substances from Heterogenous Material." Master of Criminology thesis, University of California, Berkeley, 1960.
(P2) Parker, K. D., and Kirk, P. L. *Anal. Chem.* **33**, 1378 (1961).
(P3) Pasich, B. *Nature* **190**, 830 (1961).
(P4) Patel, T. B., and Rao, V. N. *Brit. Med. J.* i, 919 (1958).
(P5) Payn, D. S. *Chem. & Ind.* (London) p. 1090 (1960).
(P6) Peare, E. M. *J. Chromatog.* **2**, 108 (1959).
(P7) Phang, S. E., Dutt, M. C., and Thng Soon Tee, *J. Pharm. Pharmacol.* **13**, 319 (1961).
(P8) Powell, H. Personal communication.
(R1) Rieders, F. Proc. Am. Acad. Forensic Sci., Chicago Meeting, 1959.
(R2) de Ropp, R. S. *J. Am. Pharm. Assoc. Sci. Ed.* **49**, 756 (1960).
(R3) Rutter, E. Personal communication.
(S1) de Salva, S. J., Clements, G. R., and Ercoli, N. J. *J. Pharmacol. Exptl. Therap.* **126**, 318 (1959).
(S2) Scaringelli, F. *J. Assoc. Offic. Agr. Chemists* **44**, 296 (1961).
(S3) Schiebel, E. *Arch. Toxicol.* **17**, 357 (1958).
(S4) Schmidt, G. *Arch. Toxicol.* **17**, 93 (1958).

(S5) Schreiner, G. E., Berman, L. B., Kovach, R., and Bloomer, H. A. *A.M.A. Arch. Internal Med.* **101**, 899 (1958).
(S6) Selby, G., and Jones, A. T. *Med. J. Australia* i, 417 (1960).
(S7) Sheppard, H., Mowles, T. F., and Plummer, A. J. *J. Am. Pharm. Assoc. Sci. Ed.* **49**, 722 (1960).
(S8) Siang, S. C. *Brit. Med. J.* i, 1412 (1960).
(S9) Sniper, W. *Brit. Med. J.* ii, 96 (1961).
(S10) Sobolewski, G. S., and Nadeau, G. *Clin. Chem.* **6**, 153 (1960).
(S11) de Souza, L. P. *Brit. Med. J.* ii, 635 (1959).
(S12) Spector, E., and Shideman, F. E. *Biochem. Pharmacol.* **2**, 182 (1959).
(S13) Spector, E. *Nature* **189**, 751 (1961).
(S14) Stegawski, T., and Lawrynowicz, R. *Przeglad. Lékarsky* **14**, 20 (1958); *Chem. Abstr.* **55**, 15725c (1961).
(S15) Stevanovic, V. *Acta Pharm. Jugoslav.* **9**, 151 (1959).
(S16) Stevenson, G. W. *Anal. Chem.* **32**, 1522 (1960).
(S17) Stevenson, G. W. *Anal. Chem.* **33**, 1374 (1961).
(S18) Stevenson, J. S. K. *Brit. Med. J.* ii, 1223 (1961).
(S19) Stewart, C. P., and Stolman, A., eds. "Toxicology: Mechanisms and Analytical Methods," Vol. I. Academic Press, New York, 1960.
(S20) Street, H. V., and Niyogi, S. K. *Nature* **190**, 337 (1961).
(S21) Street, H. V., and Niyogi, S. K. *Nature* **190**, 1199 (1961).
(S22) Street, H. V. "Application of Modern Methods of Analysis to the Determination in Biological Material of Drugs of Interest in Forensic Chemistry." Ph.D. Thesis, University of Edinburgh, Scotland, 1961.
(S23) Street, H. V. *J. Forensic Sci. Soc.* **2**, 118 (1962).
(S24) Street, H. V. *Acta Pharmacol. Toxicol.* **18**, 281 (1961).
(S25) Sunshine, I., and Curry, A. S. *Toxicol. Appl. Pharmacol.* **2**, 602 (1960).
(S26) Svensmark, O., Schiller, P. J., and Buckthal, F. *Acta Pharmacol. Toxicol.* **16**, 331, (1960).
(S27) Sweeley, C. C., and Horning, E. C. *Nature* **187**, 144 (1960).
(T1) Thomsen, A. C., and Dalgaard, O. Z. *Am. J. Med.* **25**, 484 (1958).
(T2) Tompsett, S. L. *J. Pharm. Pharmacol.* **11**, 32 (1959).
(T3) Tompsett, S. L. *J. Pharm. Pharmacol.* **12**, 62 (1960).
(T4) Tompsett, S. L. *J. Pharm. Pharmacol.* **13**, 747 (1961).
(U1) Umberger, C. J., and Adams, G. *Anal. Chem.* **24**, 1309 (1952).
(U2) Urone, P., and Smith, J. E. *Am. Ind. Hyg. Assoc. J.* **22**, 36 (1961).
(V1) Vanden Heuval, W. J. A. *J. Am. Chem. Soc.* **82**, 3481 (1960).
(V2) Vidic, E. *Arch. Toxicol.* **17**, 373 (1959).
(W1) Walker, G. W. Personal communication.
(W2) Weinig, E. *Deut. Z. Ges. Gerichtl. Med.* **47**, 410 (1958).
(W3) Wollish, E. G., Schmall, M., and Hawrylyshyn, M. *Anal. Chem.* **33**, 1138 (1961).
(Z1) Zaar, B., and Gronwall, A. *Scand. J. Clin. Lab. Invest.* **13**, 225 (1961).
(Z2) Zirkle, G. A., McAtee, O. B., King, P. D., and Van Dyke, R. *J. Am. Med. Assoc.* **173**, 1823 (1960).
(Z3) de Zoeten, E. *Pharm. Weekblad* **95**, 174 (1960).
(Z4) Zweifler, A. J. *New Engl. J. Med.* **262**, 1229 (1960).

# Ataraxics and Nonbarbiturate Sedatives

Arthur J. McBay

Chemical Laboratory, Massachusetts State Police, and Department of Legal Medicine,
Harvard University Medical School, Boston, Massachusetts

and Elvera J. Algeri*

Department of Legal Medicine, Harvard University Medical School,
Boston, Massachusetts

* Present address: Department of Biological Chemistry, Harvard University
Medical School, Boston, Massachusetts.

157

# I. Introduction

Classification of the many psychopharmacological agents available since the introduction of the first synthetic tranquilizer, chlorpromazine, in 1952, is a difficult task. This is due to the lack of clinical data for many of these compounds and to the confusion that exists even when data are available. Reliable analytical methods are often lacking. Difficulties also arise because of the overlapping of effects produced by compounds relegated to different groups. All these factors hinder adoption of accepted terminology and strict categorization. Obviously, classification based on chemical structure alone is impossible.

The choice of agents to be discussed in this chapter is based on their frequency of use in the United States on the assumption that those agents most frequently dispensed are those most likely to be encountered by medicolegal investigators. Information governing the selection was derived from a National Prescription Audit for the period covering the fourth quarter of 1961 (G4).

From the many designations in use, we have chosen the terms "ataraxics" and "nonbarbiturate sedatives," because they seem best to describe, in the broadest sense, the group of drugs assembled.

Formulation of new techniques and the increased application of the methods available for the detection and estimation of these agents by the forensic toxicologist, who has quantities of biological material from humans at his disposal, will do much to dispel some of the confusion.

# II. Derivatives of Phenothiazine

The derivatives of phenothiazine constitute the largest single group of the ataractic drugs. Chemically these compounds may be divided into three main groups: (1) those that most closely resemble chlorpromazine and contain a 3-carbon straight chain grouping attached to the nitrogen of the nucleus; (2) those that contain a piperazine ring on the 3-carbon straight chain; and (3) those that contain a piperidine group on the side chain. In each group, some structures differ only in alterations involving halogen on the phenothiazine nucleus at the 2 position.

A classification presented in Table 1 includes those compounds most commonly used at the present time. It will be noted that Group II can be considered a subgroup of Group I in that the main differences occur in the choice of groups attached to the terminal nitrogen of the 3-carbon straight chain.

The fundamental presence of the phenothiazine nucleus confers upon these compounds related properties that make their separation and characterization difficult. New compounds are constantly being introduced and must be dealt with. Of the many derivatives now available, chlorpromazine has been the most extensively studied. Although more methods exist for its determination and thus more is known about its metabolic fate in the human body, there is still a great lack of data concerning its concentration in the blood of humans after both therapeutic and toxic doses. Such data are necessary in the investigation and consideration of any drug dispensed. Until there is more information available regarding levels, not only in blood but in tissues, evaluation of the phenothiazines, especially of those prescribed in low dosage, is distinctly hampered.

### A. Detection and Identification

There are many reports dealing with the qualitative and quantitative determination of the phenothiazines in pharmaceutical preparations, and, since many of the techniques discussed in them may be applied in the forensic laboratory, a general consideration of some of them will be made. The task of identification of these compounds in such preparations is simpler than when one deals with complex biological media. Adequate amounts of material are available for study, direct testing is possible, and some clues do exist that may aid in the identification. The determination of melting point and of mixed melting point is sometimes possible, and, to be sure, is a decisive means of identification.

### 1. Titrimetry

Several titrimetric procedures are available involving argentometric, bromometric, and nonaqueous techniques (B5, M8, M9, S4) as well as polarographic methods (C5, K1).

### 2. Precipitating and Color Reagents

The individual phenothiazines behave like alkaloids towards the common alkaloidal precipitating and color reagents. Some nonphenothiazine antihistamines also react in the same way, so that application of many of these reagents is not very useful for absolute differentiation (A6, A7, C6, F9, F10, H1, N3) [see ref. (S9), Volume II, Chapter 7]. A

TABLE I

Common Derivatives of Phenothiazine

| Generic name | Chemical name (phenothiazine) | Oral dose (mg/day) | $R_1$ | $R_2$ |
|---|---|---|---|---|
| **I. *Chlorpromazinelike*** | | | | |
| Chlorpromazine (Thorazine®) | 2-Chloro-10-(3-dimethylamino-propyl)- | 75-400 | —Cl | —$(CH_2)_3$—$N(CH_3)_2$ |
| Promazine (Sparine®) | 10-(3-Dimethylaminopropyl)- | 50-600 | —H | —$(CH_2)_3$—$N(CH_3)_2$ |
| Triflupromazine (Vesprin®) | 10-(3-Dimethylaminopropyl)-2-(trifluoromethyl)- | 30-150 | —$CF_3$ | —$(CH_2)_3$—$N(CH_3)_2$ |
| Methoxypromazine (Tentone®) | 10-(3-Dimethylaminopropyl)-2-methoxy- | 30-1500 | —$OCH_3$ | —$(CH_2)_3$—$N(CH_3)_2$ |
| Promethazine (Phenergan®) | 10-(2-Dimethylaminopropyl)- | 25-50 | —H | —$CH_2CH(CH_3)N(CH_3)_2$ |
| Trimeprazine (Temaril®) | 10-(2-Methyl-3-dimethylamino-propyl)- | 10-40 | —H | —$CH_2CH(CH_3)CH_2N(CH_3)_2$ |
| **II. *Piperazine ring on side chain*** | | | | |
| Prochlorperazine (Compazine®) | 2-Chloro-10-[3-(1-methyl-4-piperazinyl)propyl]- | 15-40 | —Cl | —$(CH_2)_3$—N◯N—$CH_3$ |
| Trifluoperazine (Stelazine®) | 10-[3-(1-Methyl-4-piperazinyl)propyl]-2-trifluoromethyl- | 2-30 | —$CF_3$ | —$(CH_2)_3$—N◯N—$CH_3$ |

TABLE I (*Continued*)

Common Derivatives of Phenothiazine

| Generic name | Chemical name (phenothiazine) | Oral dose (mg/day) | $R_1$ | $R_2$ |
|---|---|---|---|---|
| II. *Piperazine ring on side chain* | | | | |
| Perphenazine (Trilafon®) | 2-Chloro-10-{3-[1-(2-hydroxyethyl)-4-piperazinyl]propyl]- | 6–24 | —Cl | $-(CH_2)_3-N$ (piperazine) $N-CH_2CH_2OH$ |
| Fluphenazine (Permitil®, Prolixin®) | 10-[3-((1-β-Hydroxyethyl-4-piperazinyl)propyl]-2-(trifluoromethyl)- | 0.5–10 | —CF$_3$ | $-(CH_2)_3-N$ (piperazine) $N-CH_2CH_2OH$ |
| III. *Piperidine ring on side chain* | | | | |
| Mepazine (Pacatal®) | 10-[(1-Methyl-3-piperidyl)methyl]- | 75–500 | —H | $-CH_2-$ (piperidine) $N-CH_3$ |
| Thioridazine (Mellaril®) | 2-Methylmercapto-10-[2-(N-methyl-2-piperidyl)ethyl]- | 30–500 | —SCH$_3$ | $-(CH_2)_2-$ (piperidine) $N-CH_3$ |

detailed study of the microchemical identification of a large number of antihistamines includes crystal and color tests applied to microgram quantities of some phenothiazines in pure form (C6). The slightly soluble picrate and reineckate derivatives of chlorpromazine, diethazine, mepazine, ethopropazine, promethazine, and thiazinamium are good crystalline products with sharp melting points (B5, T2). The quantitative determination of chlorpromazine and diethazine has been accomplished by dissolving their reineckate derivatives in acetone and obtaining their absorbance. About 10 mg of original compound are necessary (B5).

The ability of the parent compound to form a blue-purple complex with palladium chloride has long been known (O2); this reaction has served as a means of determining promazine, promethazine, and chlorpromazine in pharmaceutical preparations (C4, R11). That the 10-dialkylaminoalkylphenothiazines form chloroform-soluble complexes with bromthymol blue has been established and used for their determination (K9).

### 3. Oxidizing Agents

Detection of the phenothiazines as a group may be accomplished by treating with an oxidizing agent such as sulfuric acid, nitric acid, ammonium persulfate, bromine water, or the like which produce a red color (A6, A7, F9, F10, N3). This red color also appears after oxidation of solutions by exposure to light and air. Many investigators have determined the phenothiazine derivatives after their extraction from biological material using this oxidative reaction, which, although sensitive, lacks specificity and is often unreliable. An excess of strong oxidizing agent can destroy the color.

### 4. Ion-Exchange Resins

The ability of Amberlite IRC-50, a weak cation-exchange resin, to fix the phenothiazines was first reported by Berti and Cima (B3). Chlorpromazine and promazine are completely separated from their neutral solutions using this carboxylic acid–type resin (B3, C2, E1). Elution of adsorbed material has not been successful, and final quantitation has been by treatment of the resin with 12 N sulfuric acid. All products containing the phenothiazine nucleus will, of course, produce the color reaction.

Adsorption onto natural inorganic silicates from dilute hydrochloric acid solutions of chlorpromazine (carmine to violet color), promethazine, and mepazine (rose or brown colors) with detection of at least 5 $\mu$g of material has been reported (M7).

5. PAPER CHROMATOGRAPHY

Paper chromatography offers good possibilities for the separation of various phenothiazines (B3, F11, N2, T1, T2) [see ref. (S9), Volume II, Chapter 7, Table LXII]. Although a variety of mixtures for the solvent system has been proposed, many of the $R_f$ values reported for the individual compounds are similar or too high in value for useful differentiation (B3, T1), although they might serve in a negative sense by ruling out the presence of certain compounds.

The use of paper impregnated with citric acid–phosphate buffer at pH 4.0 and a mobile phase of ether saturated with water permits good separation of diethazine, promethazine, thiazinamium, ethopropazine, chlorpromazine, and mepazine (T2).

A mobile solvent consisting of 5% ammonium sulfate and isobutanol (equal volumes) produces good resolution of diethazine, promethazine, promazine, chlorpromazine, trifluoperazine, and levopromazine (N2).

The use of circular paper chromatography is described for separating nine possible metabolites of chlorpromazine (E2). The solvent system is a mixture of 1,2-dichloroethane, benzene, formic acid (88%), and water (3:1:4:2) with the organic phase used as the mobile solvent. The preference is for Whatman 3 MM paper to which are applied 20-$\mu$g quantities of material. Location of zones is by examination under short wavelength ultraviolet light and by spraying with the alkaloidal reagent, potassium iodoplatinate. As little as 1–2 $\mu$g of each compound is detected.

Paper chromatography has also been used to study the metabolic products of chlorpromazine in human urine (F3, G3). The authors describe different solvent systems for resolution, various color reagents for the specific detection of certain chemical entities, and results of ultraviolet spectrophotometric study of eluates.

Many of the alkaloidal reagents such as Dragendorff and potassium iodoplatinate (M10) may be used for the location of zones after resolution. Utilization of the color reaction produced by treatment with oxidizing agents such as sulfuric acid also permits recognition (B3, S3).

Colorimetry of the phenothiazines isolated by paper chromatography has been described (N2). Duplicate samples of test material are applied to paper. After location of material following resolution, the corresponding untreated zone is eluted. Potassium iodoplatinate is added to the eluate, and the absorbance of the blue complex is determined.

6. PAPER IONOPHORESIS

Paper ionophoresis permits differentiation of phenothiazines having slight differences in structure. Chlorpromazine, which differs from promazine only by the presence of chlorine on the phenothiazine nucleus, exhibits a much greater mobility and is easily separated (C1, C2). Although this technique offers good possibilities for initial screening (F3, S5), it has been little used.

### 7. INFRARED SPECTROPHOTOMETRY

The infrared spectra of diethazine and promethazine have been used for their determination in pharmaceuticals (S1). The infrared spectra of promazine, mepazine, and chlorpromazine are available [see ref. (S9) Volume I, Chapter 13B,4].

### 8. ULTRAVIOLET SPECTROPHOTOMETRY

A study of the ultraviolet absorption spectra (M3) of the common derivatives of phenothiazine shows that the configuration of the curves is quite similar and can be considered characteristic of these compounds. All of these compounds exhibit a slight maximum at 300–310 m$\mu$. The principal absorbances are at much shorter wavelengths with the maxima

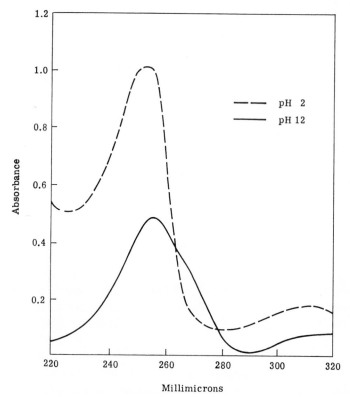

FIG. 1. The ultraviolet absorption spectra of chlorpromazine (10 $\mu$g/ml).

at acidic pH changing with variation of the substituents in the 2 position of the nucleus ($R_1$). When $R_1$ is unsubstituted (promazine, promethazine, trimeprazine, mepazine, methadilazine) or contains a methoxy substituent (methoxypromazine), the maxima are between 249 and 252 m$\mu$. When $R_1$ contains a chlorine atom (chlorpromazine, prochlorperazine, perphenazine), the maxima are at 254 m$\mu$. When $R_1$ contains a trifluoromethyl group (triflupromazine, trifluoperazine, fluphenazine), the maxima are at 255 m$\mu$. With a methylmercapto substituent (thioridazine), there is a shift of the maximum to 261 m$\mu$. In alkaline solution, the maxima shift to the longer wavelengths: the majority shifts 2 m$\mu$; with promethazine and trimeprazine, the shift is 4 m$\mu$; with triflupromazine, 8 m$\mu$; thioridazine, 11 m$\mu$. The absorbances of the acidic and basic solutions are approximately the same except for chlorpromazine, the acidic solution of which absorbs almost twice as much as the basic. The ultraviolet spectra of chlorpromazine and promazine are given in Figs. 1 and 2. It has been suggested that differential spectrophotometry for the

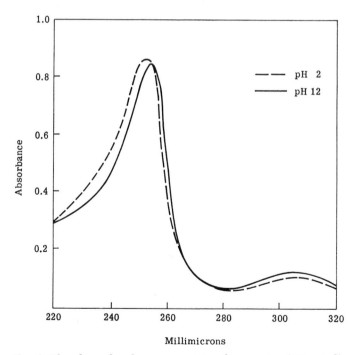

FIG. 2. The ultraviolet absorption spectra of promazine (10 $\mu$g/ml).

determination of chlorpromazine is possible, based on changes in its spectrum due to pH [see (S9), Volume I, Chapter 13,B,1].

9. Spectrophotofluorometry

The advantages of using the spectrophotofluorometer (B4) for the identification and determination of the phenothiazines at the submicrogram level should be emphasized. An instrument developed in 1955 provides for an extremely useful extension of fluorescence analysis (B4). It permits excitation of compounds and measurement of the resulting fluorescence in the ultraviolet and visible ranges. The specificity is heightened by the utilization of the wavelengths of maximal activation and of the fluorescence. Instruments are available that deliver high intensity monochromatic activation from 220 to 800 m$\mu$ and automatically analyze the fluorescence for the same range.

Chlorpromazine is included in a study (U1) that compared recoveries of submicrogram quantities of a representative group of organic compounds using this instrument with those obtained by conventional spectrophotometry necessitating the presence of considerably greater amounts of material. The results are comparable, and it is suggested in that report that a quantitative extraction procedure outlined would be useful for analysis of biological media.

The activation and fluorescence spectra of a great number of phenothiazines have been studied (R1). Like the ultraviolet absorbance of these compounds, here, also, the spectral characteristics depend on the nature of the substituents in the 2 position ($R_1$). As little as 0.05 $\mu$g/gm of sample (thioridazine) can be determined, and the method was successfully applied to the analysis of blood and tissue. The advantages of this method for the analysis of the phenothiazines of high potency are obvious. Details are not available.

## B. Determination in Biological Media

Routine application of color reactions is used in the monitoring of mental patients receiving phenothiazines specifically prescribed in certain dosages. These tests are applied directly to urine; particular reagents are used that, under defined conditions, yield semiquantitative results. Before proceeding with the analysis of tissue or blood, the medicolegal investigator can make good use of these tests for initial screening if urine is available.

### 1. Semiquantitation of Urine

Of the great number of reports dealing with rapid and simple testing of urine for proof of the ingestion of phenothiazines, many have been devised by Forrest and co-workers who have consolidated their 4 years' experience with this problem in a recent review (F7). Routine application of a minimum number of tests using few reagents is possible. To establish the presence of any phenothiazine, a single test, designated as the "FPN" Universal,[1] is applied. Depending on the results, this can then be followed by more specific, semiquantitative tests. For all the tests, 1 ml of urine is mixed with 1 ml of reagent, and the resulting color evaluated by reference to a color chart. For routine hospital testing, morning urine is usually used except that, for low dosage ranges, optimum results are obtained $1\frac{1}{2}$–3 hours after ingestion, when as little as 5 mg of a single dose can be detected. It is not possible to distinguish, however, between a recently ingested small dose and a high dose ingested several days before. Color formation is due to the unoxidized compounds excreted in the urine and certain intermediary metabolites. The sulfoxides and sulfones do not take part in the reaction. False negatives have not been encountered, and many of the false positives, which have a low incidence, can be circumvented by preliminary treatment with an anion-exchange resin. For details and discussion of these factors, the reader is referred to the original review in which there is also a critical survey of the many color tests that have been devised and applied to the testing of urine by other investigators.

*a. "FPN" Universal Test for Phenothiazines.* The reagent consists of 5 parts of 5% ferric chloride, 45 parts of 20% perchloric acid and 50 parts of 50% nitric acid. Within 10 seconds after mixing with the urine, comparison is made with a color chart. The colors depend on the dosage and combination of drugs.

*b. Chlorpromazine, Promazine, and Mepazine.* The reagent consists of 20 parts of 5% ferric chloride and 80 parts of 10% sulfuric acid. If the test is evaluated promptly, daily doses of from 100 to 300 mg of chlorpromazine produce a pale violet coloration that deepens to a dark purple for daily doses of 300 mg or more. For the same range, promazine and mepazine yield initially a pink color that intensifies to a deep purple for higher amounts.

*c. Thioridazine.* The reagent consists of 2 parts of 5% ferric chloride and 98 parts of 30% sulfuric acid. For low doses, the maximum color may not develop before 20 seconds. For 75–150 mg/day, the color is pale purplish pink deepening to intense purple or violet shades for amounts of 800 mg or more per day.

*d. Estimation Using Impregnated Strips.* An interesting modification of some of the tests developed by Forrest and co-workers (F5, F6) permits estimation of phenothiazines using 1 drop of urine (H4). A drop of specimen is applied to paper strips of Whatman 3 MM impregnated with a solution of 0.001 $M$ mercuric nitrate or of 0.001 $M$ uranyl nitrate.

[1] The "FPN" designation is from the first letters of the reagents used.

Ammonium persulfate can also be added to these solutions (90 gm/liter). After application of urine to the paper, a drop of 3% hydrogen peroxide is added to the same spot followed in a few moments by a drop of concentrated hydrochloric acid. When ammonium persulfate is used, the hydrogen peroxide is not necessary. If phenothiazines are absent, no color forms. With a positive result, a violet color forms that can be graded using a color chart. If overdosage is suspected, the acid is placed next to the test spot after the addition of peroxide. A positive result with unmetabolized urine is red to red-brown. The lower limits of detection in micrograms of each phenothiazine per milliliter in a drop of urine are: 19, triflupromazine; 24, chlorpromazine; 31, trifluoperazine; 38, prochlorperazine; 39, perphenazine; 48, promazine.

### 2. DETERMINATION IN BLOOD, TISSUE, AND URINE

Most procedures follow the same basic plan for the isolation of the phenothiazines. The material is extracted from alkaline media with an organic solvent which is then treated in various ways depending on the system adopted for final quantitation. Solvents used are ether, *n*-heptane, isobutanol, and ethylene dichloride.

Of importance is the finding (K9) that the phenothiazines possess the ability to form complexes with organic and inorganic anions, such as phthalate or chloride. With buffer solutions of pH 1.1–6.6, there is partitioning of more than 95% of the phenothiazine compounds in the chloroform phase. The usefulness of this unique property for the separation of phenothiazines from other bases is apparent. The derivatives of phenothiazine, moreover, are not extracted from chloroform into acidic solution as are most organic bases.

In colorimetric procedures, which are nonspecific, color formation is effected by the addition of concentrated mineral acids or of oxidizing agents such as dilute acid and ferric iron to the isolated material. In procedures involving ultraviolet spectrophotometry, the organic solvent may be differentially extracted to separate unchanged drug from its metabolites. The separation of unchanged drug from metabolites and hydrolysis of conjugated compounds are important aids to particular identification of the compound originally ingested.

*a. Determination of Chlorpromazine.* In the colorimetric procedure of Dubost and Pascal (D4, D5) for the determination of chlorpromazine in blood and urine, final quantitation is by measurement of the absorbance of the red color produced by the reaction of the drug in dilute sulfuric acid upon addition of an equal volume of concentrated sulfuric acid. Initial extraction of the drug is with ether from alkaline media. Free components can be determined or total components following hydrolysis.

Many of the other colorimetric procedures in the literature (B2, B3, G5, K6, L2), some of them modifications of this method, still retain the serious inherent defect: there is no means of distinguishing between unchanged drug and its metabolic products.

The procedure of Salzman and Brodie (S3) is specific, but, because of insufficient sensitivity (1 $\mu$g/ml), cannot be used for the analysis of plasma of humans receiving usual therapeutic doses. In the procedure as outlined for plasma and urine, the specimens are made alkaline and extracted with heptane containing 1.5% isoamyl alcohol. Tissue homogenized with 0.1 N hydrochloric acid is treated in the same way. The solvent phase is washed with acetate buffer at pH 5.6. Unchanged drug is then isolated by shaking the solvent with 0.1 N hydrochloric acid. Ultraviolet spectrophotometry is used for final quantitation. Proof of specificity was by paper chromatography. Only free components are determined by this method. It has been noted (G3), in regard to the acetate extract obtained from human urine, that the monomethyl and the completely demethylated sulfoxides of chlorpromazine, the predominant sulfoxide metabolites, are excreted together with minor amounts of chlorpromazine sulfoxide and are also included in the assay (see Section II,C). The recoveries of chlorpromazine added to brain are low (40%), although those from other tissues are adequate (85–95%). Complete recovery of drug from all tissues has been achieved by a procedure (W2) that incorporates some of the steps just outlined. The extracted chlorpromazine, however, is oxidized to its sulfoxide with final quantitation by spectrophotometry of the converted amount together with sulfoxide originally present.

The method of Flanagan and co-workers (F4) was devised for the determination in biological media of the free and bound forms of chlorpromazine and chlorpromazine sulfoxide. Extraction of alkaline media with ether is first carried out. Then the solvent is shaken with 1 N sulfuric acid. The extracted compounds contained in this extract are subjected to ultraviolet spectrophotometry. The conjugated constituents are obtained by alkaline hydrolysis of the aqueous residue. The hydrolyzate is then subjected to the same procedure as above with spectrophotometry of the final extracts giving the amount of conjugated material present. Paper chromatography established specificity. The procedure has been applied to the analysis of bile, urine, plasma, and gastric contents. It has not been evaluated experimentally for the other phenothiazines. The comment above regarding other sulfoxides extracted also applies here.

Mention should be made regarding the instability of chlorpromazine in N sodium hydroxide (F1). There are no changes if the final concentration of sodium hydroxide is 0.05 N. The recoveries of chlorpromazine added to biological material indicate the decomposition is inhibited in some way in such media, since the results differ from those obtained using aqueous media (F4).

Enzymatic hydrolysis of the urine of humans receiving chlorpromazine has been reported (L5, N1). A small specimen of urine at pH 4.5 is incubated with β-glucuronidase at 37°C for from 18 to 24 hours. After incubation, Nadeau and Sobolewski (N1) extract the alkalinized hydrolyzate with isobutanol. The isolated material is taken up in buffer (pH 3) during evaporation of the solvent. Final quantitation is by colorimetry of the blue complex formed after addition of potassium iodoplatinate. Such enzymatic hydrolysis may be applied to the analysis for promazine, promethazine, trifluoperazine, and prochlorperazine (N1). Lin (L5) used enzymatic hydrolysis with β-glucuronidase in his study of the metabolic fate of chlorpromazine in humans.

*b. Determination of Promazine* (W3). Promazine in urine, whole blood, plasma, and tissue can be extracted with *n*-heptane from a solution adjusted to pH 6.8 with phosphate buffer (see Section II,B,2). After addition of a little capryl alcohol to an aliquot, a saturated solution of arsenic pentoxide in concentrated hydrochloric acid is added. The absorbance of the aqueous layer is measured at 565 m$\mu$ after 90 minutes. A 2-ml sample is analyzed with a sensitivity of 8 $\mu$g/ml. Chlorpromazine and promethazine can be similarly analyzed. The possible presence of metabolites is not discussed.

*c. Determination of 10-Dialkylaminoalkylphenothiazines Using Bromthymol Blue.* In a sensitive and selective method, colorimetry is accomplished after treatment of isolated material with bromthymol blue (K9). A chloroform-soluble complex forms in the molecular ratio of 1:1. When separation from other bases is necessary, selectivity is conferred by formation of the chloroform-soluble complexes of phenothiazines with chloride and phthalate ion (see Section II,B,2). A method outlined for the analysis of urine can be applied to other biological media. Standard curves of chlorpromazine, promazine, promethazine, and diethazine were determined. Analysis in the presence of metabolites is not discussed.

## C. Metabolic Fate

Chlorpromazine is rapidly absorbed and localized in the various tissues (S3). The metabolite, chlorpromazine sulfoxide, has been isolated from the urine of dogs and identified (S2, S3). It exerts but a weak, sedative effect in man (D1). In humans, negligible amounts of unchanged drug are excreted in the urine (G3, S3). Goldenberg and Fishman (G3) have compared the metabolic fate of chlorpromazine in man and dog after oral administration. They found that in marked contrast with the dog, man excretes chlorpromazine sulfoxide as a minor metabolite accounting for less than 0.5% of the administered dose.

Demethylation of chlorpromazine also takes place (R10). Rats administered chlorpromazine(N-methyl)-$C^{14}$ metabolized the dimethylaminopropyl side chain with extensive expiration of $C^{14}O_2$ during the first 6 hours following administration. In man, there are good indications that the major urinary metabolites are the completely demethylated sulfoxide (about 3.7% of the dose) and the monomethyl sulfoxide (about 1.8% of the given dose) of chlorpromazine (F3, G3).

Hydrolysis of the urine of humans with $\beta$-glucuronidase releases increased amounts of metabolic products of chlorpromazine (L5, N1). There is strong evidence that hydroxylation of the phenothiazine nucleus occurs followed by conjugation with glucuronic acid (L5).

The presence of chlorpromazine sulfone as a metabolic product has been sought but not found. This compound is known to be rapidly degraded by liver microsomes (K2).

Like chlorpromazine, promazine is also metabolized by sulfoxidation and demethylation. Administration of promazine-$S^{35}$ to dogs resulted in the formation of promazine sulfoxide, monomethyl promazine, and monomethylpromazine sulfoxide (W1). About 2 to 3% of the administered dose is excreted unchanged in the urine, 3 to 5% as its sulfoxide, whereas their monomethyl derivatives account for about 4.5%. As is the case with chlorpromazine, the sulfone derivative has not been detected.

The formation of the sulfoxide of mepazine has also been reported on the basis of paper chromatographic evidence (H5).

Following intravenous administration of chlorpromazine, 20 mg/kg to dogs, the concentration in the plasma is found to be about 0.2 mg% within 30 minutes. After one hour this level has dropped to about 0.1 mg%, remaining the same at the end of 3 hours (S3). The drug is rapidly localized and attains high concentrations in tissue, in which the drug can be found in substantial amount after 7 hours. These workers determined unchanged drug only. Dubost and Pascal (D5) reported that only small amounts of conjugated material are present in blood after oral or subcutaneous administration of chlorpromazine to rabbits. Thirty minutes after intravenous injection of mepazine to rats, 25 mg/kg, the pattern is similar to that observed for chlorpromazine. The blood attains a concentration of about 0.2 mg%, while concentrations in tissue are high (H2).

When $S^{35}$ promazine is administered intraperitoneally to dogs, a peak concentration of promazine together with its metabolites that contain sulfur is equal to 1.5 mg% of blood after 15 minutes; 0.8 mg% of this is unchanged drug (W1). Only 25% of the promazine remains after one hour, in contrast with more than 70% of the metabolic products. Promazine disappears within 24 hours, while a level of about 0.2 mg% of its metabolites still remains. This concentration dropped to 0.07 mg%, 4 days after injection. In rats receiving the labeled drug, the concentration in blood 30 minutes after intraperitoneal administration was 0.25 mg%; after oral administration, 0.1 mg%. Labeled sulfur was detected 48 hours after administration.

A study of the results of analysis of labeled sulfur of chlorpromazine in tissue following both oral and intraperitoneal administration to rats led to consideration of the possibility that high concentration of unchanged drug may be present in the brain, while concentration of the metabolites is high in the lung, liver, kidney, and spleen. Such a supposition would account for the reports of others, who determined unchanged drug only, that the brain contains high concentrations of chlorpromazine (G5, H2, S3).

Patients receiving thioridazine excreted an average of 10.4% of the administered dose in 24-hour urine (N4). The method does not distinguish between the drug and its metabolic products.

## D. Overingestion

The literature contains few cases of fatalities due to overingestion of the phenothiazines. A review (A3) that discusses twenty-five such cases involving chlorpromazine in amounts ranging from about 7 to 140 mg/kg lists only two deaths. A 13-month-old child succumbed on the fourth day after ingestion of about 75 mg/kg of drug. Blood obtained at autopsy contained 0.1 mg of free chlorpromazine per 100 ml. In the second fatality, a 40-year-old psychotic woman ingested an unknown amount and was found dead 3 days after disappearing. Her blood level was 0.3 mg%. The review includes case histories, symptoms, and therapeutic measures adopted.

Nonfatal poisoning due to the ingestion of 2–6.5 mg of fluphenazine by children has occurred (K8, S8). Two children survived after ingestion of 4–6 mg/kg of perphenazine. Anuria was observed and it is emphasized that convulsions began after a latent period of 24 hours following intake (R5).

## III.  *d*-Propoxyphene

*d*-Propoxyphene hydrochloride (Darvon®, α-*d*-4-dimethylamino-1,2-diphenyl-3-methyl-2-propionoxybutane hydrochloride) is an analgesic that resembles codeine pharmacologically. In adults the average daily dose is approximately 50 mg. Although single doses of from 3 to 5 gm have been tolerated, ingestion of such amounts may be fatal. Symptoms of overdosage include nausea and vomiting, cyanosis, respiratory depression, and depression of the central nervous system. That there also may be stimulation of the central nervous system is indicated by the observation of convulsive seizures. Cases of overdosage of the drug by children and adults have been reported (C3).

## A. Metabolic Fate

A study of the metabolic fate of the *α-dl* form shows that mono-*N*-demethylation occurs (L3). When *N*-$C^{14}H_3$-propoxyphene hydrochloride was administered intravenously to rats, there was significant expiration of $C^{14}O_2$. The half-time is 130 minutes. Production of radioactive carbon dioxide is also effected by incubation of the labeled drug with slices of rat liver. From the urine of humans receiving the drug orally, the demethylated product was isolated in the form of its dinitrophenyl derivative and identified. Absolute measurement was not possible due to the limitations of the methyl orange colorimetric method used for analysis (B6) [see ref. (S9), Volume I, Chapter 18].

## B. Determination in Biological Media

There is no method specifically used for the determination of propoxyphene in biological media. In addition to the methyl orange procedure just mentioned, the colorimetric method of Rickards (R7) has been suggested (L4). This procedure was devised for the estimation of Methadone in biological media and depends on the ability of basic compounds containing phenyl groups to form the *meta*-dinitro compounds. Nitration follows separation of the basic compound in ether, and color formation is effected by treatment with ethylmethyl ketone. This method has been modified and adapted for the determination of Darvon® in urine or gastric washings (L4). Experimental data are not available; in the original procedure, the sensitivity is 1 μg of Methadone.

The ultraviolet absorption spectrum of propoxyphene is characteristic of compounds containing the phenyl group.

# IV. Chlordiazepoxide

Chlordiazepoxide (Librium®, methaminodiazepoxide, 7-chloro-2-methylamino-5-phenyl-3*H*-1,4-benzodiazepine-4-oxide hydrochloride) is an anticonvulsant, tranquilizing agent that acts as a muscle relaxant after low dosage, as a sedative after high. The average daily dose for adults is about 50 mg; however, 400–600 mg daily for as long as 6 months have been tolerated. After such prolonged administration in the higher dosage range, the concentration in plasma reached between 2 to 4.5 mg% (H6). Upon abrupt withdrawal of the drug, the level dropped to below 1 mg%

within $1\frac{1}{2}$ to 6 days. With oral administration of 150 mg/day to humans, the level remains below 1 mg/100 ml of plasma (R4).

Patients have recovered after ingestion of 2250 mg as a single dose (Z1); fatalities due to misuse of the drug are not found in the literature. The most common symptoms of overingestion are drowsiness, sedation, impairment of speech, and ataxia. Concentrations of 0.73 mg of chlordiazepoxide per 100 ml of urine and 0.8 mg/100 ml of blood were found 72 hours after ingestion of 1850 mg (J1).

### A. Determination in Biological Media

The classic Bratton–Marshall procedure may be applied to its determination after acid hydrolysis (R2). The extraction excludes interference due to the sulfonamides. To 5 ml of plasma or urine is added 0.5 gm of potassium carbonate. The mixture is shaken for 30 minutes with 15 ml of ether. After centrifuging, the ether phase is removed and washed twice with 2 ml of water. The solvent is then dried with sodium sulfate, and a 10-ml aliquot obtained by filtration is shaken with 3 ml of 6 N hydrochloric acid for 10 minutes. The aqueous phase is separated and heated for 30 minutes at 125°C. After cooling, the volume is made up to 5 ml with water and 0.5 ml of 0.1% sodium nitrite added; after 3 minutes, 0.5 ml of 0.5% ammonium sulfamate is added followed after 10 minutes by 0.5 ml of 0.1% N-(1-naphthyl)ethylenediamine dihydrochloride. The absorbance is determined at 550 m$\mu$. With 2 $\mu$g of the drug, an absorbance of 0.03 results. A blank consists of a specimen treated as above with omission of the hydrolysis.

### B. Use of Ultraviolet Spectrophotometry

The absorption spectra (M3) of chlordiazepoxide in acidic and basic solution are shown in Fig. 3; the possibility of identification and quantitation of this compound by means of ultraviolet spectrophotometry is suggested.

# V. Glutethimide

Glutethimide ($\alpha$-phenyl-$\alpha$-ethylglutarimide, Doriden®) is a drug with sedative-hypnotic properties. The usual dose is 0.25–0.50 gm. Although humans have survived overdoses of as much as 15 gm, death has occurred with the ingestion of 10 gm (A3, M4).

The blood of an adult reached a maximum of 0.66 mg% $3\frac{1}{2}$ hours after ingestion of 1 gm of glutethimide (A4). This level gradually decreased and 48 hours after intake was 0.13 mg%. The concentration of total metabolite in urine after 1-gm doses is about 10 mg% (M4).

In a study of six clinical cases, Schreiner and co-workers (S6) state that if the patient can be aroused by painful stimuli and deep tendon reflexes and blood pressure are normal, the concentration in blood will probably be from 0.5 to 1.0 mg%; with shallow or abdominal breathing, hypotension, absent or variable deep reflexes, from 1 to 3 mg%, and the use of bemegride may be indicated; with deep coma, hypotension, areflexia, above 3 mg%; bemegride should be given and external hemodialysis may be necessary. It should be pointed that the "deteriorating clinical condition" of one patient necessitated dialysis 16 hours after ingestion when the blood level was about 1.3 mg%. The authors state that "anoxemia worsened the coma" and that without hemodialysis the patient might have died.

In eight adults who succumbed to overingestion of glutethimide (A4, M3), the blood levels in two cases were 1.1 and 1.4 mg%; in the remaining cases, the levels ranged from 4.0 to 8.5 mg%. Concentrations in liver of five of these cases were from 4 to 19 mg%. Total urinary metabolites determined for four of these cases were from 24 to 48 mg% (M4).

It should be emphasized that in interpreting blood levels, factors such as time, disease, or personal differences must be evaluated.

## A. Metabolic Fate

The drug has not been detected unchanged in the urine of dogs after oral administration (K3, S7). The metabolite $\alpha$-phenylglutarimide, the dealkylated derivative, is excreted in the urine, the free form accounting for less than 2% of the administered dose, the conjugated form approximately 5% (K3, S7). Another metabolite isolated from dog urine in the free form is the oxidized product, $\alpha$-phenyl-$\alpha$-ethylglutaconimide (K4). Most of the administered glutethimide is rapidly excreted in urine in the form of its metabolites conjugated with glucuronic acid. A mixture of glucuronides isolated from the urine of dogs yielded 3 aglucones that were characterized. The results of this work are significant, since it is shown that hydroxylation occurs not only on the imido-ring itself, but also on the ethyl side chain.

## B. Determination in Biological Media

### 1. URINE

A colorimetric method has been described for the analysis of urine (S7). After acid hydrolysis, the urine is extracted with benzene. The extracted material is adsorbed onto alumina and elution carried out using a mixture of chloroform and methanol. The eluate is evaporated to dryness and the residue dissolved in methanol. Quantitation is by colorimetry of the purple complex formed when ferric chloride reacts with the hydroxamic acid derivative of isolated imidic material.

## 2. Urine and Serum

A much more sensitive and less cumbersome method employing ultraviolet spectrophotometry is available for the analysis of urine and serum (G2). In this procedure, the rate of hydrolysis of the drug in alcoholic alkaline solution is followed spectrophotometrically. As little as 1 ml of specimen is extracted with chloroform. After washing the separated solvent phase with alkali and with acid, the solution is evaporated to dryness. The residue is dissolved in ethanol; then an aliquot is mixed with potassium hydroxide. The rate of the alkaline hydrolysis is followed by noting the decrease in absorbance at 235 m$\mu$, the maximum, with time. By extrapolation, the amount originally present is calculated. The characteristic ultraviolet spectrum of glutethimide is also determined by scanning the wavelengths between 225 and 280 m$\mu$ immediately after adding the alkali.

## 3. Whole Blood and Tissue

The method of Goldbaum and Williams (G2) just discussed was modified to permit analysis of whole blood, hemolyzed blood, and tissue (A2, A4). A 5-ml sample of blood is extracted with 30 ml of ethyl acetate which is then separated and washed first with alkali and then with acid. After boiling the ethyl acetate with Norit, the solution is filtered, and the filtrate evaporated to dryness. The residue is dissolved in ethanol, and the procedure of Goldbaum and Williams is then followed. If liver is analyzed, 5 gm are homogenized with 20 ml of water. After heating on a boiling water bath, the mixture is filtered. The filtrate is then extracted with an equal volume of ethyl acetate and the analysis continued as outlined for blood.

## VI. Hydroxyzine

Hydroxyzine (1-($p$-chlorobenzhydryl-4-[2-(2-hydroxyethoxy)ethyl] piperazine, Atarax®, Vistaril®) is a well-known tranquilizing agent. In adults, the usual dosage is from 75 to 400 mg/day, but daily doses of 800 mg have been administered for several weeks without harmful effects. After receiving 50 mg/kg for a few days, dogs exhibited toxic symptoms of retching, clonic convulsions, and prostration; some of them died (B7). Fatalities in humans have not been reported. Concentrations of the drug in biological material and methods of detection are not available in the literature.

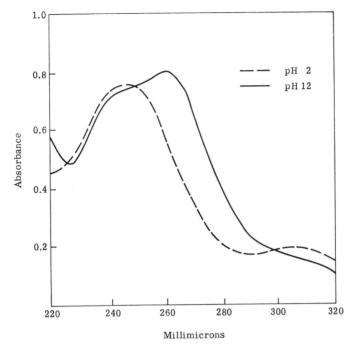

FIG. 3. The ultraviolet absorption spectra of chlordiazepoxide HCl (8 μg/ml).

## VII. Methapyrilene

Methapyrilene  (2-[(2-dimethylaminoethyl)-2-thenylamino]pyridine, Thenylene®, Dormin®, Histadyl®, Sominex®, Tranquil®) is an antihistamine used for the treatment of allergies both local and systemic. Commercial preparations containing this compound are sold without prescription and are often seen advertised as safe, nonnarcotic, nonbarbiturate sedatives. The average adult dose is about 25 mg. Ingestion of 1 gm as a single dose produces anxiety, nervousness, hyperactive reflexes, and convulsions.

Fatalities due to overingestion have been reported. A 16-month-old child ingested 100 mg and became drowsy and nauseated, and then vomited. Tremors, convulsions, and finally death ensued (R9). After ingestion of more than 700 mg, a 19-year-old woman died in a hospital 45 minutes after being admitted cyanotic and convulsing, and 1½ hours after being found in convulsions. Serum obtained at autopsy contained 1.2 mg of methapyrilene per 100 ml (O1). In another suicide by massive ingestion of an unknown amount of this compound, the concentration in serum was 3 mg% (M3).

Determination in Serum

A method for the quantitative determination of this drug in serum has been reported that makes use of ascending paper chromatography and ultraviolet spectrophotometry (O1). The extraction procedure is similar to that of Goldbaum [see ref. (S9), Volume I, Chapter 11, p. 385]. For the ascending paper chromatographic study, a solvent system consisting of a mixture of n-butanol and glacial acetic acid (10:1) saturated with water is used. The $R_f$ value of methapyrilene is 0.66. Location of the zone is by spraying with Dragendorff reagent (M10). Elution with dilute hydrochloric acid of the material on an adjacent untreated strip and observation of its characteristic ultraviolet spectrum further confirm its presence. The absorption spectra in acidic and basic solution are shown in Fig. 4.

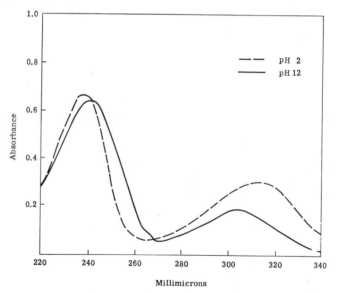

Fig. 4. The ultraviolet absorption spectra of methapyrilene (10 μg/ml).

## VIII. Ethchlorvynol

Ethchlorvynol (ethyl-β-chlorovinylethynylcarbinol, Placidyl®) a chlorinated acetylenic carbinol, is a hypnotic drug with anticonvulsant properties. The usual therapeutic dose for adults is from 200 to 600 mg. Adults have survived ingestion of 10–15 gm with coma of 5–7 days (A1, D3). A male adult succumbed 2 days after ingestion of 49.5 gm with death attributed to "bronchopneumonia." Following oral ingestion of single 1-gm doses by adults, the blood contained a maximum concentration of 1.4 mg% within 1 to $1\frac{1}{2}$ hours (A5). This level gradually decreased, reaching zero 4 hours after ingestion. In two fatalities (A5) due to deliberate overdosage of the drug by adults, the blood contained 13.8 and 14.8 mg%, the liver 26.8 and 28.0 mg%. The amounts actually ingested could not be determined, but in one case a total of 9–15 gm of drug was found in the stomach contents, in which the characteristic odor of ethchlorvynol was distinct. Pulmonary congestion and edema were the main pathological findings. There is no knowledge of the metabolism of ethchlorvynol in the body.

### Determination in Biological Media

In the determination of the unsaturated carbinol, methylparafynol, colorimetry is accomplished after the formation of its silver acetylide (M2, P1, P2). Ethchlorvynol can be determined by this same means; however, sensitivity and specificity are lacking.

A procedure utilizing near-infrared spectrophotometry can be used for qualitative purposes. The method requires milligram quantities of material (R8).

The following colorimetric method for the quantitative analysis of ethchlorvynol in blood and tissue is simple, sensitive, and reliable (A5). It is based on the ability of some compounds possessing the allyl group to form a red or yellow color upon treatment with phloroglucinol and concentrated hydrochloric acid (K5).

To 2 ml of whole blood are added 15 ml of water, 2 ml of 20% sulfuric acid (w/w), and 1 ml of 50% sodium tungstate. For liver, 2 gm are homogenized by hand using a glass tissue grinder, the water being added in small amounts. The mixture is shaken, then filtered by suction. A 14-ml aliquot of filtrate is extracted with 4 ml of ethyl acetate. The solvent extract is dried by pouring it through sodium sulfate on a plug of glass wool; 2 ml of the dried filtrate is transferred to a 10-ml volumetric flask. After addition of 0.4 ml of a freshly prepared solution of 10% phloroglucinol in 95% ethanol followed by 3.6 ml of concentrated hydrochloric acid, the flask is placed on a boiling water bath for 30 minutes. A reagent blank is run at the same time and consists of 2 ml of ethyl acetate and the phloroglucinol–hydrochloric acid reagent. When ethchlorvynol is present, a pale green color forms within a few minutes that gradually changes to orange. After rapid cooling under running tap water, the solutions are diluted to 10 ml with water and mixed, and the spectrum from 470 to 560 m$\mu$ is determined within 15 minutes after transferring to 1-cm cells. The concentration of ethchlorvynol present is determined from the absorbance at 508 m$\mu$, the maximum of the curve. Calculations are based on a standard solution of pure material at different concentrations in ethyl acetate subjected to the same treatment with the color-producing reagents. An expected recovery of 3.5 ml of ethyl acetate rather than 4 ml is used, since losses of the solvent occur due to its solubility during the extraction procedure. The procedure should be followed as outlined using reagent grade chemicals. Recoveries of 25–500 μg of ethchlorvynol added to 2 ml of blood or 2 gm of liver were 94 and 95%. Salicylate and barbiturates including secobarbital do not interfere. The procedure, however, cannot be applied in the presence of formaldehyde (fixed tissue) or lignin-containing material (paper, cork).

## IX. Methyprylon

Methyprylon (3,3-diethyl-2,4-dioxo-5-methylpiperidine, Noludar®) is a sedative-hypnotic that exerts a depressant action on the central nervous system. The therapeutic dose is from 150 to 400 mg. Although recoveries have followed overingestion of as much as 20 gm, death has occurred after ingestion of 6 gm (R6). It is interesting that while toxic amounts do not cause respiratory depression, severe hypotension is produced.

### A. Metabolic Fate

In man and dog, dehydrogenation of methyprylon occurs with the formation of 2,4-dioxo-3,3-diethyl-5-methyltetrahydropyridine that has been isolated from urine (B1, P3). In man, about 3% of the administered dose is excreted as this metabolite in the urine (P3). Metabolic studies (B1) show that hydroxylation of this product takes place, the hydroxymethyl derivative being isolated from the urine of dogs. When these 2 metabolites are fed to dogs, they were excreted partly as such and partly oxidized to a carboxylic acid derivative, 4,6-dioxo-5,5-diethyltetrahydronicotinic acid. This product and the hydroxylated derivative are also excreted in urine as the glucuronides. Decarboxylation of the carboxylic acid product also takes place, and the resulting compound is excreted in the urine.

The pooled plasma of three adults contained from 0.6 to 1.0 mg of methyprylon per 100 ml and 0.02 to 0.09 mg of the dehydrogenated derivative per 100 ml 1–4 hours after oral ingestion (R3).

### B. Determination in Plasma and Urine (R3)

Quantitation is by determining the absorbance of the blue color produced by the reaction between methyprylon and the classic Folin–Ciocalteu reagent. To 5 ml of plasma or urine are added 1 ml of 5 N sodium hydroxide and 40 ml of chloroform. The mixture is shaken for 1 hour after which the solvent is separated and washed by shaking for

10 minutes with 4 ml of 0.5 N sodium hydroxide. The chloroform phase is then dried over sodium sulfate and filtered. After evaporation to dryness of an aliquot of filtrate, the residue is dissolved in 3 ml of water. Then 1 ml of the color-producing reagent is added. After mixing, 1 ml of 0.8 N sodium hydroxide is added. The absorbance is determined at 600 m$\mu$ within 10 minutes. The sensitivity is 50 $\mu$g/ml; the reaction is linear for 50–500 $\mu$g. The dehydrogenated metabolite does not interfere. Methyprylon added to blood or to urine is recovered with an accuracy of ±6%.

## C. Detection by Paper Chromatography

In their study of the metabolism of methyprylon, Bernhard and coworkers (B1) have outlined a method for the paper chromatographic separation of the drug from its metabolic products. The descending technique is used with a mobile solvent consisting of dibutyl ether, isopropyl ether, methylcellosolve, and 5% acetic acid (10:1:1:1). Amounts of material applied to Whatman No. 1 paper are 30–40 $\mu$g/0.005 ml. The paper is conditioned in an atmosphere saturated with 5% acetic acid and the solvent mixture. Location of zones is by spraying with a solution containing 20 ml of 5 N potassium hydroxide and 100 ml of ethanol. The spots exhibit a light blue to green fluorescence. The presence of methyprylon is confirmed by spraying with a solution of 1.6% potassium ferricyanide and 2 N potassium hydroxide; a white-blue fluorescence results. Methyprylon has an R$_f$ value of 0.50, the dehydrogenated derivative 0.72. The R$_f$ values of the other metabolites are also given.

## D. Use of Ultraviolet Spectrophotometry (P3)

As can be predicted, methyprylon does not absorb in the ultraviolet. However, the oxidation product, 2,4-dioxo-3,3-diethyl-5-tetrahydropyridine, has a characteristic absorbance due to the alteration of the piperidine ring. Specimens of urine are adjusted to pH 6 and extracted with chloroform. The separated solvent extract is filtered, and the ultraviolet absorption spectrum determined. The maximum absorbance is at 305 m$\mu$.

## X. Ethinamate

Ethinamate (1-ethynylcyclohexylcarbamate, Valmid®) is a depressant of the central nervous system. The usual dose is 0.5 or 1 gm. In animals, sedation, narcosis, and death by respiratory failure have been produced by increased doses. The drug is considered to be relatively safe, and as much as 28 gm have been ingested by adults without fatal outcome (G6). Death, however, has followed ingestion of about 15 gm (D2).

## A. Metabolic Fate

The metabolic fate of ethinamate has been studied using carboxyl-$C^{14}$–labeled drug administered to rats (M5). Hydrolytic cleavage of the carbamate occurs, but the main change is by hydroxylation to hydroxyethinamate. This compound is excreted in the urine in the free form with about the same amount conjugated with glucuronic acid. The hydroxylated compound was isolated from the urine of humans and identified. It has been proved to be 1-ethynyl-4-hydroxycyclohexylcarbamate (M6). The acetylenic group remains intact. Unchanged ethinamate has been found in the blood, liver, and urine of humans after overingestion of the drug (P4).

## B. Determination in Biological Media

Like other such compounds, ethinamate can be determined colorimetrically after formation of its insoluble silver acetylide (M2, P1, P2). As is recognized, this method is nonspecific and insensitive, and the drug usually is present in amounts too small to permit its determination in blood and tissue. It is noteworthy that the major urinary metabolite, hydroxyethinamate, does not form an insoluble silver complex due to the presence of the hydroxyl group (M5).

## C. Detection by Paper Chromatography

In one procedure (L4), urine or homogenates of tissue are brought to pH 8 or 9 and extracted with chloroform or ether. The solvent is separated, evaporated to a small volume, and then applied to paper. Ascending chromatography is used with a solvent system of *n*-butanol saturated with $5 N$ ammonium hydroxide. After resolution, the sheet is dried and then immersed in a saturated solution of mercuric nitrate that reveals location of the material by formation of black zones. Ethinamate is separated from its metabolites and appears at $R_f$ 0.80–0.85. Potassium permanganate ($0.02 N$) can also be used to locate zones. By comparing results obtained when known amounts of ethinamate are subjected to the same treatment, an approximation may be made.

Pruess and Meyer (P4) have also used paper chromatography in their study of ethinamate and its metabolic products. The dialyzates of biological media as well as extracts obtained by the treatment of blood and tissue according to the Stas procedure were applied to paper.

## XI. Phenaglycodol

Phenaglycodol (2-*p*-chlorophenyl-3-methyl-2,3-butanediol, Ultran®) is a tranquilizing agent with anticonvulsant activity. The usual adult daily dose is from 600 to 1200 mg; in children, 2400 mg/day have been tolerated for as long as 2 months without adverse effects. Fatalities have not been reported, although ingestion of single doses of about 6–15 gm by adults have produced coma and, in one case, deep sleep for as long as 60 hours (L4). In animals, massive amounts caused death by respiratory paralysis.

## Determination in Biological Media

At present, there is no method available that permits the detection of this compound in fluids or tissue, but the following procedure has been successfully used for determining the drug in artificial gastric juice (L4).

A sample of gastric content is extracted with four 50-ml portions of ether. The combined ether extracts are washed with three 25-ml portions of water. The wash solutions are combined and extracted with two 25-ml portions of ether. All the extracts of ether are combined, dried over sodium sulfate, then filtered. The filtrate is evaporated almost to dryness on a steam bath with the aid of a current of air. The final remnants of ether are allowed to evaporate spontaneously. The residue is dissolved in 10 ml of chloroform, and the absorbance is determined using infrared spectrophotometry. The amount present is calculated by comparison with the known spectrum of phenaglycodol.

## XII. Captodiamine

Captodiamine ($p$-butylmercaptobenzhydrol-$\beta$-dimethylaminoethyl sulfide, Suvren®, Covatin®) is similar in structure to diphenhydramine. A sedative and antispasmodic, it exerts its depressant effect mainly on the central nervous system. It appears to potentiate the anesthetic effect of the barbiturates as well as the analgesic action of several other drugs. The usual daily dose is about 400 mg. Two mental patients received daily doses of 1000 mg (about 15 mg/kg) for 18 months without adverse effects. In four attempted suicides, adults survived the ingestion of between 2000 and 2500 mg (F2, K7). Prominent symptoms, which generally disappeared in 24 hours, included disturbances of vision and of equilibrium, excitation, dizziness, nausea, and nystagmus. In one instance an excess of alcohol was also imbibed.

The death of a 7-year-old mentally retarded girl who ingested 1550 mg (67 mg/kg) as a single dose has been attributed to this drug (M3). There were no significant pathological changes. The following procedure was adopted to permit analysis of blood, liver, and urine.

### A. Method

For blood and urine, 5-ml specimens are analyzed; for liver, 5 gm are homogenized with 5 ml of water. About 0.5 ml of 50% sodium hydroxide and 50 ml of ether are added to the specimen. The mixture is shaken for 15 minutes, centrifuged, and the aqueous phase discarded. The ether extract is washed twice with 5 ml of a buffer solution consisting of 20 gm of sodium borate and 200 gm of sodium chloride per liter. The wash solutions are discarded. After filtering, the ether is extracted with 5 ml of 1% sulfuric acid. The aqueous phase is poured through Whatman No. 5 paper; its ultraviolet spectrum is then determined. Captodiamine exhibits a single maximum at 263 m$\mu$. The same solution is made alkaline with a drop of 50% sodium hydroxide (a slight cloudiness may appear) and the spectrum again determined. In basic solution, there is a shift in the maximum to 270 m$\mu$. An acidic solution of captodiamine containing 18 $\mu$g/ml has an absorbance of 0.78 at 263 m$\mu$. The ultraviolet spectra in acidic and basic solution are shown in Figure 5.

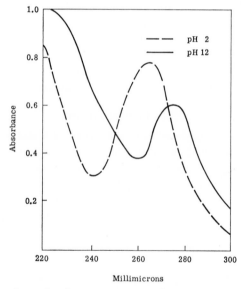

FIG. 5. The ultraviolet absorption spectra of captodiamine (18 $\mu$g/ml).

## B. Use of Paper Chromatography

Extracts of liver were applied to Whatman No. 1 paper and subjected to paper chromatography using the ascending technique and a solvent system of *n*-butanol and glacial acetic acid (10:1) saturated with water (M10). The $R_f$ value of the extracted material was the same as that of the pure drug, 0.76. Zones were located by viewing under ultraviolet light at 237 m$\mu$ and by treatment with Dragendorff reagent (M10). Material from a parallel and untreated strip was eluted with 1% sulfuric acid and the ultraviolet absorption spectra of the eluate determined.

The liver contained 3.2 mg of captodiamine per 100 gm. The spectra of the extracts of liver were the same as those of the pure drug. In the spectrum of the acidic extract of blood, there was a slight maximum at 265 m$\mu$ that could not be attributed to the drug; the quantity of drug necessary to produce this maximum is less than 0.05 mg/100 ml of blood. Captodiamine was not detected in the urine.

# XIII. Imipramine

Imipramine (N-($\gamma$-dimethylaminopropyl)iminodibenzyl hydrochloride, Tofranil®) is a most interesting antidepressant. It differs from the usual tranquilizers by effecting a return to normal state of mind—hence its designation, thymoleptic—in cases of severe depression, but it does not stimulate the central nervous system or produce euphoria in the normal individual. Structurally, it resembles chlorpromazine with the sulfur of the ring replaced by $CH_2$—$CH_2$. The usual daily dose is from 75 to 150 mg. Recovery after ingestion of 1500 mg as a single dose has been reported (L1), while fatalities have followed ingestion of more than this amount (F12, M1). Common symptoms after toxic amounts are overactivity, hypotension, arrhythmia, and convulsions. It is interesting that after massive doses both depression of the central nervous system and stimulation result, as seen in cases of intoxication by antihistamines.

The concentrations of imipramine in biological fluids and in tissues have been determined in a case of suicidal ingestion of a massive dose by an adult (F12). Imipramine was isolated from stomach contents and identified by infrared spectrophotometry. Quantitation of imipramine by the colorimetric procedure using methyl orange yielded the following results: blood contained 3 mg%; urine, 0.69 mg%; kidney, 17.9 mg%; liver, 31.7 mg%.

## A. Metabolic Fate

A study of the metabolic fate of the drug in man and in animals showed that it is rapidly absorbed and localized in the tissues (H3). In man and animals, oxidative hydroxylation in the 2 position and N-mono-demethylation occur. The hydroxy metabolite, N-($\gamma$-dimethylamino-propyl)-2-hydroxyiminodibenzyl, is excreted in the urine. Conjugation of this compound with glucuronic acid also takes place; the metabolite has been isolated from the urine of rabbits after acid and enzymatic hydrolysis of the glucuronide. The N-mono-demethylated metabolite was detected after paper chromatographic studies of extracts of urine of animals and of man and was identified as being $N$-($\gamma$-monoethylaminopropyl)iminodibenzyl. In man receiving clinical doses of imipramine, 2–4% of the administered dose is excreted, chiefly as the demethylated derivative. Unchanged imipramine is also excreted in the urine. In man, 6–10% of the administered imipramine is excreted as these compounds; in rabbit, 40 to 50%. Following oral or intravenous administration to rabbits, only small amounts, less than 0.2 mg%, are found in the plasma. In rat and mouse, high concentrations found in the tissues are of much greater magnitude than those in plasma. The demethylated product predominates in the liver, lung, and kidney. In man receiving 100 mg intravenously, the concentration in plasma drops very quickly, and only within the first 30 minutes following administration can amounts over 0.1 mg per 100 ml be measured.

### B. Detection in Urine

A rapid color test for urine allows a rough approximation of the amount of drug originally ingested (F8). For the test, 1 ml of urine is mixed with 1 ml of a solution consisting of equal parts of 0.2% potassium dichromate, 30% sulfuric acid (by volume), 20% perchloric acid, and 50% nitric acid (by volume). With a positive result, a green color appears immediately. The amount of drug ingested may be approximated by comparison of the resulting color with a chart. Ingestion of as little as 25–50 mg of imipramine daily gives a positive result.

### C. Detection by Paper Chromatography (H3)

Specimens of urine are adjusted to pH 9–10 and extracted with ethylene dichloride. The extract is applied to Whatman No. 3 paper; ascending technique is used. The solvent system consists of ammonium hydroxide (2.5%):ethanol:glacial acetic acid (200:15:3). After resolution, location of zones is by spraying with diazotized $p$-nitroaniline followed by treatment with concentrated hydrochloric acid. Unchanged imipramine ($R_f$ 0.3), the demethylated product ($R_f$ 0.45), and the hydroxylated metabolite ($R_f$ 0.6) are readily detected. [An additional zone ($R_f$ 0.8) is due to decomposition of the hydroxylated metabolite.] Upon treatment of the sheet with the color reagents, the zones that contain the hydroxy metabolite and its secondary zone appear as red spots. The zones containing imipramine and its demethylated derivative reveal themselves a few minutes later as blue-violet spots. Within 24 hours, all zones are this color. Extracts of other biological media can also be studied in this way. Elution and study of the individual zones are, of course, possible.

## D. Determination in Biological Media

### 1. SPECTROPHOTOFLUOROMETRIC PROCEDURE (G1)

An 8-ml sample of plasma and 0.2 ml of 0.2 $M$ borate buffer (pH 11) are added to 60 ml of heptane. The mixture is shaken gently for 45 minutes and then centrifuged. A 40-ml aliquot of the solvent is then shaken for 15 minutes with 2 ml of 0.1 $N$ hydrochloric acid solution. After centrifuging, 1 ml of the acid solution is separated and 0.1 ml of 2 $N$ sodium hydroxide solution is added. The concentration of drug is estimated by spectrophotofluorometric measurement. The compound fluoresces at 400 m$\mu$ when activated at 290 m$\mu$. Reagent blanks and recoveries are determined together with the test sample. The plasma of patients receiving therapeutic doses contains about 0.01–0.06 mg of imipramine per 100 ml.

### 2. COLORIMETRY AFTER TREATMENT WITH OXIDIZING AGENTS (H3)

Iminodibenzyl derivatives give a blue color upon treatment with oxidizing agents. Serial dilutions are performed using 1-ml solutions to which are added 2 ml of 5 $N$ hydrochloric acid and a drop of 1% sodium nitrite. The least dilution produces a blue-green color for amounts of about 0.5–0.7 mg%. The yellow color that results 3 hours after addition of the reagents is measured colorimetrically.

### 3. COLORIMETRY USING METHYL ORANGE

The colorimetric procedure of Brodie (B6) [see ref. (S9), Volume I, Chapter 18] involving complexing with methyl orange was modified (H3) to permit determination of imipramine alone or together with its metabolic products. After extraction of the specimens with ethylene dichloride, the solvent containing the imipramine together with its hydroxylated and demethylated products can be shaken with phosphate buffer at pH 6. In this way the imipramine can be separated and determined.

#### REFERENCES

(A1) Abbott Laboratories, Chicago, Illinois. Personal communication (1957).
(A2) Algeri, E. J. *Am. J. Clin. Pathol.* 31, 412 (1959).
(A3) Algeri, E. J., Katsas, G. G., and McBay, A. J. *J. Forensic Sci.* 4, 111 (1959).
(A4) Algeri, E. J., and Katsas, G. G. *J. Forensic Sci.* 5, 217 (1960).
(A5) Algeri, E. J., Katsas, G. G., and Luongo, M. A. *Am. J. Clin. Pathol.* 38, 125 (1962).
(A6) Auterhoff, H. *Arch. Pharm.* 284, 123 (1951).
(A7) Auterhoff, H. *Arch. Pharm.* 285, 14 (1952).
(B1) Bernhard, K., Just, M., Lutz, A. H., and Vuilleumier, J. P. *Helv. Chim. Acta* 40, 436 (1957).

(B2) Berti, T., and Cima, L. *Arch. Intern. Pharmacodyn.* 98, 452 (1954).
(B3) Berti, T., and Cima, L. *Farmaco (Pavia) Ed. Sci.* 11, 451 (1956).
(B4) Bowman, R. L., Caulfield, P. A., and Udenfriend, S. *Science* 122, 32 (1955).
(B5) Bräuniger, H., and Hofmann, R. *Pharmazie* 10, 644 (1955).
(B6) Brodie, B. B., Udenfriend, S., and Dill, W. *J. Biol. Chem.* 168, 335 (1947).
(B7) Brunten, A. M. *In* "Psychotropic Drugs" (S. Garattini and V. Ghetti, eds.), pp. 405–413. Elsevier, New York, 1957.
(C1) Calò, A., Mariani, A., and Mariani-Marelli, O. *Svensk Farm. Tidskr.* 60, 842 (1956).
(C2) Calò, A., Mariani, A., and Mariani-Marelli, O. *Pharm. Acta Helv.* 33, 126 (1958).
(C3) Cann, H. M., and Verhulst, H. L. *A.M.A. J. Diseases Children* 99, 380 (1960).
(C4) Cavatorta, L. *J. Pharm. Pharmacol.* 11, 49 (1959).
(C5) Chuen, N., and Riedel, B. E. *Can. Pharm. J.* 94, 51 (1961).
(C6) Clarke, E. G. C. *J. Pharm. Pharmacol.* 9, 752 (1957).
(D1) Davidson, J. D., Terry, L. L., and Sjoerdsma, A. *J. Pharmacol. Exptl. Therap.* 121, 8 (1957).
(D2) Davis, R. P., Blythe, W. B., Newton, M., and Welt, L. G. *Yale J. Biol. Med.* 32, 192 (1959).
(D3) Domenici, T. Personal communication.
(D4) Dubost, P., and Pascal, S. *Ann. Pharm. Franç.* 11, 615 (1953).
(D5) Dubost, P., and Pascal, S. *Ann. Pharm. Franç.* 13, 56 (1955).
(E1) Eiduson, S., and Wallace, R. D. *Federation Proc.* 17, Part I, 365 (1958).
(E2) Eisdorfer, I. B., and Ellenbogen, W. C. *J. Chromatog.* 4, 329 (1960).
(F1) Fels, I. G., Kaufman, M., and Karczmar, A. G. *Nature* 181, 1266 (1958).
(F2) Fiorentini, H., and Cardaire, G. *Ann. Méd. Légale Criminol. Police Sci. Toxicol.* 40, 67 (1960).
(F3) Fishman, V., and Goldenberg, H. *Proc. Soc. Exptl. Biol. Med.* 104, 99 (1960).
(F4) Flanagan, T. L., Lin, T. H., Novick, W. J., Rondish, I. M., Bocher, C. A., and Van Loon, E. J. *J. Med. Pharm. Chem.* 1, 263 (1959).
(F5) Forrest, F. M., Forrest, I. S., and Mason, A. S. *Am. J. Psychiat.* 115, 1114 (1959).
(F6) Forrest, F. M., Forrest, I. S., and Mason, A. S. *Am. J. Psychiat.* 116, 549 (1959).
(F7) Forrest, F. M., Forrest, I. S., and Mason, A. S. *Am. J. Psychiat.* 118, 300 (1961).
(F8) Forrest, I. S., Forrest, F. M., and Mason, A. S. *Am. J. Psychiat.* 116, 1021 (1960).
(F9) Fossoul, C. *J. Pharm. Belg.* 5, 202 (1950).
(F10) Fossoul, C. *J. Pharm. Belg.* 6, 383 (1951).
(F11) Frahm, M., Fretwurst, E., and Soehring, K. *Klin. Wochschr.* 34, 1259 (1956).
(F12) Freimuth, H. C. *J. Forensic Sci.* 6, 68 (1961).
(G1) Geigy Pharmaceuticals, Yonkers, New York. Personal communication (1960).
(G2) Goldbaum, L. R., and Williams, M. A. *Anal. Chem.* 32, 81 (1960).
(G3) Goldenberg, H., and Fishman, V. *Proc. Soc. Exptl. Biol. Med.* 108, 178 (1961).
(G4) Gosselin, R. A. "National Prescription Audit. Fourth Quarter, 1961." R. A. Gosselin and Co., Inc., Dedham, Massachusetts.

(G5) Gouzon, B., Pruneyre, A., and Donnet, V. *Compt. Rend. Soc. Biol.* **148**, 2039 (1954).
(G6) Gruber, C. M. *J. Indiana State Med. Assoc.* **49**, 35 (1956).
(H1) Haas, H. *Arzneimittel-Forsch.* **2**, 79 (1952).
(H2) Henriksen, U., Huus, I., and Kopf, R. *Arch. Intern. Pharmacodyn.* **109**, 39 (1957).
(H3) Herrmann, B., and Pulver, R. *Arch. Intern. Pharmacodyn.* **126**, 454 (1960).
(H4) Heyman, J. J., Bayne, B., and Merlis, S. *Am. J. Psychiat.* **116**, 1108 (1960).
(H5) Hoffmann, I., Nieschulz, O., Popendiker, K., and Tauchert, E. *Arzneimittel-Forsch.* **9**, 133 (1959).
(H6) Hollister, L. E., Motzenbecker, F. P., and Degan, R. O. *Psychopharmacologia* **2**, 63 (1961).
(J1) Jenner, F. A., and Parkin, D. *Lancet* **II**, 322 (1961).
(K1) Kabasakalian, P., and McGlotten, J. *Anal. Chem.* **31**, 431 (1959).
(K2) Kamm, J. J., Gillette, J. R., and Brodie, B. B. *Federation Proc.* **17**, Part I, 382 (1958).
(K3) Kebrle, J., and Hoffmann, K. *Experentia* **12**, 21 (1956).
(K4) Kebrle, J., Schmid, K., Hoffmann, K., Vuilleumier, J. P., and Bernhard, K. *Helv. Chim. Acta* **42**, 417 (1959).
(K5) Kobert, K. *Z. Anal. Chem.* **46**, 711 (1907).
(K6) Kok, K. *Acta Physiol. Pharmacol. Neerl.* **4**, 388 (1955).
(K7) Kopf, R., and Nielsen, I. M. *Arzneimittel-Forsch.* **8**, 154 (1958).
(K8) Kothari, U. C. *Current Therap. Res.* **3**, 329 (1961).
(K9) Kotionis, A. Z. *Arzneimittel-Forsch.* **11**, 108 (1961).
(L1) Lancaster, N. P., and Foster, A. R. *Brit. Med. J.* **II**, 1458 (1959).
(L2) Leach, H., and Crimmin, W. R. C. *J. Clin. Pathol.* **9**, 164 (1956).
(L3) Lee, H. M., Scott, E. G., and Pohland, A. *J. Pharmacol. Exptl. Therap.* **125**, 14 (1959).
(L4) Lilly and Company, Indianapolis, Indiana. Personal communication (1961).
(L5) Lin, T. H., Reynolds, L. W., Rondish, I. M., and Van Loon, E. J. *Proc. Soc. Exptl. Biol. Med.* **102**, 602 (1959).
(M1) Manners, T. *Lancet* **II**, 932 (1960).
(M2) Marley, E., and Vane, J. R. *Brit. J. Pharmacol.* **13**, 364 (1958).
(M3) McBay, A. J. Unpublished data (1961).
(M4) McBay, A. J., and Katsas, G. G. *New Engl. J. Med.* **257**, 97 (1957).
(M5) McMahon, R. E. *J. Am. Chem. Soc.* **80**, 411 (1958).
(M6) McMahon, R. E. *J. Org. Chem.* **24**, 1834 (1959).
(M7) Meyer, F. *Arzneimittel-Forsch.* **7**, 296 (1957).
(M8) Milne, J. B., and Chatten, L. G. *J. Pharm. Pharmacol.* **9**, 686 (1957).
(M9) Milne, J. *J. Am. Pharm. Assoc. Sci. Ed.* **48**, 117 (1959).
(M10) Munier, R., and Macheboeuf, M. *Bull. Soc. Chim. Biol.* **31**, 1144 (1949).
(N1) Nadeau, G., and Sobolewski, G. *Can. Med. Assoc. J.* **80**, 826 (1959).
(N2) Nadeau, G., and Sobolewski, G. *J. Chromatog.* **2**, 544 (1959).
(N3) Neuhoff, E. W., and Auterhoff, H. *Arch. Pharm.* **288**, 400 (1955).
(N4) Neve, H. K. *Acta Pharmacol. Toxicol.* **17**, 404 (1960).
(O1) O'Dea, A. E., and Liss, M. *New Engl. J. Med.* **249**, 566 (1953).
(O2) Overholser, L. G., and Yoe, J. H. *Ind. Eng. Chem. Anal. Ed.* **14**, 646 (1942).
(P1) Perlman, P. L., and Johnson, C. *J. Am. Pharm. Assoc. Sci. Ed.* **41**, 13 (1952).
(P2) Perlman, P. L., Sutter, D., and Johnson, C. B. *J. Am. Pharm. Assoc. Sci. Ed.* **42**, 750 (1953).

(P3) Pribilla, O. *Arzneimittel-Forsch.* **6,** 756 (1956).
(P4) Pruess, R., and Mayer, E. *Arch. Toxicol.* **18,** 243 (1960).
(R1) Ragland, J. B., and Kinross-Wright, J. *Federation Proc.* **20,** Part I, 397 (1961).
(R2) Randall, L. O., and Iliev, V. (Hoffmann-LaRoche, Inc., Nutley, New Jersey.) Personal communication (1961).
(R3) Randall, L. O., Iliev, V., and Brandman, O. *Arch. Intern. Pharmacodyn.* **106,** 388 (1956).
(R4) Randall, L. O. *Diseases Nervous System* **22,** Suppl. No. 7, 7 (1961).
(R5) Rectem, V., and Van Lierop, A. *Acta Paediat. Belg.* **14,** 47 (1960).
(R6) Reidt, W. U. *New Engl. J. Med.* **255,** 231 (1956).
(R7) Rickards, J. C., Boxer, G. E., and Smith, C. C. *J. Pharmacol. Exptl. Therap.* **98,** 380 (1950).
(R8) Rieders, F. *J. Forensic Sci.* **6,** 401 (1961).
(R9) Rives, H. F., Ward, B. B., and Hicks, M. L. *J. Am. Med. Assoc.* **140,** 1022 (1949).
(R10) Ross, J. J., Young, R. L., and Maass, A. R. *Science* **128,** 1279 (1958).
(R11) Ryan, J. A. *J. Am. Pharm. Assoc. Sci. Ed.* **48,** 240 (1959).
(S1) Salvesen, B., Domange, L., and Guy, J. *Ann. Pharm. Franç.* **13,** 208 (1955).
(S2) Salzman, N. P., Moran, N. C., and Brodie, B. B. *Nature* **176,** 1122 (1955).
(S3) Salzman, N. P., and Brodie, B. B. *J. Pharmacol. Exptl. Therap.* **118,** 46 (1956).
(S4) Sandri, G. C. *Farmaco (Pavia) Ed. Sci.* **10,** 444 (1955).
(S5) Sano, I., and Kajita, H. *Klin. Wochschr.* **33,** 956 (1955).
(S6) Schreiner, G. E., Berman, L. B., Kovach, R., and Bloomer, H. A. *A.M.A. Arch. Internal Med.* **101,** 899 (1958).
(S7) Sheppard, H., D'Asaro, B. S., and Plummer, A. J. *J. Am. Pharm. Assoc. Sci. Ed.* **45,** 681 (1956).
(S8) Steinman, I. D. Cited by Kothari (K8).
(S9) Stewart, C. P., and Stolman, A., eds. "Toxicology: Mechanisms and Analytical Methods," Vols. I and II. Academic Press, New York, 1960–1961.
(T1) Tabau, R. L., and Vigne, J. P. *Bull. Soc. Chim. France* p. 458 (1948).
(T2) Thieme, H. *Pharmazie* **11,** 332 (1956).
(U1) Udenfriend, S., Duggan, D. E., Vasta, B. M., and Brodie, B. B. *J. Pharmacol. Exptl. Therap.* **120,** 26 (1957).
(W1) Walkenstein, S. S., and Seifter, J. *J. Pharmacol. Exptl. Therap.* **125,** 283 (1959).
(W2) Wechsler, M. B., and Forrest, I. S. *J. Neurochem.* **4,** 366 (1959).
(W3) Wiser, R., Knebel, C., and Seifter, J. *Pharmacologist* **2,** 83 (1960).
(Z1) Zbinden, G., Bagdon, R. E., Keith, E. F., Phillips, R. D., and Randall, L. O. *Toxicol. Appl. Pharmacol.* **3,** 619 (1961).

# The Determination of Antiarthritics, Antihistamines, and Thymoleptics

by Fredric Rieders

Division of the Medical Examiner, Department of Public Health of the City of Philadelphia, Pennsylvania

## I. Antiarthritics

### Phenylbutazone

#### 1. Uses

Sold under the trade name Butazolidin® (Geigy), phenylbutazone, an antipyretic analgesic with anti-inflammatory properties, is used in the treatment of gout and other forms of arthritis.

#### 2. Physical Properties

Phenylbutazone (1,2-diphenyl-4-butyl-3,5-pyrazolidinedione) is white or faintly yellow, crystalline, with a slightly bitter taste and faintly fruity odor. Its molecular weight is 308.37 and its capillary melting point is 105°C. It is soluble in the common organic solvents and in alkali but not in water, acid, or bicarbonate solution.

#### 3. Extraction

*a. Stas–Otto Procedure.* In the Stas–Otto procedure, phenylbutazone

191

is isolated in the acid-ether, phenolic (intermediate acid) fraction, while its metabolites (B1) appear in the acid-chloroform fraction.

*b. Direct Extraction.* Since both phenylbutazone and its metabolites are highly bound to plasma proteins (B2), complete direct extractions of tissues require preliminary acid denaturation of the proteins; without this, only about 60% of drug and metabolites is extracted (B2).

## 4. PURIFICATION

*a. Paper Chromatography.* Tissue extracts containing phenylbutazone can be purified by paper chromatography with 8:2 benzene:cyclohexane on Whatman No. 1 filter paper impregnated with 50% alcoholic formamide containing 5% ammonium carbonate; the $R_f$ is 0.83 and the spot can be located under 254-m$\mu$ ultraviolet light or by spraying with a 1:1 mixture of 15% $FeCl_3$ and 1% $K_3Fe(CN)_6$ (K1).

*b. Thin Layer Chromatography.* Purification by ascending thin layer chromatography on Silica Gel-G with 3% methanol in chloroform as solvent, giving an $R_f$ of about 0.3, and spot location by spraying with a 1:4 dilution of household bleach, drying, spraying with 5% phenol, drying, and spraying with 2% starch/1% KI can also be effected (R4).

## 5. COLOR REACTION

Purified phenylbutazone, eluted with a 1:1 mixture of ethanol and water from paper or thin layer chromatograms, gives a color reaction: when 1 part eluate is mixed with 1 part 2.5% cupric acetate in 10% sodium acetate and the mixture is extracted with chloroform, the upper, aqueous phase is light blue, while the lower, chloroform phase is colorless (S1).

## 6. ULTRAVIOLET SPECTRA

For the detection and estimation of phenylbutazone in biologic material by direct solvent extraction and ultraviolet spectrophotometry, Burns *et al.* (B2) give the following procedure:

To 1–3 ml plasma or urine or to 2 ml of tissue homogenate (1 gm tissue and 5 ml $H_2O$), 0.5 ml of 3 N HCl and 20 ml 3% isoamyl alcohol in purified heptane are added. The mixture is shaken for 30 minutes and centrifuged. The phases are separated and 15 ml of the heptane is drawn off and extracted for 5 minutes with 5 ml 2.5 N NaOH. The optical density of the NaOH extract is determined at 265 m$\mu$ in a 1-cm quartz cuvette. The optical density is approximately 0.010 per microgram phenylbutazone carried through this procedure with 100% recoveries of 10–100 $\mu$g, tissue blanks corresponding to 3–5 $\mu$g/ml for plasma and 6–10 $\mu$g/gm for other tissues.

A direct extraction and ultraviolet procedure for phenylbutazone together with its metabolites is as follows (R4): 10 ml tissue homogenate (1 part tissue plus 3 parts 0.1 $N$ $H_2SO_4$) or 2.5 ml blood plus 0.5 ml 1 $N$ $H_2SO_4$ are shaken for 5 minutes with 100 ml chloroform. The chloroform is drawn off through a Whatman No. 1 filter paper (into 10 ml fresh 3% sodium bicarbonate to which 1 drop 10% $H_2SO_4$ was added, shaken 1 minute, drawn off through Whatman No. 1 filter paper for separation from salicylate) into 8 ml 1 $N$ NaOH and shaken 3 minutes. The NaOH layer is removed, and 2.5 ml are placed into a tube containing 0.5 ml $H_2O$ ("salt") and 2.5 ml into a second tube containing 0.2 ml 6 $N$ $H_2SO_4$ ("free acid"). The following spectra (220–350 m$\mu$) are obtained by means of a recording spectrophotometer (with the recorder pen set to 50% or 100% transmittance at 350 m$\mu$):

(1) "salt" versus 1 $N$ NaOH as reference;
(2) "free acid" versus $H_2O$ as reference;
(3) "salt" versus "free acid" as reference.

The spectra which are thus obtained are shown in Fig. 1.

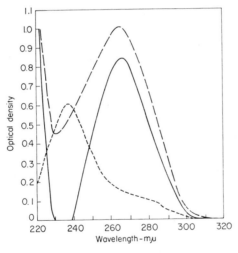

Fig. 1. Phenylbutazone, 6 mg/100 ml blood; UV spectra of extract. Key: - - - - - acid; — — — salt; ——— difference. (See text, Section I,A,6.)

## II. Antihistamines

### A. Extraction

The antihistaminic drugs [(1) carbinoxamine (Clistin®); (2) chlorpheniramine (Chlor-Trimeton®, Teldrin®); (3) dexchlorpheniramine (Polaramine®); (4) dimethpyrindene (Forhistal®); (5) diphenhydramine (Benadryl®); and (6) tripelennamine (Pyribenzamine®)] are isolated in the Stas–Otto procedure in the alkaline-ether fraction (or, more effectively, in the alkaline-chloroform fraction) as intermediate bases.

## B. Thin Layer Chromatography

Purification of the tissue extracts, detection, and preliminary identification by $R_f$ of the drugs (R4) can be effected by ascending thin layer chromatography on Silica Gel-G with methanol as the solvent. Under 254-m$\mu$ ultraviolet light the spots of the drugs appear darker than the background. Following exposure to this light, the spots of carbinoxamine, dexchlorpheniramine, and dimethpyrindene turn yellow. Further visualization of the spots can be effected by spraying with 1% iodine in methanol, Dragendorff reagent, or potassium iodoplatinate. The $R_f$ values of the drugs are: (1) 0.65; (2) 0.55; (3) 0.61; (4) 0.40; (5) 0.50; and (6) 0.46.

## C. Ultraviolet Spectra

A procedure for the direct extraction of the antihistaminics from tissues and body fluids and for their detection, identification, and quantitation is as follows (R4):

Five milliliters urine plus 7 ml 50% KOH, 10 ml blood plus 10 ml 50% KOH, or 20 ml tissue homogenate (2 parts tissue plus 3 parts 50% KOH) are shaken for 15 minutes with 100 ml of 5% ethanol in $CHCl_3$. The organic phase is drawn off through a Whatman No. 1 filter paper, washed with 10 ml 3% $NaHCO_3$, filtered as before, and extracted 5 minutes with 8 ml 1 $N$ $H_2SO_4$. The $H_2SO_4$ layer is removed and 2.5 ml are mixed with 0.5 ml 6 $N$ $H_2SO_4$ ("salt") and another 2.5 ml with 0.5 ml 6 $N$ NaOH ("free base"). The following spectra (220–350 m$\mu$) are obtained by means of a recording spectrophotometer (with the recorder pen set to 50% or 100% transmittance at 350 m$\mu$):

(1) "salt" versus $H_2O$ as reference;

(2) "free base" versus 2 $N$ NaOH as reference;

(3) "salt" versus "free base" as reference.

Spectra of chlorpheniramine and of tripelennamine obtained by this procedure are shown in Figs. 2 and 3 respectively.

# III. Thymoleptics

## A. Uses

The hydrazine derivatives isocarboxazid (Marplan®), nialamide (Niamid®), and phenelzine (Nardil®) and the diazepine derivative imipramine, so-called thymoleptics or psychic energizers, are used in the treatment of certain depressive states.

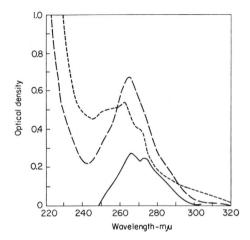

FIG. 2. Chlorpheniramine, 5 mg/100 ml blood; UV spectra of extract. KEY: - - - - base; — — — salt; ——— difference. (See text, Section II,C.)

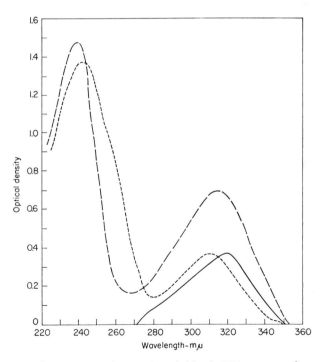

FIG. 3. Tripelennamine, 2.5 mg/100 ml blood; UV spectra of extract. KEY: - - - - - base; — — — salt; ——— difference. (See text, Section II,C.)

B. General Procedures for Extraction and Purification

1. EXTRACTION

The compounds are relatively labile and relatively strongly bound to proteins. To separate them from tissue bulk, extraction and concentration of extracts should be done as much below 50°C as possible by the use of flash evaporation at reduced pressure under mildly acid conditions (R4). All of these compounds are intermediate bases and appear in the alkaline-ether or alkaline-chloroform fraction of the Stas–Otfo procedure. Direct extraction from strongly alkalinized blood, urine, cerebrospinal fluid, and tissue homogenates and their identification and estimation by ultraviolet spectrophotometry as described for antihistamines (Section II,C) result in 50–70% recoveries (R4). The results are similar if a protein-free tissue filtrate is prepared by means of $ZnSO_4$ or trichloracetic acid, made alkaline and extracted with 5 volumes $CHCl_3$ (R4).

2. THIN LAYER CHROMATOGRAPHY

Their isolation from extracted impurities can be effected by ascending thin layer chromatography on Silica Gel-G using methanol as the solvent (R4).

C. Individual Thymoleptics

1. IMIPRAMINE

*a. Thin Layer Chromatography.* Thin layer chromatography (Section III,B,2) gives a spot at an $R_f$ of about 0.5 which is yellow under 254-m$\mu$ ultraviolet light and brown on a white background upon spraying with 1% iodine in methanol and drying (R4).

*b. Color Tests.* Imipramine gives blue to greenish colors with Froehde's, Mandelin's, Marquis', Mecke's, Reickard's, Flueckiger's, Schneider's, and Wasicky's reagents, by concentrated sulfuric and by fuming nitric acid (R1). Red colors are obtained with Vitali's reagent and by the addition of alkali to an acetone solution of the nitration product of imipramine (R1).

*c. Miscellaneous Analytical Characteristics.* Photomicrographs of crystals, X-ray diffraction data, and the ultraviolet absorption spectrum of imipramine have been published recently (R2, R3).

*d. Detection and Estimation in Urine.* Imipramine in urine can be detected and estimated by the pale olive to emerald green color and its duration which is obtained by mixing 1 ml urine with 1–2 ml of a reagent consisting of a mixture of equal volumes of 0.2% $K_2Cr_2O_7$, 30% (v/v) $H_2SO_4$, 50% (v/v) $HNO_3$, and 20% (v/v) $HClO_4$ (F1, F2). (See also the chapter by McBay and Algeri in this volume.)

2. ISOCARBOXAZIDE

*a. Paper Chromatography.* Isolation can be effected by ascending paper chromatography on Whatman No. 1 paper, pretreated with Mc-Ilvaine's phosphate-citrate buffer, pH 3.7, using butanol:methanol:water (50:40:10) (S2).

*b. Miscellaneous Analytical Characteristics.* Color reactions (S2, R1), photomicrographs of crystals (R2), X-ray diffraction data, and the ultraviolet absorption spectrum (R3) of isocarboxazide have been published recently.

3. NIALAMIDE

Rajeswaran and Kirk have reported color reactions, photomicrographs of crystals, X-ray diffraction data, and the ultraviolet absorption spectrum (R1, R2, R3).

4. PHENELZINE

*a. Thin Layer Chromatography.* Thin layer chromatography (Section III,B,2) gives a spot at $R_f$ of about 0.35 which shows blue fluorescence under 254-m$\mu$ ultraviolet light.

*b. Miscellaneous Analytical Characteristics.* Color reactions (R1), photomicrographs of crystals (R2), X-ray diffraction data, and the ultraviolet absorption spectrum of phenelzine (R3) have been reported.

*c. Colorimetric Determination.* Following isolation from tissue, either by direct extraction or by extraction from a protein-free filtrate (Section III,B,2), phenelzine can be estimated by the following procedure: the aqueous phenelzine isolate is buffered to pH 8 with 0.8 M phosphate buffer; 1/60 volume Folin–Ciocalteu reagent and 1/30 volume 5 N NaOH are added; the color is read at 750 m$\mu$ after not less than 10 or not more than 60 minutes (L1).

## REFERENCES

(B1) Burns, J. J., Rose, R. K., Goodwin, S., Reichenthal, J., Horning, E. C., and Brodie, B. B. *J. Pharmacol. Exptl. Therap.* 113, 481 (1955).
(B2) Burns, J. J., Rose, R. K., Chenkin, T., Goldman, A., Schulert, A., and Brodie, B. B. *J. Pharmacol. Exptl. Therap.* 109, 346 (1953).
(F1) Forrest, I. S., and Forrest, F. M. *Am. J. Psychiat.* 116, 840 (1960).
(F2) Forrest, I. S., and Forrest, F. M. *Am. J. Psychiat.* 116, 1021 (1960).
(K1) Konupcik, M. *Cesk. Farm.* 9, 239 (1960).

(L1) Lutz, W. H. (Warner Chilcott Labs.) Personal communication (1961).
(R1) Rajeswaran, P., and Kirk, P. L. *Bull. Narcotics, U. N. Dept. Social Affairs* **13**, 15 (1961).
(R2) Rajeswaran, P., and Kirk, P. L. *Bull. Narcotics, U. N. Dept. Social Affairs* **13**, 21 (1961).
(R3) Rajeswaran, P., and Kirk, P. L. *Bull. Narcotics, U. N. Dept. Social Affairs* **14**, 19 (1962).
(R4) Rieders, F., and Cordova, V. Unpublished data, Office of the Medical Examiner, Philadelphia, Pennsylvania, 1961.
(S1) Sahli, M., and Ziegler, H. *Arch. Pharm. Chemi* **68**, 186 (1961).
(S2) Schwartz, M. A. *Proc. Soc. Exptl. Biol. Med.* **107**, 613 (1961).

# Narcotics and Related Bases

by CHARLES G. FARMILO AND KLAUS GENEST

*Organic Chemistry and Narcotics Section, Food and Drug Directorate, Department of National Health and Welfare, Tunney's Pasture, Ottawa, Canada*

## I. General Introduction

### A. Scope and Definition

The purpose of this chapter is to review recent advances in methods for quantitative and qualitative determination of narcotics made since our recent work was published (F5). Brief reference will also be made to the methods of isolation from tissues and identification of the metabolites and unchanged narcotics in studies on metabolism. These methods are of particular interest to those engaged in analytical toxicology, and in drug control work, especially in the study of recidivism in the treatment of drug addicts.

In this chapter, any substance which is included in the list of materials under international conventions is by definition (C7) a narcotic (U1, U2). Their names are given in the conventions, or in the official notifications of the Secretary-General of the United Nations to member governments, or are the international nonproprietary names proposed or recommended by the World Health Organization. The generic names in Table I are in part the ones employed in the schedule to the Act for Control of Narcotic Drugs (E4) and in part in the work by Farmilo and Levi (F8).

Narcotic drugs may be divided into three broad classes depending on their origin:

    I. Natural narcotics
       *a.* Cannabis (marihuana)
       *b.* Coca leaf
       *c.* Opium
    II. Manufactured narcotics
       *a.* Opiates (morphine, heroin, oxycodone, etc.)
       *b.* Coca alkaloids (cocaine)
    III. Synthetic Narcotics
       Opioids (pethidine, methadone, etc.)

Synthetic narcotics are gaining importance for pain treatment in North America, while the manufactured drugs are most used elsewhere. Heroin, a manufactured drug, still the favorite North American drug of addiction, is the one most frequently isolated from police exhibits and identified in sudden death cases of poisoned addicts. The natural products are found in the international illicit narcotic traffic where opium is "the first, and still the foremost drug of addiction" (H1).

The era of synthetic narcotics started with the discovery of pethidine by Eisleb in 1939 (E3), a substance with potent analgesic effect, chemically unrelated to morphine. Such substances are called opioids (I2, I3) and are pharmacologically like morphine and other opiates. Several families of opioids have been discovered since. At the present time, eleven are under Canadian control: (1) iminoethanophenanthrofurans (morphines); (2) iminoethanophenanthrenes (morphinans); (3) benzazocines; (4) arylpiperidines (pethidine); (5) phenazepines; (6) diarylalkoneamines (methadone); (7) thiambutenes; (8) phenylalkoxams; (9) moramides; (10) ampromides; and (11) benzimidazoles. In addition (12) azabicyclooctanes (cocaine) and (13) dibenzopyrans (tetrahydrocannabinol), from the species *Erythroxylon* and *Cannabis sativa*, respectively, are controlled.

The latter two groups of drugs are included in narcotic schedules

TABLE I

FORMULAE of NARCOTICS by CHEMICAL FAMILIES

① IMINOETHANOPHENANTHROFURANS
(MORPHINES)

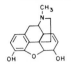

MORPHINE

② IMINOETHANOPHENANTHRENES
(MORPHINANS)

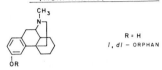

R = H
l, dl — ORPHAN

③ BENZAZOCINES

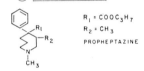

R = $CH_2CH_2C_6H_5$
PHENAZOCINE

④ ARYLPIPERIDINES

$R_1$ $R_3$ $R_6$ = H
$R_2$ = $COOC_2H_5$
$R_5$ = $CH_3$
PETHIDINE

⑤ PHENAZEPINES

$R_1$ = $COOC_3H_7$
$R_2$ = $CH_3$
PROPHEPTAZINE

⑥ DIARYLALKONEAMINES (AMIDONES)

$R_1$ = N $(CH_3)_2$
$R_2$ = $CH_3$
$R_3$ = H
METHADONE

⑦ THIAMBUTENES

$R_1$ $R_2$ = $C_2H_5$
$R_3$ = $CH_3$
DIETHYLTHIAMBUTENE

⑧ PHENYLALKOXAMS

DIOXAPHETYLBUTYRATE

⑨ MORAMIDES

d, l, & dl — MORAMIDE

⑩ AMPROMIDES

DIAMPROMIDE

⑪ BENZIMIDAZOLES

ETONITAZENE

⑫ AZABICYCLOOCTANES

COCAINE

⑬ BENZPYRANS

PYRAHEXYL

more for historic and sociological reasons than for morphinelike manifestations or addiction liability. There are thirteen separate chemical
families to consider from the analyst's viewpoint. Not all are of equal
importance in drug control; reference to some statistics may help to de-
cide the status of the individual narcotics.

## B. World Requirements for Narcotics (U3)

The most important opioids in volume of production, trade, and use
are listed in Table II in order of the estimated number of millions of
doses required. The annual consumption of pethidine has increased to

TABLE II

ESTIMATED WORLD REQUIREMENTS OF OPIOIDS
FOR 1961 IN ORDER OF NUMBER OF DOSES

| Names | | | World requirements | | |
|---|---|---|---|---|---|
| International | Trade | Source | Dosage[a] (mg) | Kg[b] | Millions of doses[c] |
| Pethidine | Demerol | Winthrop Laboratories Division of Sterling Drugs | 50[t] | 16,500 | 330.0 |
| Methadone | Dolophine | Lilly | 5[t] | 630 | 126.0 |
| Normethadone | Cophylac | Hoechst, Canada | 10[s] | 402 | 40.2 |
| Anileridine | Leritine | Merck | 25[t] | 831 | 33.2 |
| Levorphanol | Dromoran | Hoffmann La Roche | 2[t] | 40 | 20.0 |
| Phenazocine | Narphen | Smith & Nephew Pharm. | 2[i] | 29 | 14.5 |
| Dextromoramide | Palfium | Purdue Fredricks, Canada | 5[t] | 405 | 8.1 |
| Piminodine | Alvodine | Winthrop Laboratories | 50[t] | 300 | 6.0 |
| Dipipanone | Pipidone | Burroughs Wellcome | 25[i] | 74 | 3.0 |
| Alphaprodine | Nisentil | Hoffmann La Roche | 50[i] | 57 | 1.0 |
| Diphenoxylate | Lomotil | G. P. Searle Co. of Canada | 2.5[t] | 1 | 0.4 |
| Propoxyphene[d] | Darvon | Lilly | (65)[p] | (313) | (4.8) |

[a] Dosage forms available on the Canadian market: tablet dosage, *t*; injection solution, *i* (mg/ml); syrup, *s* (mg/ml); pulvule, *p*.

[b] These are the sums of the "Total of the Estimates" defined in article 5 of the 1931 Convention of all countries and territories of the world.

[c] The millions of dose values are computed by dividing the values of doses in milligrams into the total amount of drug required in kilograms.

[d] Propoxyphene was originally included on the international narcotic schedule in 1957; it was removed in 1958. The drug is still classified as a narcotic in Canada. It is sold in pulvule form. The numbers in brackets are based on Canadian requirements.

16.2 tons in 1960 from 13 tons in 1955. Per capita consumption is highest in the United States, with New Zealand and Denmark close behind. Trimeperidine, which is akin to pethidine, until 1960 was produced (1223 kg) and consumed (1107 kg) exclusively in the USSR. Consumption of methadone has declined from 464 kg in 1956 to 420 kg in 1960. In addition to the above narcotics, which have world-wide importance, ketobemidone (72,7),[1] properidine (12,2), diethylthiambutene (7,2), dimethylthiambutene (1,1), isomethadone (3,1), and etoxeridine (1,1) must also be considered important in certain countries.

These statistics are included to give the reader some idea of the drugs most likely to be encountered in the control of the illicit traffic. It is of some encouragement to note that of the fifty synthetic narcotic drugs now under international control not even one half have gone beyond the experimental stage. The reason for this is that governments have agreed to the limitation of the number of narcotics to be used. The efficacy of world control depends on effective national control laws, for the enforcement of which sound physicochemical methods for drug detection are required. The advances in narcotic analytical methodology are the subject of this chapter which is divided into two main parts; the work reported in the literature, and work completed in this laboratory.

## II. Literature Review

### A. Introduction

This review outlines some of the significant developments in analytical chemistry of narcotics and related bases. The years 1959–61 are covered including earlier papers not mentioned in our Chapter 7 of *Toxicology*, Volume II (F5). Special attention is given to new or improved methods not previously used in narcotics analysis such as thin layer chromatography and gas chromatography. The scope of compounds comprises narcotics and their metabolites and related compounds which are found associated with them as impurities or adulterants. Also compounded drugs in pharmaceuticals and those reported to be used as substitutes for narcotics are included. Revitch and Weiss (R2), for example, report on the illicit use of the antihistamine, tripelennamine hydrochloride, as a substitute for narcotics in penal institutes. No systematic literature coverage for all related drugs such as antihistamines or phenothiazines is made.

---

[1] The number in parentheses before the comma is kilograms consumed while the number after the comma is the number of consuming countries.

## B. Qualitative Methods

### 1. Extraction Methods

Morgan (M15) describes a method for the rapid detection of organic bases in urine on the 1 ppm level. The method was later modified (M16) to accommodate larger amounts (several 100 $\mu$g) for subsequent IR spectrophotometry in microcells. The general technique to detect morphine and other alkaloids is as follows:

The urine sample is adjusted to pH 9 with sodium hydroxide. It is then extracted once by a conventional technique with about one fifth of its volume of chloroform and transferred after filtration to a test tube so that the height of liquid is 5–7 cm. A strip of chloroform/water–washed Whatman 3 MM paper, 7 × 1.5 cm, is spotted 2 cm from one end with drops of 0.25 and 0.5 N sulfuric acid and placed in the chloroform extract. The extract is agitated with a stream of dry oxygen-free nitrogen. After some time the strip is removed from the chloroform. Plots of time required vs concentration of caffeine, morphine, cocaine, and nicotine for a variety of solvents are given in the original. After drying the strip is briefly exposed to ammonia vapors, treated in a current of air, and developed paper chromatographically in solvents such as BuOH:HCl,-conc.:H$_2$O (50:10:20) or isobutylmethylketone:AcOH:H$_2$O (20:10:5).

Makisumi *et al.* (M3) investigate the extraction of morphine with ether in the Stas–Otto procedure. They find maximal extraction at pH 10 whereas 100% recovery for apomorphine and cocaine is achieved at pH 7 and for procaine at pH 9. Niyogi *et al.* (N5) report on the recovery of codeine and strychnine from animal tissue extracts by means of a Dowex-50 ion-exchange column.

### 2. Microcrystal and Color Tests

Microchemical crystal and color tests for the newer synthetic narcotics, phenazocine and trimeperidine, were reported. Ternikova (T6) describes color and precipitation reactions of trimeperidine as given in Table III. The best reagent is said to be Marquis' (T5). The sensitivity towards this reagent is found to be 0.3 mg in alkaline extracts of tissue. The sensitivity can be increased when dichloroethane instead of chloroform is used for the extraction. Five mg% of trimeperidine can be detected in decomposing cadaver material up to 1 month old, whereas in 2- and 3.5-months-old material these limits are increased to 10 and 100 mg%, respectively.

Microchemical data on another pair of new synthetic narcotics, phenazocine and metazocine, are given by Clarke (C4). Suitable color

## TABLE III
### Precipitation Tests for Trimeperidine (T6)

| Reagent | Reaction |
|---|---|
| $BiI_3$-KI | White precipitate |
| $HgI_2$-KI | White precipitate |
| Phosphomolybdate | White precipitate |
| Chloraminic acid | Yellow precipitate |
| Bromine water | Brilliant yellow |
| $H_2SO_4$/HCHO | Red-purple, brown on heating |
| $H_2SO_4$/vanadic acid | Red-purple, deep blue on heating |
| 1 part $NH_4NO_3$ + 3 parts $H_2SO_4$ | Yellow |

tests for phenazocine are: Marquis'[2] (brown), Fröhde's[2] (bright blue→ yellow→ green), and the diazo test with $p$-nitroaniline[3] as coupling agent brown, turning bluish grey on drying). Microcrystal tests which distinguish the optical isomers of phenazocine from one another and from metazocine are tabulated in Table IV. Microcolor and crystal tests of phenazocine hydrobromide which distinguish it from morphine, codeine, and pethidine are described by Latshaw and MacDonnell (L1). Sodium tungstate (1% in $H_2O$) gives a reddish violet and $p$-dimethylamino-benzaldehyde (10% in glacial acetic acid) gives a violet changing to reddish violet color. Mercuric-potassium iodide is recommended as a microcrystal reagent.

## TABLE IV
### Microcrystal Tests for Benzazocines (C4)

| Compound | KI | $Na_2CO_3$ | Picrolonic acid |
|---|---|---|---|
| (+) Phenazocine | Oily rosettes | Bunches of irregular prisms | Oily precipitate |
| (−) Phenazocine | Oily amorphous precipitate | Fans of oily needles | Shell-like rosettes |
| Metazocine | No precipitate | Dense rosettes of prisms | Curving blades |

Publication of tests for the older narcotics continues. Wachsmuth (W1) tabulates results on color tests with eighteen reagents and ten narcotics of the morphine type. The following two new tests for morphine and heroin are suggested.

[2] F5, p. 546, Table LIX.
[3] F5, p. 573, Table LXXIII.

*Micro color test for morphine and derivatives* (Y1): A small amount of morphine is dissolved in 1–2 drops of sulfuric acid, 1 drop of nitrobenzene is added, and the mixture is heated until it just boils. After cooling it is diluted with 3–4 drops of water, and shaken with 1–2 drops of butanol. A violet color (max 552 m$\mu$) develops in the butanol layer. Limit is 2 $\mu$g morphine hydrochloride.

*Color test for heroin* (L4): Ten drops of a nitric/phosphoric acid mixture (12 ml HNO$_3$, concentrated, and 38 ml H$_3$PO$_4$, 85%) are placed in a 5-ml glass-stoppered centrifuge tube and 3.25 ml chloroform added. The heroin is washed into the tube with a little chloroform. The tube is shaken vigorously for 30 seconds. The bottom layer acquires a color which is a function of the amount of heroin present. The colors produced after 10 minutes are shown in Table V. Of twenty-five other narcotics and possible diluents or adulterants only antipyrine has a positive reaction. The latter substance, however, gives a negative Marquis reaction.

TABLE V
COLOR TEST FOR HEROIN ACCORDING TO LERNER (L4)

| Amount of heroin | Color |
| --- | --- |
| 10 $\mu$g | Light yellow |
| 1 mg | Yellow-brown |
| 10 mg | Dark red-brown |
| Blank | Light green |

3. PAPER CHROMATOGRAPHY

This technique is now used, mainly for qualitative sample-screening purposes. Büchi's system (toluene:isobutanol:water) is applied to the separation of opium alkaloids in poppy extracts (I5) and to commercial morphine and codeine preparations such as injectable solutions of morphine, with or without atropine, opium tinctures, and codeine in sirups on paper soaked with calcium hydroxide solution (G5). Systems suggested earlier by Goldbaum and Kazyak (G8) are used by Hilf *et al.* (H5) the study R$_f$ values and behavior under UV light of fifteen alkaloids and related compounds, including five narcotics. Procaine is found frequently as an adulterant in heroin seizures. It can be detected by Sanchez' reagent (10 ml of aqueous furfural, 5 drops glacial acetic acid) on the chromatogram. It is the only nonnarcotic compound among twenty narcotics which gives a positive reaction when tested (A15). Other impurities in heroin seizures were investigated by Nakamura (N1) who suggests three solvent systems (BuOH:H$_2$O:AcOH, 10:5:1; isoamyl OH:H$_2$O:AcOH, 10:5:1; isoamyl OH:H$_2$O:NH$_4$OH, 10:5:1) to separate

$O^3$- and $O^6$-monoacetylmorphine from heroin and $O^6$-acetylcodeine from codeine. Paper with a content of 9–16% succinyl groups is reported to yield good separations of opium alkaloids with conventional solvents (M9).

Some attention is given to the paper chromatography of cannabis: Asahina (A3, A16), Davis and Farmilo (D2a), Korte and Sieper (K16, K17), De Ropp (D4), Schultz and Mohrmann (S13a), and Kolšek *et al.* (K11a) suggest various solvent systems and sprays for the identification of the cannabinols in cannabis.[4] Genest and Farmilo (G4) describe solvent systems for the separation of the most important natural and synthetic narcotics.[5] Separations of toxicologically important bases by centrifugally accelerated paper chromatography can be achieved in 5–15 minutes. Dal Cortivo *et al.* (D1) use a Hi Speed Chromatograph at 750–1200 rpm and separate basic constituents of narcotic seizures and preparations of urine and bile extracts on phosphate (pH 5) impregnated paper with butanol, saturated with buffer. The $R_f$'s by this procedure are slightly higher than those obtained by the ascending method. Paper chromatography is used to detect alkaloids in toxicological analysis of foods. Added amounts of codeine, veratrine, quinine, and narcotine (0.1 gm drug/100 gm food) in a variety of foods may be detected by paper chromatography on formamide-impregnated paper with chloroform as mobile phase (K11). Street (S24) describes systems in which a mixture of morphine, nalorphine, and codeine can be separated (see Table VI).

TABLE VI

SYSTEMS FOR SEPARATION OF MORPHINE, NALORPHINE, AND CODEINE (S24)

| | $R_f$ value in system | | |
|---|---|---|---|
| Compound | 1 | 2 | 3 |
| Morphine | 0.0 | 0.57 | 0.80 |
| Nalorphine | 0.0 | 0.41 | 0.38 |
| Codeine | 0.84 | 0.58 | 0.62 |

*System 1.* Mobile phase: 0.2 N ammonia on Whatman Ecteola cellulose anion-exchange paper, 4 × 4½ inches; ascending; time, 5 minutes.

*System 2.* Mobile phase: $M/15$ phosphate buffer, pH 7.4, on Whatman No. 1 treated with glycerol monoricinoleate (10% in acetone); horizontal; time, 90 minutes.

*System 3.* Mobile phase: $M/15$ phosphate buffer, pH 7.4, on What-

---

[4] For details of procedure see Section V,B,2 of this chapter.
[5] For details of procedure see Section III,B,8 of this chapter.

man No. 1 treated with tributyrin (10% in acetone); ascending at 86° in incubator; time, 20 minutes.

## 4. ELECTROPHORESIS

Electrophoresis is found to be a useful tool in the toxicologists' laboratory. Willner (W8) studied the electrophoretic properties of pure morphine, hydromorphone, codeine, oxycodone, hydrocodone, thebacon, pethidine, ketobemidone, atropine, and cocaine at 2 ma and 110 volts. Glycine/NaOH buffers of various pH's are used to separate several binary mixtures. A six-component mixture (morphine, ketobemidone, oxycodone, codeine, cocaine, and atropine) separates at pH 11.1–11.2 during the usual 15 hours running time. The mixture morphine/hydromorphone could not be separated. Pholcodine in tablets, sirups, or suppositories can be differentiated from morphine, codeine, and ethylmorphine by electrophoresis within 30–60 minutes in 1% acetic acid as electrolyte (R4). A rapid method requiring 25 minutes using a pH 3 agar gel medium for separation of alkaloids from tissue extracts under a high potential gradient (250 volts at about 100 ma) is described by Williams *et al.* (W7). Spengler (S19) investigates analgesics in urine by high voltage electrophoresis. Niyogi *et al.* (N6) describe the detection of added morphine, codeine, brucine, strychnine, quinine, and atropine in serums by electrophoresis.

## 5. THIN LAYER CHROMATOGRAPHY (TLC)

This technique which is an application of chromatographic principles based on adsorption phenomena rather than solvent distribution, as in paper chromatography, evolves from the work of Izmailov and Schraiber (I4), who, in 1938, separated organic compounds on aluminum oxide scattered over glass plates. Later, Kirchner *et al.* (K7) introduced the "Chromatostrip" technique, using narrow glass strips on which adsorbent was glued with starch adhesive. However, the difficulty of preparing good quality adsorbents and obtaining a uniform layer of adsorbent prevented a universal acceptance of the method. These problems were overcome by Stahl (S20) who devised a commercially useful standardized adsorbent (silica gel and aluminum oxide containing about 5% calcium sulfate as a binder) which gives reproducible results. TLC has quickly found wide application to many groups of organic compounds (W11, S21).

The main advantages of TLC as compared with paper chromatography are:

(*i*) Great speed—most chromatograms require only 20–30 minutes of separation time;

(*ii*) Corrosive spray reagents can be applied;

(*iii*) The developed plate can be subjected to temperatures which may be deleterious to filter paper;

(*iv*) Frequently sharper separations can be achieved;

(*v*) Lower limits of detection have been reported compared with paper chromatography.

Attempts to apply TLC (then called "surface chromatography") to narcotics analysis were made by Borke and Kirch (B17) who, using 1,4-dioxane as solvent, separated some opium alkaloids on glass plates covered with a composite, buffered, fluorescent paste. Recently several workers have successfully applied Stahl's procedure. Nürnberg (N7) reports on the separation of a mixture of basic drugs. In increasing order of $R_f$, parabromdylamine, codeine, methylephedrine, and phenyldimethylpyrazolone may be separated on Silica Gel G layers with methanol:acetate buffer pH 4.62 (3 + 7) as solvent. Machata (M1) applies Stas–Otto extracts directly to TLC. For the acid extracts chloroform with 15% ether is a suitable solvent, whereas bases can be chromatographed with methanol. Plate I contains $R_f$ values for a variety of toxicologically important compounds in these solvents. A good reproducibility of $R_f$'s is reported. All experiments were made on 250-$\mu$ layers of Silica Gel G. The front of 14 cm was obtained in 1 hour. The same author reports a suicide case caused by opium tincture. One hundred and eight milligrams of opium alkaloids are found in the stomach contents. A clear separation of morphine, codeine, and narcotine is observed in spite of the high concentration of the alkaloids. The spray reagent for bases is Dragendorff's and acetic iodine/potassium iodide solution [5% iodine in 10% KI (5 ml)] are mixed with water (3 ml) and 2 N acetic acid (5 ml). In cases where no suitable reagent can be found the author recommends heating of the developed plates to about 500°. The substances then appear as charred spots. Bäumler and Rippstein (B13) recommend TLC for alkaline/ether extracts of stomach contents, stomach washes, blood, and urine. The time of development of the chromatograms for a distance of 10 cm is 30 minutes for basic material and for barbiturate-like substances 45 minutes on Silica Gel G plates. For the latter chloroform:acetone (9:1) is recommened as mobile phase. Methanol or methanol:acetone (1:1) is found to be useful for most alkaloids. Rauwolfia alkaloids and phenothiazines, however, give tailing spots. The solvent methanol:acetone:triethanolamine (1:1:0.03) was more generally useful for basic compounds. Results obtained in this system for narcotics are shown in Table VII. Other mobile phases recommended for the separation of morphine and its derivatives are: chloroform:ethanol (9:1 or 9:2) on Silica Gel G layer, dimethylformamide:diethylamine:ethanol:

R_f   VALUES

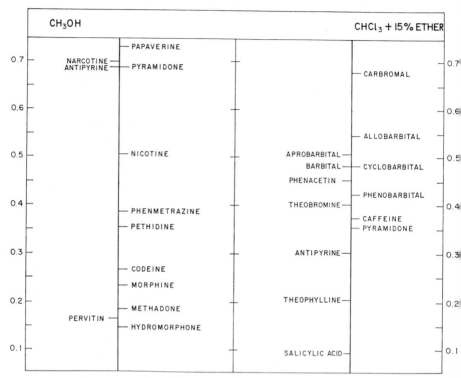

PLATE I. R_f values for toxicologically important compounds on thin layer chromatograms according to Machata (M1).

ethylacetate (5:2:20:75) on layers of cellulose powder, and benzene: heptane:chloroform:diethylamine (6:5:1:0.02) on the same material impregnated with formamide (T3).

Waldi *et al.* (W2) report on a systematic analysis of fifty-four alkaloids by TLC. For development on Silica Gel G layers the mobile phase has to contain a basic component in order to free the base and bind the acidic groups to avoid tailing. Basic layer material such as Aluminum Oxide G or Silica Gel G pretreated with sodium hydroxide can also be used, but the Silica Gel G plates in conjunction with a basic mobile phase generally produce sharper separations. The following solvents are recommended:

1. Chloroform:acetone:diethylamine (5:4:1)
2. Chloroform:diethylamine (9:1) (for morphine, hydromorphone, codeine, dihydrocodeine, hydrocodeinone)

TABLE VII

R$_f$ Values of Narcotics and Related Alkaloids from Thin Layer
Chromatograms According to Bäumler and Rippstein (B13)

| Compound | R$_f$ Values | Color in UV light | Color with Dragendorff's reagent |
|---|---|---|---|
| Narceine | 0.22–0.24 | Blue | Violet |
| Dextromethorphan | 0.22–0.24 | — | Red |
| Levorphanol | 0.27–0.29 | — | Red |
| Hydromorphone | 0.27–0.29 | Dark | Yellow |
| Hydrocodone | 0.28–0.30 | — | Orange |
| Thebacon | 0.29–0.33 | Yellowish | Orange |
| Ethylmorphine | 0.36–0.38 | — | Red |
| Morphine | 0.39–0.41 | Dark | Orange |
| Thebaine | 0.40–0.42 | Dark | Red |
| Codeine | 0.42–0.44 | — | Red |
| Methadone | 0.47–0.49 | — | Red |
| Ketobemidone | 0.55–0.57 | Dark | Orange |
| Pethidine | 0.55–0.57 | — | Red |
| Cocaine | 0.60–0.62 | — | Orange |
| Narcotine | 0.81–0.83 | Bright light blue | Orange |
| Papaverine | 0.81–0.83 | Bright yellow | Orange |
| Dextromoramide | 0.86–0.88 | — | Orange |

3. Cyclohexane:chloroform:diethylamine (5:4:1) (for cocaine)
4. Cyclohexane:diethylamine (9:1)
5. Benzene:ethylacetate:diethylamine (7:2:1)

On Aluminum Oxide G layers:

1. Chloroform
2. Cyclohexane:chloroform (3:7) + 0.05% diethylamine (3 drops)

On Silica Gel G layers pretreated with 0.1 N NaOH:

Methanol

TLC on Silica Gel G layers is also used by Vidic (V4) for six narcotics and atropine. Dextromoramide (R$_f$ 0.85) can be separated from its metabolite in urine (0.57) and from dextromethorphan (0.26), methadone (0.42), and normethadone (0.59) in 0.1 N methanolic ammonia. Cochin and Daly (C5) report R$_f$ values of analgesic drugs after extraction from pH 9.0 urine with ethylene chloride:isoamylalcohol (9:1) on Silica Gel G and Aluminum Oxide G with various mobile phases. Their results can be found in Table VIII.

TABLE VIII

R$_f$ VALUES OF IODOPLATINATE POSITIVE COMPOUNDS
EXTRACTABLE FROM URINE AT pH 9.0[a] (C5)

| Compound | R$_f$ values Silica Gel | | | | R$_f$ values Alumina | |
|---|---|---|---|---|---|---|
|  | S1 | S2 | S3 | S4 | A1 | A2 |
| Chlorpromazine | 0.48 | 0.79 | 0.93 | 0.35 | 0.80 | 0.98 |
| Cocaine | 0.74 | 0.45 | 0.98 | 0.39 | 0.61 | 0.96 |
| Codeine | 0.40 | 0.52 | 0.46 | 0.32 | 0.72 | 0.65 |
| Diacetylmorphine | 0.47 | 0.54 | 0.80 | 0.43 | 0.72 | 0.83 |
| Levorphanol | 0.34 | 0.75 | 0.62 | 0.29 | 0.76 | 0.91 |
| Mescaline | 0.18 | 0.81 | 0.30 | 0.30 | 0.36 | 0.53 |
| Methadone | 0.53 | 0.78 | 0.96 | 0.20 | 0.78 | 0.98 |
| Morphine | 0.40 | 0.55 | 0.17 | 0.34 | 0.59 | 0.18 |
| Nalorphine | 0.82 | 0.71 | 0.34 | 0.75 | 0.72 | 0.20 |
| Nicotine | 0.58 | 0.27 | 0.90 | 0.44 | 0.72 | 0.90 |
| Normorphine | 0.14 | 0.76 | 0.05 | 0.16 | 0.33 | 0.11 |
| Pethidine | 0.51 | 0.64 | 0.90 | 0.44 | 0.77 | 0.98 |
| Phenazocine | 0.90 | 0.93 | 0.93 | 0.59 | 0.86 | 0.98 |
| Propoxyphene | 0.80 | 0.82 | 0.97 | 0.53 | 0.84 | 1.00 |
| Tripelennamine | 0.50 | 0.46 | 0.93 | 0.28 | 0.76 | 0.98 |

[a] Solvent systems:

S1 = ethyl alcohol:pyridine:dioxane:water (50:20:25:5);
S2 = ethyl alcohol:acetic acid:water (60:30:10);
S3 = ethyl alcohol:dioxane:benzene:ammonium hydroxide (5:40:50:5);
S4 = methyl alcohol:butanol:benzene:water (60:15:10:15);
A1 = butanol:butyl ether:acetic acid (40:50:10);
A2 = butanol:butyl ether:ammonium hydroxide (25:70:5).

## 6. GAS-LIQUID PARTITION CHROMATOGRAPHY (GLPC)

Despite the impact of GLPC on many other fields of analytical chemistry, studies on narcotics were rare, until recently. Most narcotics have a relatively high boiling point or are solids. Stainier and Gloesener (S22) made use of the fact that some narcotics are esters of lower alcohols. They hydrolyze cocaine and pethidine in 3.5% potassium hydroxide and gas-chromatographed the resulting methyl and ethyl alcohols, respectively, on a 1-meter Carbowax 1500 column using triethanolamine as stationary phase and hydrogen as carrier gas at 70°. The direct analysis of narcotics was possible only after column material for high boiling substances became available. Lloyd *et al.* (L9) separate alkaloids on a 6 ft × 4 mm Chromosorb W (80–100 mesh) column containing 2–3% of the silicone rubber SE-30 as stationary phase. The retention times for a number of alkaloids at 204° using an ionization detector and argon gas (pressure 15 psi) are given in Table IX.

The same column material was later used by Kingston and Kirk (K6)

TABLE IX

RETENTION TIME VALUES OF OPIUM ALKALOIDS ACCORDING TO LLOYD *et al.* (L9)

| Compound | RT values (min) |
|---|---|
| Codeine | 8.2 |
| Neopine | 9.1 |
| Morphine | 11.0 |
| Thebaine | 13.2 |
| Laudanosine | 21.0 |
| Papaverine | 35.3 |
| Gnoscopine | 90.6 |

and by Farmilo and Davis (F9)[6] for the analysis of phenolic compounds in cannabis resin.

## 7. UV SPECTRA

UV absorbance curves which can be helpful in the identification of marihuana in organic solvents (A3, A13) and in 0.01 N acid and base are reported (S8). The latter paper describes a purification procedure in which the petrol ether extract is washed consecutively with 5% sulfuric acid, 50% ethanol, and 10% sodium hydroxide to avoid background absorbance due to accompanying material from other herbs. Characteristic maxima and minima for marihuana identification are shown in Table X.

TABLE X

UV MAXIMA AND MINIMA OF MARIHUANA ACCORDING TO SCARINGELLI (S8)

| Media | Maximum (m$\mu$) | Minimum (m$\mu$) |
|---|---|---|
| Acid | 275–280 | 250 |
| Base | 285; 320–325 | — |
| Differential | 245; 335 | 270 |

Gautier *et al.* (G1) give data on UV curves and extinction coefficients of alkaloids precipitated as tetraphenylborides, including those for cocaine, codeine, ethylmorphine, morphine, and pholcodine. Weijlard reports UV data for anileridine (W6).

## C. Quantitative Methods

## 1. EXTRACTION

A method which is based essentially on liquid/liquid extraction was

---

[6] For details of method see Section V,B,4 of this chapter.

214          *Charles G. Farmilo and Klaus Genest*

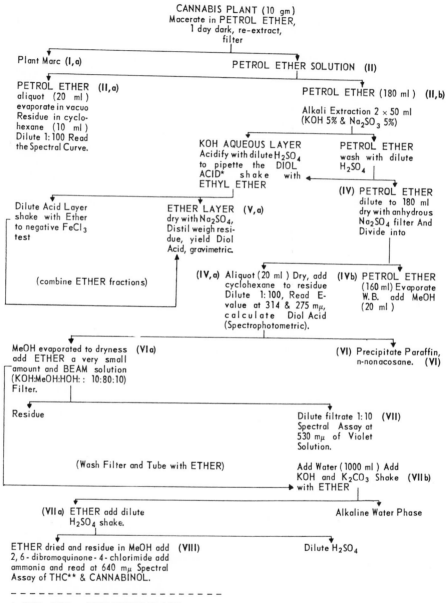

PLATE II. Flow sheet of procedure for extraction of cannabinols and *n*-non-
acosane from cannabis according to Schultz and Haffner (S13).

published by Schultz and Haffner (S13) for the analysis of cannabinols in marihuana. A flow sheet of the extraction procedure is given in Plate II.

*Procedure.* The fairly finely divided drug (10 gm) is macerated with sufficient petrol ether, kept for 1 day in the dark, decanted, and the marc re-extracted. The combined solvents are diluted to 200 ml. An aliquot (20 ml) is taken and evaporated at reduced pressure to dryness. The residue is dissolved in spectrally pure cyclohexane (10 ml) and diluted 1:100. The extinction value of this solution is obtained at 314 m$\mu$.

The remaining petrol ether solution (180 ml) is shaken with an aqueous solution (2 × 50 ml) of potassium hydroxide (5%) containing sodium sulfite (5%). The alkaline aqueous phase is immediately separated and acidified with dilute sulfuric acid. Rapid work is required at this stage. The petrol ether layer is shaken with dilute aqueous sulfuric acid and separated and the etheric layer dried over anhydrous sodium sulfate, then diluted to 180 ml. An aliquot (20 ml) is dried at reduced pressure and the residue dissolved in cyclohexane (10 ml) and diluted 1:100. The extinction values are measured at 314 m$\mu$ and 275 m$\mu$ and the acid content calculated as follows:

$$\text{acid content} = \frac{\Delta E \times 10^4}{1.9 \times 10^3} \text{ gm}/100 \text{ gm}$$

where $\Delta E$ = difference in the extinctions.

The dilute aqueous sulfuric acid solution from above is now shaken with ethyl ether repeatedly until a negative test with methanolic-ferric chloride (5%) is obtained. The combined etheric phases are dried over anhydrous sodium sulfate, filtered, the ether solution evaporated at reduced pressure, and the residue weighed. The extraction can be hastened by the addition of a small amount of petrol ether to the ethyl ether. The weight obtained is multiplied by 11.1 and the resulting value is then equivalent to the weight of the diol acid in gm/100 gm [on Plate II, see (V,a)].

The remaining petrol ether extract (160 ml) is evaporated on a water bath. The residue is taken up in methanol (20 ml) [in Plate II see (IVa)], which causes a paraffin hydrocarbon (*n*-nonacosane) to precipitate. The filtrate is evaporated, dried, and weighed. The final weight multiplied by 12.5 gives the quantity of phenols and ballast substances in gm/100 gm [Plate II see (VIa)].

The residue is taken up in ether (several drops) and Beam's reagent (5 ml, KOH:HOH:CH$_3$OH; 10:10:80) is added then allowed to stand in the air for 18 hours. The violet-colored solution is filtered, the filter washed with methanol, and the solution diluted with methanol to a volume of 10 ml. The whole is diluted to 1:10. The extinction value is obtained at 530 m$\mu$. The cannabidiol content is calculated using the extinction coefficient of 3.88. Allowing for the fact that out of 200 ml only 160 ml are employed for the assay, the factor then becomes 3.1. The following equation is employed [in Plate II see (VII)]:

$$\text{cannabidiol content} = \frac{E \times 100}{3.1 \times 100} \text{ gm}/100 \text{ gm}$$

The filter and tube are washed with ether. The violet solution (Plate II, VIIb) is then diluted with water (1000 ml) and after the addition of KOH (15 gm) and $K_2CO_3$ (10 gm) is shaken with ether, with which the above wash ether is then combined. The collected ether solution is washed with dilute sulfuric acid and then the ether evaporated on a water bath. The residue is dissolved in methanol (10 ml). An aliquot (0.5 ml) is taken and to it is added 2,6-dibromoquinonechlorimide (0.5 ml, 0.1%) in methanol. Ammoniacal methanol (1%) is added to make a solution of 10 ml. After $\frac{1}{2}$ hour the extinction value at 640 m$\mu$ is determined using a blank of the dibromoquinonechlorimide in ammoniacal methanol (0.5 ml with ammoniacal methanol, 9 ml) [in Plate II see (VIII)].

The amount of tetrahydrocannabinol and cannabinol is calculated in terms of phenol using the extinction value as 2.63, in which the dilution factor 1:200 is included. The factor 2.1 is based on 160 ml of petrol ether extract.

$$\text{remaining phenols} = \frac{E}{2.1} \text{ gm}/100 \text{ gm}$$

## 2. Spectrophotometry

Sakurai (S1, S2, S3, S4, S5) describes several color reactions for the opium alkaloids morphine, codeine, thebaine, narcotine, and papaverine and after partition in solvents their colorimetric application. The Pride and Stern method (P18) is found to give satisfactory results for morphine analysis in galenical preparations (J3). Another colorimetric method makes use of the violet color (maximum, 490 m$\mu$) which codeine develops with ferric chloride in presence of a mixture of sulfuric and acetic acids after heating. The reaction is also positive for morphine, heroin, and ethylmorphine. Ethylmorphine can be analyzed in presence of codeine by adding sodium arsenate and measuring at 530 m$\mu$ (W1). Vacek and Tyrolova (V1) report the assay of trimeperidine and ketobemidone. Both narcotics can be eluted from Amberlite IRA 400 columns with 0.1 N HCl. Trimeperidine can then be estimated in the ultraviolet region at 258 m$\mu$, whereas ketobemidone is assayed by colorimetry with diazotized sulfanilic acid. Both methods are applied to injectable solutions of the narcotics. A spectrophotometric assay of morphine in opium and paregoric is described by Milos (M10). The method consists of extraction of opium with boiling dilute acetic acid, treatment of the extract with barium acetate, and final extraction with chloroform:isobutanol from ammoniacal solution. The quantation is made by differential UV spectrophotometry in acid vs alkaline solutions at 300 m$\mu$. The results of a collaborative study of the simultaneous determination of heroin and quinine in powdered samples containing inert material are reported by Pro (P20). Heroin is measured at 297.5 m$\mu$ and quinine at 330 m$\mu$ in alkaline solution. Five collaborators found values for both bases within a 10% range of the theoretical values. Vidic (V3) developed a microprocedure in which the sensitivity of the UV spectrophotometric quantation of morphine derivatives after elution from paper chromatograms is increased 3.5 to 9 times over the UV assay of the free bases by treatment with 72% sulfuric acid. The acid treatment causes a dehydration reaction to form apomorphine-type compounds in case of morphine, codeine, and dihydrocodeine, whereas compounds containing a ketone group and levorphanol are changed to a lesser degree.

*Procedure (V3) for Morphine, Hydromorphone, and Levorphanol.* Chromatography is carried out by an ascending technique on paper washed with 0.1 N HCl. After chromatography the spot is cut to form a pointed edge, layed on a HCl-wetted paper strip of the same width, and the base eluted with 0.1 N HCl in a capillary apparatus (M8). In the course of 2 hours 1–2 ml of eluate are collected and transferred to a 50-ml stoppered flask and the pH adjusted to 9.0 by addition of 0.05 gm of a $Na_2CO_3/NaHCO_3$ mixture (31:100). The eluate is then extracted for 3 minutes with 30 ml chloroform:isopropanol (90:10), and the extract separated and evaporated to dryness. The residue is treated with 5 ml 72% sulfuric acid, transferred into a 25-ml volumetric flask, stoppered, and heated for 1 hour to 85°C. After cooling, the UV absorbance is measured against a similarly treated blank and compared with standard curves. An average yield of 92% is reported. The maxima are: morphine 276 m$\mu$, hydromorphone 280 m$\mu$, and levorphanol 288 m$\mu$.

*Procedure for Codeine, Dihydrocodeine, Hydrocodone, and Oxycodone.* The procedure is the same except that unwashed paper is employed for chromatography. The capillary elution is carried out for 3 hours and the average recovery is 95%. The maxima are: codeine 245 and 272 m$\mu$, dihydrocodeine 251 m$\mu$, and hydrocodone and oxycodone 280 m$\mu$. Also the ratios between the maxima and minima in case of morphine (276/252 m$\mu$) and dihydrocodeine (251/232 m$\mu$) can serve to control background absorbance. A colorimetric method for thebaine based on its conversion in acidic solution to thebenine (A12) and the mechanism of the diazo reaction of thebaine and codeine are reported (P10).

A fluorometric method applied for pharmaceutical preparations of codeine and ethylmorphine is reported by Balatre *et al.* (B8): 0.25 to 2.5-$\mu$g amounts of the compounds are heated with concentrated sulfuric acid, then treated with water and ammonia and their fluorescence spectra measured in a colorimeter equipped with 365-m$\mu$ filter. The maximum for codeine is 478 m$\mu$, and for ethylmorphine 499 m$\mu$. Another fluorometric method for the simultaneous estimation of pure morphine and codeine is based on the observation that both morphine and codeine show a fluorescent maximum at 350 m$\mu$ in 0.1 N sulfuric acid. At pH 10–12, however, the fluorescence of morphine is negligible whereas that of codeine remains unchanged (B33). Pro (P19) reports the determination of methadone in tablets by UV and IR spectrophotometry.

### 3. CHROMATOGRAPHY

Several authors applied quantitative chromatographic methods to the analysis of opium alkaloids. Baerheim-Svendsen and Bergane (B1, B2) compare results for the morphine assay in opium by paper chromatography with those obtained by electrophoresis. The opium extract is chromatographed in BuOH:AcOH:$H_2O$ (4:1:5), the morphine spot is cut out and eluted, and the color produced by the nitroso reaction is measured. Electrophoresis is carried out in 10% acetic acid for 3 hours at 500 volts. The morphine-containing area is treated in a similar fashion as in the paper chromatographic procedure. The morphine results for four opium samples are appreciably higher by the electrophoretic procedure. The authors conclude that the paper chromatographic procedure gives better separations. Ion-exchange separations are used for the colorimetric microdetermination of tropane alkaloids in the presence of morphine (S18) on Dowex 1 columns. Quantitative partitions on Celite columns are reported for codeine and its derivatives from ephedrine (K14, K15). Secondary alkaloids in opium are separated by Büchi and Huber (B37) after elution from an alumina column on a Celite/pH 4.8 phosphate buffer into three fractions. Papaverine/narcotine and thebaine are eluted with ether:benzene (3:1) and codeine with chloroform containing 1% ethanol, saturated with ammonia. The final determination of the alkaloids after separation of the papaverine/narcotine fraction is made gravimetrically or titrimetrically as reineckates. In the field of cannabis analysis chromatographic methods are used by several authors. Korte and Sieper (K16) succeed in isolating crystalline cannabidiol and tetrahydrocannabinol from *Cannabis sativa* by purification of hemp extracts on a neutral alumina column and subsequent 138- and 188-stage countercurrent distribution of the eluate. De Ropp (D4) isolates tetra-hydrocannabinol and cannabinol from a methanolic extract of the flowering tops of *Cannabis sativa* after purification over a Florisil column and partition chromatography on a Celite column using cyclohexane as the mobile and *N,N*-dimethylformamide as the stationary phase for the fractionation.

## 4. OTHER METHODS

Several papers deal with critical studies of the morphine assay in opium by various pharmacopoeial methods (T4, R3, B35, B36). The four authors highly recommend the Mannich method, in which morphine dinitrophenyl ether is precipitated, and volumetrically or gravimetrically assayed, after purification of the opium extract by acidic alumina column chromatography. A nephelometric method for the determination of morphine in ripe poppy capsules has been developed (K13). Morphine can also be determined by oxidation to pseudomorphine and potentio-metric titration with zinc sulfate (P16) or by nonaqueous titration in presence of codeine with isopropanol/potassium hydroxide (W10). The polarographic quantation of morphine as 2-nitrosomorphine in small samples of blood plasma is described by Milthers (M11). The method permits determination of morphine in blood at concentrations of 1 $\mu$g/ml with an average recovery of 96 $\pm$ 5%. The assay of methadone is also investigated by polarography (J1). Several methods for the analysis of dextromoramide in its dosage form are reported by Demoen (D3). Solutions for injection, compressed tablets, and suppositories of this narcotic can be assayed by UV spectrophotometry (at 261.5 m$\mu$), by nonaqueous titration (0.02 N HClO$_4$ in glacial acetic acid and $\alpha$-naphthol-benzein as indicator), or gravimetrically after a chloroform extraction from sodium hydroxide solution. Ethylmorphine hydrochloride and codeine phosphate can be determined by coulometry after bromination in quantities of 2–5 mg (K1) whereas trimeperidine can be titrated in glacial acetic acid with perchloric acid using crystal violet as indicator (C3).

## D. Metabolism

### 1. INTRODUCTION

The number of narcotic drugs placed under international control by the Protocol of 1948 was twelve morphine derivatives (opiates), two synthetic narcotics, methadone and pethidine (opioids). By 1957 this number jumped to twenty-one opiates and thirty-nine opioids, and another three of the former and sixteen of the latter group were added by 1960. The research on metabolic transformation for narcotics lagged far behind the organic chemists' production. During the period of report more metabolic data on the older narcotics like morphine, heroin, cocaine, pethidine, and methadone became available, but only a few of the newer synthetics—propoxyphene, anileridine, dextromoramide, and ketobemidone—were of interest to laboratories studying metabolism. Also a valuable metabolic study was carried out on ethoheptazine. These studies should be encouraged and expanded even though data on pure narcotics are available; most narcotics are metabolized and excreted in changed form. Knowledge of metabolic pathways is therefore valuable for the biochemist and the practical toxicologist. A recent extensive review of the metabolism of morphine and its surrogates and its pharmacological significance was published by Way and Adler (W4).

## 2. Narcotics in General

The inhibition of human cholinesterase by narcotics and their antagonists is investigated by Foldes *et al.* (F17). For aliphatic substrates (acetylcholine and butyrylcholine) inhibitory effects are found for morphine, nalorphine, levorphanol, levallorphan, dihydrocodeine, oxycodone, 14-hydroxydihydromorphinone, pethidine, alphaprodine, and allylprodine. The allyl derivatives give more inhibition than the methyl-substituted parent compounds for plasma cholinesterase but not for red cell cholinesterase. The most potent inhibitors for the latter enzyme are narcotics of the morphinan series. With aromatic substrates [procaine and benzoylcholine (E6)], however, an accelerating effect of narcotics on the hydrolysis is observed. This effect is studied for human plasma cholinesterase and hydrocodone and hydromorphone in addition to the ten compounds mentioned above. With these substrates allyl substitution decreases the accelerating effect. The decreased N-demethylation of morphine, levorphanol, cocaine, and pethidine in tolerant rats with liver microsomes is found by Herken *et al.* (H4) not to be related with the tolerance phenomenon. Axelrod and Inscoe (A19) contribute more data on the glucuronide formation of narcotics. An enzyme in liver microsomes of guinea pigs formed glucuronides of morphine, nalorphine, levorphanol, and codeine. In urine, unchanged (7, 5, 16, and 8%) and conjugated drug (39, 12, 53, and 18%) are found. With the exception of codeine, all conjugates are present as glucuronides.

## 3. Morphine, Heroin, and Morphinans

The metabolic demethylation of morphine and morphinans, a process which also takes place in the poppy plant (S23, K8), is investigated by Mannering and Takemori (M4, T1, T2). They study the kinetics of the enzyme reactions in a mouse liver microsome system for morphine and several morphinan derivatives and find that a free $O^3$-hydroxy group in the molecule retards the $N$-demethylation. Also the effect of repeated administration of levorphanol, dextorphan, and morphine on the capacity of rat liver preparations to demethylate these and other related compounds is studied. Morphine and levorphanol are found to be very effective in depressing $N$-demethylation while dextrorphan, a nonnarcotic, is relatively ineffective. In a study of excretion of $C^{14}$-labeled morphine the following amounts of urinary $N$-$C^{14}$-methylmorphine and pulmonary $C^{14}O_2$ are found after subcutaneous injection (2 mg/kg) in dogs: free morphine, 13–15%; conjugated morphine, 48–52%; exhaled $C^{14}O_2$, 0.2%; in monkeys for the same entities: 6–14%, 55–71%, and about 1% (M7). Paerregaard (P1) studies the excretion of morphine in the urine of nonaddicts. After injection of 5–20 mg morphine 40–50% is found in urine after 48 hours, more than half of it in the first 8 hours. Eight to 10% of the amount excreted is recovered as free morphine. Way *et al.* (W5), in a study of the biotransformation of heroin in mice, confirm its rapid metabolism *in vitro* and *in vivo*. Deacetylation to $O^6$-monoacetylmorphine (MAM) and morphine occurs most rapidly in the liver. The paper chromatographic separation of the metabolites in chloroform—10% butanol tissue extracts, after concentration, is carried out by an ascending isoBuOH:HCOOH:$H_2O$ (70:30:50) system. The $R_f$'s for heroin, MAM, and morphine are 0.67, 0.59, and 0.46, respectively. Also, methods for the estimation of free and total phenols (Folin–Ciocalteu) and of MAM by the methyl-orange method after countercurrent separation are described. Eisenman *et al.* (E2) observes that addiction to morphine caused a significant decrease of the urinary level of 17-ketosteroid excretion.

Rapoport and associates (R1) study the morphine metabolism in addicts and nonaddicts with labeled morphine. The excretion patterns in nonaddicts (after injection of 10 mg morphine-$N$-$C^{14}H_3$) and addicts (after stabilization on 180 mg/24 hours) in urine are similar. In addicts 70% of the injected dose is excreted in urine in 24 hours, in nonaddicts 63%; during the same period, 8% is free and 49% bound morphine. This pattern is essentially the same in an experiment with nonaddicts using nuclear-$C^{14}$-morphine. In both groups about 6% of the injected dose is found as expired $C^{14}O_2$. Practically no normorphine could be discovered. This fact weakens the demethylation and tolerance hypotheses in morphine metabolism and dependence mechanisms. The method developed for the analysis of morphine and normorphine in urine includes successive hydrolysis with different portions of acid until the pH remains below 1; there is an extraction procedure going from liquids of greater polarity to those of less polarity: butanol–chloroform/ethanol–chloro-form–methylene chloride. Morphine is found in the methylene chloride fraction after extraction from pH 8.4 and normorphine in the same solvent after morphine removal and extraction from pH 9.2. The final isolation of crystalline material is made by microsublimation.

4. PETHIDINE, METHADONE, AND COCAINE

A paper chromatographic system for pethidine and its decomposition products by liver homogenates (K20, K21) is devised and changes in the metabolism of pethidine in rats are explored after irradiation with 600 r for 6 days. The level of pethidine in irradiated rats increases in blood and decreases in brain. The amount of unchanged drug found in urine is lowered. The capability of the liver homogenate and of the whole organism to metabolize the narcotic is diminished (G19). The dialytic mobility of pethidine in blood of irradiated rats is also lowered. This finding cannot be explained by changes of plasma proteins, but pH changes of the plasma due to the irradiation may be the cause (G20). A method for the extraction of pethidine from biological material with ethylene dichloride is given by Kazyak (K5). Data on the metabolic fate of methadone are reported by Schaumann (S9, S10, S11). The author shows that discrepancies in the results of earlier studies are partially due to the methylation to a quaternary base, methylmethadone, as a metabolite.

*Three methods for separating the methylated compound for methadone:*
    (*i*) *Paper chromatography.* MeOH (70%):ammonia (25%) (9:1); methylmethadone, $R_f$ 0.74; methadone, 0.37.
    (*ii*) *Liquid/liquid extraction.* The aqueous medium is extracted at pH 5 with benzene. The benzene phase is washed with 5 ml buffer and twice with water and can be used for the estimation of unchanged methadone and nonquaternary metabolites. To the combined aqueous solutions 0.5 ml methyl-orange solution, according to Brodie, and 5 ml pH 5 buffer solution are added and the methylmethadone–methyl-orange complex is extracted with 20 ml ethylene chloride or benzene and measured colorimetrically. Eighty-two per cent of methylmethadone added to organs was recovered.
    (*iii*) *Column chromatography.* The neutral aqueous solution containing metabolites is chromatographed through a basic alumina (10 gm) column which is washed four times with 15 ml water. The filtrate contains methylmethadone. Nonquaternary bases are then eluted with $4 \times 15$ ml alcoholic sulfuric acid (2%). Both fractions are determined by the methyl-orange method. Of added methadone and methylmethadone, in presence of liver tissue, 84% and 76%, respectively, were recovered.

Evidence is also found for the presence of a demethylated metabolite of methadone. The amount of unchanged methadone is studied in organs, urine, and bile of rats by a biological method using the isolated intestine of guinea pigs. After feeding 20 mg/kg *d,l*-methadone, 5, 10, and 50% of the unchanged narcotic are found in bile, organs (liver, lungs, kidney), and urine, respectively, 1 hour after the administration.

Elliot and Elison (E5) investigate the influence of some adrenal and pituitary hormones on the metabolism of methadone-2-$C^{14}$ in rats. Cortisone treatment enhanced absorption, and Vasopressin® treatment depressed it. Tissue distribution was most affected by cortisone: brain and spinal cord $C^{14}$ levels were low, intestinal levels indicated a more rapid excretion; muscle, liver, and urinary levels were not changed. Countercurrent distribution studies of bile indicate the presence of methadone and two metabolites.

Men habitually chewing 30–40 gm coca leaves daily are found to eliminate ecgonine at a urine level of 2.44–7.74 mg/100 gm (S6). The process was followed paper chromatographically in a $BuOH:AcOH:H_2O$ (100:4:50) system.

## 5. Propoxyphene

The metabolic degradation of *α-dl*-propoxyphene in rats and humans is examined by Lee *et al.* (L2). With rats and N-$C^{14}H_3$-labeled propoxyphene after i.v. injection of 4 mg/kg, 37.5% is found as pulmonary $C^{14}O_2$, and 15.4% excreted in the urine and 34.9% in the feces after 48 hours. The excretion of unlabeled propoxyphene in human urine after administration of 400 mg narcotic per day for a total of 2 days reveals the major metabolite to be de-*N*-methylpropoxyphene. The latter could be isolated from pooled urine of six persons as the dinitrophenyl derivative. Only a small fraction of the drug is extracted unchanged in urine. With the unspecific methyl-orange method (extracting from pH 11.0) the authors find "apparent" propoxyphene amounting to 2.9–9.7 mg during 24 hours after a 400-mg dosage. In one case the extraction is made from pH 9.0, which technique extracts the metabolite but prevents its rearrangement to compounds that do not form complexes with methyl-orange. This procedure gives 18 mg instead of 3.1 mg in the urine.

## 6. Dextromoramide

Attisso (A17, A18) and Vidic (V4) published methods for the identification and estimation of dextromoramide in biological material. Attisso's method consists of solubilization of dextromoramide in ethanol in presence of tartaric acid, double extraction with ether:chloroform (4:1) from pH 9, and purification to give the tartrate in chloroform solution. Quantation is made by direct UV spectrophotometry in iso-PrOH:0.1 N HCl (9:1). The method is applied to biological fluids and tissue of rats after prolonged treatment. Administration of 5 mg/day for up to 40 days causes accumulation of dextromoramide in the order of 200–600 $\mu$g in the liver, kidney, and brain. Vidic shows that the spectrophotometric method can be considerably improved by nitration of dextromoramide. This leads to about 30-fold increase of sensitivity as compared with the direct UV method. The author also gives paper chromatographic methods for the identification of dextromoramide and its metabolites.

*a. Extraction of Urine* (V4). Ten to 50 ml urine are brought to pH 10 with $Na_2CO_3$ solution and twice extracted with $1\frac{1}{2}$–2 volumes of cyclohexane. The washed cyclohexane extracts are re-extracted with 15% acetic acid (2–3 ml). The solvent is evaporated and the residue taken up in methanol and applied to Schleicher and Schüll 2045 b M paper.

*b. Paper Chromatography.* Chromatography reveals the presence of two metabolites and unchanged dextromoramide in human urine. The $R_f$'s for these compounds and for some other synthetic narcotics and their metabolites are shown in Table XI.

*c. Spectrophotometric Determination.* The isolated material is dissolved in concentrated $H_2SO_4$ (1 ml) and concentrated $HNO_3$ (1 ml)

TABLE XI

$R_f$ VALUES OF DEXTROMORAMIDE AND RELATED NARCOTICS AND THEIR METABOLITES ACCORDING TO VIDIC (V4)

| Name of narcotic | $R_f$ in System[a] | | |
|---|---|---|---|
| | 1 | 2 | 3 |
| Dextromoramide | 0.69–0.75 | 0.62 | 0.71 |
| Metabolites of dextromoramide | 0.65–0.70 | 0.31 and 0.23 | 0.75 and 0.59 |
| Methadone | 0.66–0.72 | 0.34 | 0.26 |
| Metabolite of methadone | — | Close to start | 0.04 |
| Normethadone | — | 0.54 | 0.60 |
| Metabolite of normethadone | — | Close to start | 0.08 |
| Dextromethorphan | — | — | 0.39 |
| Pethidine | 0.60–0.65 | 0.16 | 0.81 |
| Metabolite of pethidine | — | — | 0.13 |

[a] System 1: ethylene dichloride:AcOH:$H_2O$ (10:4:1);
System 2: chloroform:toluene:cyclohexane:AcOH:$H_2O$ (70:70:70:63:42);
System 3: mobile phase: MeOH:$H_2O$:25% ammonia (60:30:10).
Stationary phase: impregnation with olive oil (15% in toluene)
Chromatography was carried out after blotting and air drying of the impregnated paper. Identification was made with Dragendorff's and nitraniline sprays (F5, p. 573).

in a small glass dish and heated on the boiling water bath for 1 hour. After cooling it is transferred with water to a 5-ml volumetric flask. The spectrum is then measured from 220 to 350 mμ against a similarly treated blank. For quantation the maximum at 278 mμ ($\epsilon = 13340$) is suitable. The minimum is at 236 mμ. The shape of the curve is different from that obtained for methadone. In 10 ml urine or blood 0.2 mg/100 ml could still be estimated. Curves obtained from urine of addicts show a maximum of 272–274 mμ and a minimum at 242 mμ probably due to the presence of metabolites.

In seventy-three samples of urines originating from addicts who took 69–552 mg dextromoramide daily, 0.2–2.1 mg/100 ml of metabolized narcotic is found.

## 7. KETOBEMIDONE

A report on a fatal ketobemidone poisoning is published by Schmidlin-Mészáros and Hartmann (S12). Ketobemidone is identified in organs and body fluids after Stas–Otto extraction by paper chromatography in $BuOH:HCOOH:H_2O$ (12:1:7), UV spectrophotometry, vacuum sublimation, Marquis' test, microcrystals with chloroplatinic acid, and a biological test (Straub's tail phenomenon). Semiquantitative estimation by paper chromatography shows that after a massive dose of 100–150 mg of ketobemidone the highest accumulation is found in the stomach contents, urine, and kidneys. Intermediate levels are found in liver and brain and traces only in blood and spleen. The liver and kidney fractions show evidence of the presence of metabolites, whereas glucuronides of ketobemidone are suspected in the urine.

## 8. ETHOHEPTAZINE

Although ethoheptazine (4-carbethoxy-1-methyl-4-phenylhexamethyleneimine) is not listed as a narcotic under international control, it belongs to the same chemical group as proheptazine, a controlled narcotic. The metabolic fate is explored by Walkenstein *et al.* (W3) with 4-$C^{14}$-labeled ethoheptazine in dogs and rabbits after injection of 35 mg/kg and in rats after 50 mg/kg. The metabolic patterns differ from those anticipated from the findings on pethidine. The following metabolites are found by paper chromatography of dog urine ($R_f$ values in brackets): unchanged ethoheptazine (0.89), probably hydroxyethoheptazine (0.73), two unknown metabolites (0.38 and 0.35), hydrolyzed ethoheptazine (0.22), and hydroxyethoheptazine (0.11). The solvent system is butanol, saturated with $1 M$ ammonium acetate (pH 7.0). Identification sprays include Dragendorff's and diazotized *p*-nitraniline [see (F5), p. 573, Table LXXIII]. A method for the estimation of ethoheptazine and its hydroxy and hydrolyzed metabolites is described. The method is based on liquid/liquid extraction and Brodie's methyl-orange technique. None of the metabolites appear as conjugates and no pulmonary $C^{14}O_2$ is found. The amounts of metabolites excreted in terms of per cent of dose in dogs are: unchanged, 3.45%; hydroxylated, 9.34%; and hydrolyzed metabolites, 7.91%.

## 9. ANILERIDINE

Porter (P17) investigates the absorption and metabolism of anileridine in guinea pigs, rats, and man. The narcotic is rapidly absorbed by the tissues of rats following parenteral administration. Highest concentrations are found in the lungs, kidneys, and brain. Analysis of the urine of men reveals that only 5% of orally taken drug remains unchanged. The major pathway lies in the destruction of the isonipecotic acid moiety. Fifteen to 35% of the dose could be accounted for as unidentified diazotizable substances, probably $p$-acetylaminophenylacetic acid or related compounds, whereas only about 20% of the metabolites are made up of unchanged anileridine or its close relatives: unchanged, 7–14%; acetylanileridine acid, 1–2%; acetylanileridine, 0.5–2%. The following methods for extraction and determination of metabolites are given:

*a. Anileridine and Acetylanileridine.* Plasma (3 ml), tissue homogenate (10 ml containing 1–2 gm of tissue), or urine are extracted twice at pH 7–8 with 2 volumes of ethylene chloride. The extracts are evaporated to dryness and dissolved in 1 N $H_2SO_4$ (2.5 ml). Two 1-ml aliquots are taken and one of them autoclaved (15 lb pressure, 30 minutes). To each aliquot is added 1 ml of water, then, at 3-minute intervals, 0.1% $NaNO_2$, 0.5% ammonium sulfamate, and 0.5% N-(1-naphthyl)ethylenediamine·2HCl (0.5 ml each). Absorbancies are measured at 510 m$\mu$ at about 30 minutes after the final addition of reagent.

*b. Anileridine Acid and Acetylanileridine Acid.* Urine samples which had been extracted with ethylene chloride are extracted at pH 7–11 with benzyl alcohol. Samples are also autoclaved, then treated similarly as above.

Recovery of anileridine and acetylanileridine from aqueous solutions is 93–99%, while recovery of the acid forms is about 87%.

## 10. $d$-$\alpha$- AND $l$-$\alpha$-ACETYLMETHADOLS

Sung and Way (S25) also used Brodie's method for the determination of $d$-$\alpha$- and $l$-$\alpha$-acetylmethadol in rats. After injection of 20 mg/kg of the levorotatory isomer, it was found that between 40 and 50% of the drug was still present after 12 hours. Study of distribution of the drug in tissues showed the highest concentration in the lung. Kidney, spleen, liver, and fat contained appreciable levels whereas low levels were present in heart, brain, and blood. Only negligible amounts (less than 3% of dose) were found in feces and urine, which finding leads to the conclusion that the drug is being disposed of by biotransformation.

# III. Physicochemical Methods for the Identification of Narcotics and Related Bases

## A. Introduction

Seven years have passed since the first article in our series was printed in the Bulletin on Narcotics (F1, F8, B9, B10, F10, O1, H6, L6, G2, G3). The demand for methods for narcotic identification has continued with the growth of new families of narcotics. In this section recent results by Martin *et al.* (M5) on some of the more important opioids shown in Table I are reported and their physical constants discussed in relation to other individual narcotics in these families.

## B. Methods

### 1. WATER ANALYSIS

A Karl Fischer titration method (F16, P11) was used. The electrometric titrimeter is equipped with a miniature electron ray tube visual indicator. An opening for 10 seconds of the "electric eye" visual indicator is taken as the end point. Pholcodine is dried in an Abderhalden pistol (C2) under reduced pressure to a constant weight for determination of water.

### 2. MELTING POINTS

A Fisher–Johns microfusion apparatus is used to determine the melting points according to the procedure given for Class I compounds (P11).

### 3. DISSOCIATION CONSTANTS

The acid coefficients ($pK_a$ values) of the twelve compounds are determined by fractional neutralization. Titration curves of the salts of the narcotics are obtained in aqueous ethanol (50%) whenever possible, but aqueous propanol (75%) is used when solubility in the former solvent is low. The salts are titrated electrometrically with 0.01 N NaOH and the free bases with 0.01 N HCl. Saunders and Srivastava (S7) describe the method of calculation which is applied to the simple halide salts. Levallorphan tartrate, ethoheptazine citrate, and pholcodine results (Plate III) require more complex calculations which are discussed in Section III,C,1.

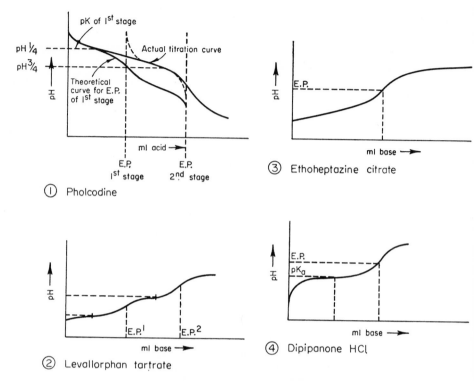

PLATE III. Titration curves of narcotics.
Fig. 1. Pholcodine free base versus acid.
Fig. 2. Levallorphan tartrate versus base.
Fig. 3. Ethoheptazine citrate versus base.
Fig. 4. Dipipanone hydrochloride versus base.

## 4. Nonaqueous Titrations

The details of the method have been previously described (L5) using perchloric acid in glacial acetic acid as a titrant and crystal violet as the end point indicator. Some determinations were confirmed potentiometrically in glacial acetic acid using a pH meter equipped with glass and calomel electrodes.

## 5. Ultraviolet Spectrophotometry

Absorbance curves (Plates IV, V, and VI) are obtained over the range 205–360 m$\mu$ using a Beckman DK-2 automatic ratio-recording spectrophotometer equipped with 1-cm silica absorption cells, a hydrogen lamp source, and a photo multiplier detector. The following instrument settings are used: sensitivity, 30; time, 5; time constant, 0.1; initial

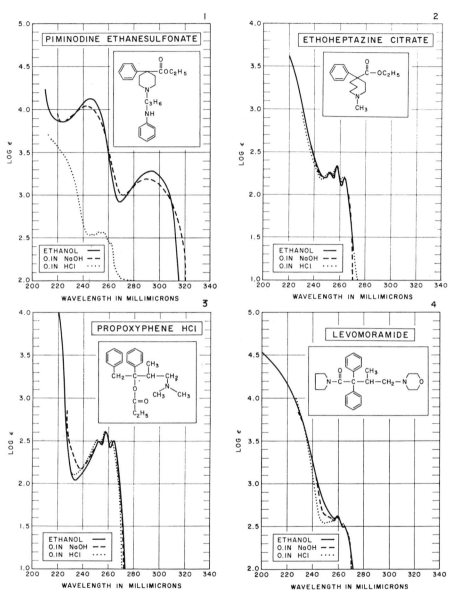

PLATE IV. Ultraviolet curves of narcotics in three solvents.
Fig. 1. Piminodine ethane sulfonate.
Fig. 2. Ethoheptazine citrate.
Fig. 3. Propoxyphene hydrochloride.
Fig. 4. Levomoramide.

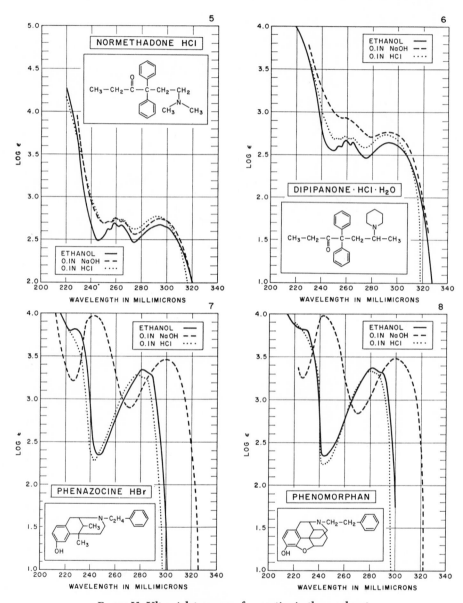

PLATE V. Ultraviolet curves of narcotics in three solvents.
Fig. 5. Normethadone hydrochloride.
Fig. 6. Dipipanone hydrochloride.
Fig. 7. Phenazocine hydrobromide.
Fig. 8. Phenomorphan.

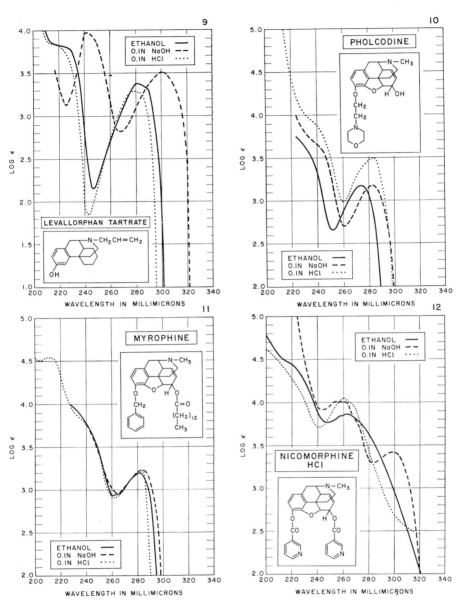

PLATE VI. Ultraviolet curves of narcotics in three solvents.
Fig. 9. Levallorphan tartrate.
Fig. 10. Pholcodine.
Fig. 11. Myrophine.
Fig. 12. Nicomorphine hydrochloride dihydrate.

absorbance range, 0–1. The solvent is placed in cuvettes in both the reference and sample beams and the wavelength set at 360 m$\mu$, the instrument set at zero calibration, and the baseline scanned over the range with solvent only.

Approximately 25-mg samples of the drug are weighed accurately and dissolved in 0.1 N sodium hydroxide, 0.1 N hydrochloric acid, and ethanol, respectively. Each determination is carried out in replicate. The solutions are transferred to 50-ml volumetric flasks and made up to volume. All of the compounds are soluble in alcohol. The narcotics which are insoluble in aqueous sodium hydroxide are dissolved in ethanol (25 ml) to which is then added 0.1 N sodium hydroxide (25 ml). A similar procedure is used for the hydrochloric acid solutions of insoluble compounds. Dilutions are carried out when required to bring the absorbance into a suitable range.

For purposes of plotting, the individual absorbances are obtained from the sample spectrum by subtraction of the baseline absorbance and the recorded absorbances. From these data the molecular extinction coefficients ($\epsilon$) are calculated using the molecular weights corrected for water content (Table XII, column 7). The log $\epsilon$ values are plotted as ordinates against wavelengths in m$\mu$ along the abscissas.

### 6. X-RAY POWDER DIFFRACTION

The samples are ground (250-mesh sieve) and loaded into a glass capillary tube (0.2 mm ID, 0.01 mm wall thickness). Myrophine is put into a capillary at 40°F in a cold room since it tends to melt at normal temperatures. The uniformity of packing and absence of foreign particles are checked microscopically. Diffraction patterns are obtained using Philips' Debye–Scherrer powder cameras (diameter 114.83 mm) and cobalt k$\alpha$ radiation. The film exposure times vary from 10 to 18 hours at 28 kvp and 10 ma. The center of each line on the negatives is determined using a standard powder film–measuring device and the position of the line calculated from it. When variations greater than 0.1 mm in the position of the centers of successive lines on a film are observed, the centers are remeasured. Line positions are corrected for film shrinkage, and converted from a table (S26) into $d$ values, $\lambda = 1.78890$ Å. Relative intensities are estimated visually on a scale of 100.

At least four X-ray diffraction powder photographs of each compound are used as a basis of the measurements reported here. One photograph of each substance in its original state is taken to determine the effect of grinding on the pattern (Plate VII).

TABLE XII

PHYSICAL DATA FOR AUTHENTICATION OF TWELVE NARCOTICS (M5)

| International name | Source and other identification numbers | Empirical formula | Formula weight calculated | Water analysis Per cent | Water analysis Moles | Formula weight + $H_2O$ found | Melting point found (°C) | Acid coefficient found (pKa) | Nonaqueous titrations (% recovery) |
|---|---|---|---|---|---|---|---|---|---|
| Dipipanone hydrochloride monohydrate | Burroughs Wellcome Co. Ltd., 78828 | $C_{24}H_{34}ClNO_2$ | 403.98 | 4.87 | 1.09 | 405.69 | 112–116 | 8.7 | 102.1 |
| Ethoheptazine citrate[N,N a] | John Wyeth, Bros. Co. Ltd., Walkerville, Ont., Canada, RR18746 | $C_{22}H_{31}NO_9$ | 453.46 | 0.24 | 0.06 | 454.56 | 138.5 | 8.45[b] | 100.4 |
| Levallorphan tartrate | Roche Ltd., London, England, RO-1-7700 | $C_{23}H_{31}NO_7$ | 433.49 | 0.35 | 0.08 | 435.01 | 178–179 | 8.3 | 98.5 |
| Levomoramide (free base) | Smith, Kline, & French, Philadelphia, Pa., 15157, NIH 7579 | $C_{25}H_{32}N_2O_2$ | 392.52 | 0.09 | 0.02 | 392.87 | 190 | 6.6 | 99 |
| Myrophine (free base) | USPHS, NIH 5986A | $C_{38}H_{51}NO_4$ | 585.81 | 1.55 | 0.51 | 595.18 | 33–34 | 6.8[c] | 100 |
| Nicomorphine hydrochloride dihydrate | Lannacker, Heilmittel, Wien, Austria | $C_{29}H_{30}ClN_3O_7$ | 567.5 | 5.9 | 1.86 | 567.5 | 172–177 | 7.0 | 100.3 |
| Normethadone hydrochloride | Hoechst, Germany, NIH 2820 | $C_{20}H_{26}ClNO$ | 331.88 | 1.21 | 0.22 | 335.92 | 175–177 | 6.0 | 101 |
| Phenazocine hydrobromide | Mallinckrodt, St. Louis, Mo., J259, NIH 7519 | $C_{22}H_{28}BrNO$ | 402.37 | 1.04 | 0.235 | 406.60 | 164.5 | 8.5 | 103.5 |
| Phenomorphan hydrobromide | Roche Ltd., London, England, RO-1-1955 | $C_{24}H_{30}BrNO$ | 428.40 | 1.09 | 0.262 | 433.16 | 289–292 | 7.3 | —[d] |
| Pholcodine monohydrate | Allen & Handbury Co. Ltd., Toronto, Canada | $C_{23}H_{32}N_2O_5$ | 416.53 | 4.77[e] | 1.10 | 418.45 | 69.70 | 5.3[b] 6.9[c] | 99 |
| Piminodine ethane sulfonate | Winthrop, Canada Ltd., 14-098-2, NIH 7590 | $C_{23}H_{36}N_2O_5S$ | 476.63 | 0.59 | 0.157 | 479.46 | 135.5 | 6.9 | 101 |
| Propoxyphene hydrochloride[N,N a] | Eli Lilly & Co., Indianapolis, Ind. | $C_{22}H_{30}ClNO_2$ | 375.93 | 0.504 | 0.105 | 377.83 | 169–170 | 6.3 | 102.9 |

[a] *NN*, not under international narcotic control.
[b] pKa of *free base* in 50% aqueous ethanol.
[c] pKa determined in 75% propanol.
[d] Phenomorphan did not dissolve in glacial acetic acid.
[e] Moisture content confirmed by determination in Abderhalden apparatus.

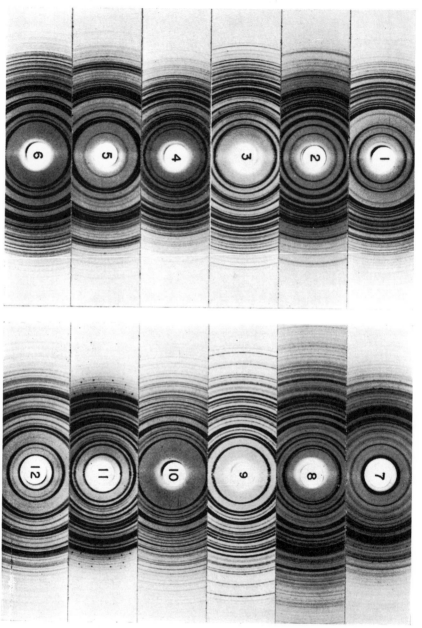

PLATE VII. X-ray powder diffraction patterns of narcotics.
Fig. 1. Piminodine ethanesulfonate.
Fig. 2. Ethoheptazine citrate.
Fig. 3. d-Propoxyphene hydrochloride.

7. INFRARED SPECTROPHOTOMETRY

Two types of IR spectra are obtained:

*a. Potassium Bromide Pressed Disc Spectra.* The compound (5 mg) and potassium bromide (495 mg) are weighed separately and mixed in a dental amalgamator. The mixture (203 mg) is transferred to a die and pressed at 15,000 psi for 2 minutes to yield a pellet (200 mg) using a Carver Press. A similar pure potassium bromide disc is made for use as a reference. (See Plates VIII, IX, and X.)

*b. Spectra in Carbon Tetrachloride.* Myrophine gives opaque potassium bromide discs, and is dissolved in carbon tetrachloride (1%), in which the spectrum is obtained. Measurements are made in a sodium chloride cell (1 mm path length) using "spec-pure" carbon tetrachloride in the reference beam. (See Plate X, Fig. 11.)

8. PAPER CHROMATOGRAPHY

*System 1.* IsoBuOH:AcOH:$H_2O$ (100:10:24) on paper impregnated with 0.5 $M$ $KH_2PO_4$ (pH 4.2).

*System 2.* IsoBuOH:AcOH:$H_2O$ (100:10:24) on paper impregnated with $(NH_4)_2SO_4$ (2%, pH 5.3).

*System 3.* Butylacetate:AcOH:$H_2O$ (35:10:3) on paper impregnated with 0.5 $M$ $KH_2PO_4$ (pH 4.2).

*System 4.* PrOH:$H_2O$:diethylamine (1:8:1) on paper impregnated with 4% light paraffin (BP 1948) in hexane.

*System 5.* Ammonium formate (10%) in water, saturated with *sec*-octanol on paper impregnated with 20% *sec*-octanol in acetone.

*System 6.* Light paraffin (BP 1948):diethylamine (9:1) on paper impregnated with 20% formamide in acetone.

C. Results and Discussion

1. DISSOCIATION CONSTANTS

Saunders and Srivistava (S7) make use of the fact that in sufficiently dilute solutions (weak electrolytes) of acids or bases pH $=$ p$K_a$ at the

Fig. 4. Levomoramide (free base).
Fig. 5. Normethadone hydrochloride.
Fig. 6. *dl*-Dipipanone hydrochloride monohydrate.
Fig. 7. Phenazocine hydrobromide.
Fig. 8. *d*-Phenomorphan hydrobromide.
Fig. 9. Levallorphan tartrate.
Fig. 10. Pholcodine monohydrate (free base).
Fig. 11. Myrophine (free base).
Fig. 12. Nicomorphine hydrochloride dihydrate.

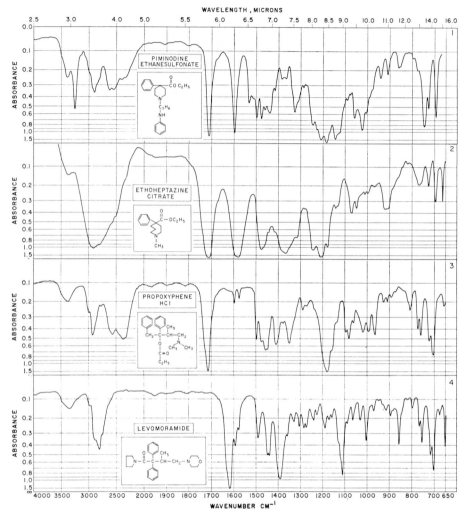

PLATE VIII. Infrared spectra of narcotics.
Fig. 1. Piminodine ethanesulfonate.
Fig. 2. Ethoheptazine citrate.
Fig. 3. Propoxyphene hydrochloride.
Fig. 4. Levomoramide.

half-neutralization point, i.e., when the ratio [acid]/[base] = 1. This relationship holds when a monobasic acid or monoacidic base is titrated with a similarly simple base or acid. Not all of the twelve compounds shown in Tables XII and XIII and Plate II fall into this category; in fact they can be discussed under four headings as follows:

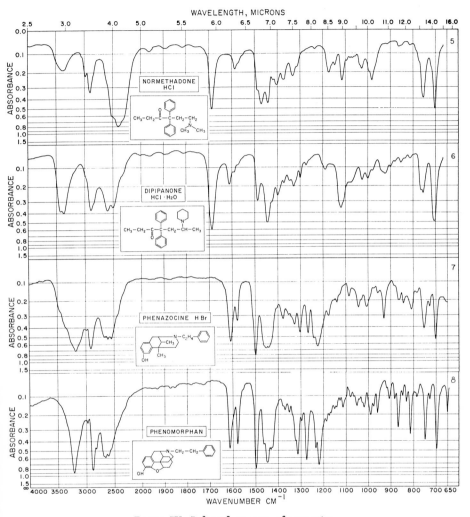

PLATE IX. Infrared spectra of narcotics.
Fig. 5. Normethadone hydrochloride.
Fig. 6. Dipipanone hydrochloride dihydrate.
Fig. 7. Phenazocine hydrobromide.
Fig. 8. Phenomorphan.

*a. Salts of the Type* $[RNH]^+X^-$. In this class one basic function is combined with a monobasic acid. For practical purposes it includes compounds having more than one nitrogen atom of which only one can be titrated in aqueous solution. Examples are the hydrochloride salts of dipipanone, normethadone, propoxyphene, and nicomorphine; phenazo-

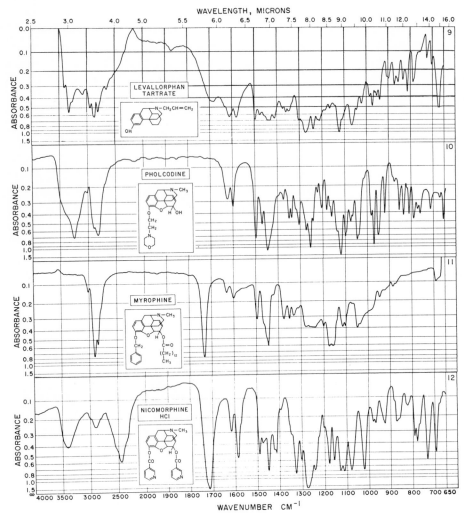

PLATE X. Infrared spectra of narcotics.
Fig. 9. Levallorphan tartrate.
Fig. 10. Pholcodine.
Fig. 11. Myrophine.
Fig. 12. Nicomorphine hydrochloride dihydrate.

cine hydrobromide; and piminodine ethane sulfonate (e.g., Plate IV, Fig. 3).

*b. Free Bases with One Titratable Basic Function.* Myrophine and levomoramide are the two narcotics in this class.

*c. Free Bases with Two Titratable Basic Functions.* Pholcodine is the only example in this class.

*d. Salts in Which a Monoacidic Base Combined with a Polybasic Acid.* Ethoheptazine citrate and levallorphan tartrate are examples of compounds of this type.

*e. Individual Compounds.* Two equivalents of acid are required to neutralize 1 mole of pholcodine free base, but the titration curve (Plate III, Fig. 1) showed only one point of inflexion at the endpoint, indicating the equal strength of the nitrogens. This is illustrated in Plate III, Fig. 1 by the titration curve of pholcodine.

Levallorphan tartrate shows two clear-cut end points (Plate III, Fig. 2) one of which results from the second stage of tartaric acid ionization and the other from the base. Confirmation is obtained by titrating tartaric acid in which the second stage of tartaric acid neutralization coincides with the first step in the neutralization of levorphanol tartrate.

Ethoheptazine citrate, more correctly named ethoheptazine dihydrogen citrate, is a more complicated substance being a salt of a tribasic acid and a monoacidic base. The following titratable ionic species are present in solutions: second and third stage ionization of citric acid, and ethoheptazinium acid. In the titration 2 moles of base are used before an inflexion point is observed, but no indication of the third species is obtained (Plate III, Fig. 3). The pK's of citric acid are known and it appeared that the point of inflection obtained corresponds to that of neutralized citric acid; i.e., the titration curve provides no information regarding ethoheptazine, except to show that it belongs to the group of stronger bases in comparison with the other narcotics studied. Preparation of the free base, ethoheptazine, and subsequent titration in 50% ethanol yields a $pK_a = 8.45$.

In some similar cases of a salt of this type the $pK_a$ of the $BH^+$ ion lies between the two end points of the acid with which it is combined. To demonstrate this case codeine phosphate was titrated: the second and third dissociation constants of phosphoric acid are 7.2 and 12.3. Values for the base dissociation constant of codeine range from 6.1 (K12)—from titration of codeine hydrochloride with aqueous sodium hydroxide—to 6.7–6.9 (B5)—from titration of the free base with sodium hydroxide in 50% aqueous ethanol. The range of $pK_a$ values corresponding to these are 8.2–7.5 (where $pK_a = pK_w - pK_b$) which values may be seen to lie between the second and third dissociation constant exponents of phosphoric acid. Two moles of sodium hydroxide are required to reach the point of inflection for codeine phosphate, and applying the procedure outlined above the pK's for the two species are 7.0 and 8.2, respectively.

According to these experiments, therefore, the $pK_a$ of codeine is 8.2, while the value 7.0 corresponds to the second pK of phosphoric acid.

From the experimentally determined pK values the theoretical end point pH value and the salt solution pH value (prior to titration) are calculated, and compared with the values found experimentally. These data are listed in Table XIII and it can be seen that reasonable agreement is obtained, which confirms the $pK_a$ values determined.

TABLE XIII

ACID COEFFICIENTS, END POINT pH VALUES, AND
SOLUTION pH VALUES OF NARCOTICS (M5)

| Compound | $pH_a$ | Theoretical pH at end point | Actual pH at end point | pH of salt solutions Calculated | Found |
|---|---|---|---|---|---|
| Dipipanone HCl[a] | 8.7 | 10.3 | 10.15 | 5.8 | 6.1 |
| Levallorphan tartrate | 8.3 | 10.0 | 10.1 | 5.6[b] | |
| | | | | (5.1) | 4.8 |
| Levomoramide[c,d] | 6.6 | 9.2 | 8.5 | 4.54 | 4.5 |
| Myrophine[c] | 6.8 | 9.5 | 8.8 | 4.9 | 4.4 |
| Nicomorphine HCl[a] | 7.0 | 9.4 | 9.5 | 4.65 | 4.8 |
| Normethadone HCl[a] | 8.1 | 9.95 | 10.15 | 5.2 | 5.4 |
| Phenazocine HBr[a] | 8.5 | 10.15 | 10.2 | 5.4 | 5.7 |
| Phenomorphan HBr | 7.3 | 9.6 | 9.5 | 4.65 | 4.85 |
| Piminodine ethanesulfonate | 7.2 | 9.35 | 9.0 | — | — |
| Propoxyphene HCl[a] | 7.8 | 9.8 | 10 | 5.1 | 5.6 |

[a] Salt of strong acid and weak base.

[b] When calculating pH of salt solution using formula for salt of weak acid and weak base the value (5.6) differs appreciably from that found. This expression does not include a term for concentration, and is valid only at concentrations 0.01 N where $pK_a = pK_b$. This is clearly not the case here (G7). Considering the compound as a salt of a strong acid and a weak base a value of 5.1 is calculated.

[c] Free bases. Position is reversed here: "end point" is pH of 0.01 N solution of compound in solvent. pH of salt solution is at point of inflection obtained. Differences between found and calculated initial pH may be due to carbon dioxide absorption or trace impurities.

[d] Demoen (D3) reported $pK_a = 7.05$ in 50% MeOH for d form.

*f. Summary.* Summarizing the discussion of the dissociation constant it may be stated that in using the Henderson–Hasselbach (H3, G7) equation to approximate the acid dissociation constant $pK_a$, and applying it as an identification constant especially where salts of polybasic acids are concerned, their titration curves should be obtained with that of the free acid with which the base is combined. The weaknesses of the method lie in the lack of control of temperature which affects the value of $pK_w$, the use of an insensitive pH meter, and the difficulty of obtaining exactly reproducible conditions.

## 2. ULTRAVIOLET SPECTRA

The spectra of narcotics grouped according to chemical structure show clearly the influence of the major and minor chromophores (Plates IV–VI). The details are discussed elsewhere (F1, O1, M5, G6).

*Influence of pH Changes on Spectra.* pH is an important factor in the ultraviolet spectral identification of certain narcotics. In the present study ethoheptazine and propoxyphene show no significant change in their spectra obtained in ethanolic, acidic, or basic solutions, while levomoramide, normethadone, dipipanone, and myrophine spectra have minor changes. The first and last compounds in this set have spectral peaks at 253 and 260 m$\mu$ which are suppressed in acid and base, respectively. The second and third compounds show small increases in absorbances in acid and base compared with ethanolic solution. On the other hand, substantial changes in the spectra of piminodine, phenomorphan, levallorphan, phenazocine, and nicomorphine are produced by changing the pH of the media. Piminodine shows complete suppression of the aniline-type spectrum in HCl solution (Table XIV).

The phenols, phenazocine, phenomorphan, and levallorphan (Figs. 7, 8, and 9 in Plates V and VI) show identical shifts of their spectra by approximately 20 m$\mu$ to higher wavelengths in alkaline solution. A hyperchromic effect from 2000 to 3000 units is observed (G6).

Nicomorphine (Plate VI, Fig. 12) is an ester, dinicotinylmorphine, whose spectrum in ethanolic and acidic solution is essentially the same as the nicotinic acid spectrum. Hydrolysis produces morphinate and nicotinate ions, which yield an ultraviolet spectrum similar to that of a mixture of morphine and nicotinic acid. To prove that hydrolysis occurs in alkaline medium, and not in ethanolic solution, they are chromatographed in isoBuOH:AcOH:H$_2$O (10:1:2.4) on ammonium sulfate–treated paper (G3). The ethanolic solution shows one spot ($R_f = 0.68$) which is detected by its absorbance at 2537 Å ultraviolet light and as an orange spot with a modified König's reagent (H7) which is used for the detection of pyridine derivatives in paper chromatography. On the other hand, the alkaline solution gave two spots. The first with the lowest $R_f$ (0.13) is identified by UV light, potassium iodoplatinate spray reagent (G3), and Kieffer's (M12) reagent as morphine. The second spot has a dark absorbance under UV light (2537 Å), a red-purple color with König's reagent, and an $R_f$ value of 0.51, properties identical with those produced by a known nicotinic acid. Another hydrolysis product, probably O$^6$-mononicotinylmorphine, $R_f = 0.33$, is found when the

TABLE XIV

Ultraviolet Spectral Data of Twelve Narcotics in Acidic, Basic, and Ethanolic Solvents (M5, K4)

| Wave length (mμ) | Solvent 0.1 N HCl | | | | Solvent 0.1 N NaOH | | | | Solvent ethanol (50%) | | | | Wave length (mμ) |
|---|---|---|---|---|---|---|---|---|---|---|---|---|---|
| | Compound maximum | Molar extinction | Compound minimum | Molar extinction | Compound maximum | Molar extinction | Compound minimum | Molar extinction | Compound maximum | Molar extinction | Compound minimum | Molar extinction | |
| 204 | — | — | — | — | — | — | — | — | — | — | Myrophine | 33,000 | 204 |
| 210 | — | — | — | — | — | — | — | — | Myrophine | 35,400 | — | — | 210 |
| — | — | — | — | — | — | — | — | — | — | — | — | — | — |
| 223 | — | — | — | — | — | — | Piminodine | 1735 | — | — | Phenazocine | 6600 | 223 |
| — | — | — | — | — | — | — | — | — | — | — | — | — | — |
| 226 | — | — | — | — | — | — | Levallorphan | 1317 | — | — | Piminodine | 7130 | 226 |
| 227 | — | — | — | — | — | — | Phenazocine | 1645 | — | — | Phenazocine | 6860 | 227 |
| — | — | — | — | — | — | — | Phenomorphan | 1800 | — | — | — | — | — |
| 232 | — | — | Propoxyphene | 129 | — | — | — | — | — | — | — | — | 232 |
| 234 | — | — | — | — | — | — | — | — | — | — | — | — | 234 |
| 238 | — | — | — | — | Phenazocine | 9590 | Propoxyphene | 153 | — | — | Propoxyphene | 111 | 238 |
| — | — | — | — | — | — | — | — | — | — | — | — | — | — |
| 240 | — | — | Nicomorphine | 5360 | — | — | Nicomorphine | 8600 | — | — | Ethoheptazine | 156 | 240 |
| 241 | — | — | Levallorphan | 78 | — | — | — | — | — | — | — | — | 241 |
| 243 | — | — | Phenomorphan | 202 | — | — | — | — | — | — | — | — | 243 |
| — | — | — | — | — | — | — | — | — | — | — | — | — | — |
| 244 | — | — | Piminodine | 340 | — | — | — | — | Piminodine | 13,320 | Phenomorphan | 221 | 244 |
| 245 | — | — | — | — | — | — | — | — | — | — | Normethadone | 313 | 245 |
| 246 | — | — | — | — | — | — | — | — | — | — | Phenazocine | 230 | 246 |
| 247 | Piminodine | 348 | — | — | — | — | — | — | — | — | Levallorphan | 144 | 247 |
| — | — | — | — | — | — | — | — | — | — | — | Nicomorphine | 5960 | — |
| 248 | — | — | Ethoheptazine | 153 | — | — | — | — | — | — | — | — | 248 |
| 249 | — | — | Levomoramide | 340 | — | — | Ethoheptazine | 160 | — | — | Dipipanone | 360 | 249 |
| — | — | — | — | — | — | — | — | — | — | — | — | — | — |
| 250 | — | — | Piminodine | 346 | Propoxyphene | 319 | — | — | Propoxyphene | 315 | — | — | 250 |
| — | — | — | Dipipanone | 491 | — | — | — | — | — | — | — | — | — |
| 251 | Ethoheptazine | 179 | Normethadone | 503 | — | — | Normethadone | 486 | — | — | Ethoheptazine | 178 | 251 |
| 252 | Propoxyphene | 331 | Piminodine | 260 | — | — | Ethoheptazine | 188 | — | — | Pholcodine | 494 | 252 |
| — | — | — | — | — | — | — | — | — | — | — | — | — | — |

| No. | Ref. 1 | | Ref. 2 | | Ref. 3 | | Ref. 4 | | Ref. 5 | | Ref. 6 | | No. |
|---|---|---|---|---|---|---|---|---|---|---|---|---|---|
| 253 | Dipipanone | 495 | | | | | | | Dipipanone | 410 | Ethoheptazine | 153 | 253 |
| — | Levomoramide | 358 | | | | | | | Normethadone | 427 | Propoxyphene | 287 | — |
| — | Normethadone | 522 | | | | | | | | | | | — |
| — | Piminodine | 392 | | | | | | | | | | | 254 |
| 254 | | | Ethoheptazine | 168 | Normethadone | 515 | Propoxyphene | 294 | | | Ethoheptazine | 153 | 255 |
| 255 | | | Propoxyphene | 312 | | | Ethoheptazine | 168 | | | Propoxyphene | 287 | — |
| — | | | Dipipanone | 486 | | | | | | | | | — |
| — | | | Levomoramide | 353 | | | | | | | | | 256 |
| 256 | | | Normethadone | 526 | Nicomorphine | 10,410 | | | | | Dipipanone | 402 | 257 |
| 257 | Ethoheptazine | 216 | Piminodine | 364 | | | Levomoramide | 361 | | | Levomoramide | 377 | — |
| — | Piminodine | 369 | | | | | Dipipanone | 877 | | | Normethadone | 425 | 258 |
| — | Propoxyphene | 413 | | | | | Normethadone | 513 | | | | | — |
| 258 | Dipipanone | 533 | Ethoheptazine | 219 | Ethoheptazine | 219 | | | Ethoheptazine | 210 | | | 259 |
| — | Levomoramide | 399 | Propoxyphene | 400 | Propoxyphene | 400 | | | Levomoramide | 401 | | | — |
| 259 | Normethadone | 580 | Dipipanone | 883 | Dipipanone | 883 | | | Dipipanone | 478 | | | — |
| — | | | Levomoramide | 400 | Levomoramide | 400 | | | Levomoramide | 400 | | | 260 |
| — | | | | | | | | | Normethadone | 510 | | | 261 |
| 260 | | | Pholcodine | 1000 | Normethadone | 566 | Pholcodine | 527 | | | | | — |
| 261 | Nicomorphine | 11,760 | Ethoheptazine | 153 | | | | | | | Ethoheptazine | 127 | — |
| — | | | Myrophine | 797 | | | | | | | Myrophine | 865 | 262 |
| — | | | Propoxyphene | 294 | | | | | | | Propoxyphene | 266 | — |
| 262 | | | Levomoramide | 327 | | | | | | | | | 263 |
| — | | | Propoxyphene | 269 | | | | | | | | | — |
| 263 | Ethoheptazine | 163 | | | Ethoheptazine | 160 | Ethoheptazine | 143 | Ethoheptazine | 154 | Dipipanone | 425 | 264 |
| — | Propoxyphene | 324 | Dipipanone | 502 | Propoxyphene | 315 | | | Nicomorphine | 7610 | Normethadone | 456 | — |
| — | Piminodine | 264 | Normethadone | 551 | | | | | | | | | 265 |
| 264 | Levomoramide | 336 | | | Levomoramide | 306 | Levomoramide | 304 | Propoxyphene | 321 | Levomoramide | 306 | — |
| — | | | | | | | Normethadone | 523 | | | | | 268 |
| 265 | Dipipanone | 511 | | | | | | | Dipipanone | 460 | | | 270 |
| — | Normethadone | 482 | | | Normethadone | 427 | | | Levomoramide | 308 | | | 271 |
| — | | | | | | | | | Normethadone | 530 | | | 272 |
| 268 | | | | | | | Levallorphan | 668 | | | | | |
| 270 | | | | | | | Phenomorphan | 695 | Piminodine | 823 | | | |
| 271 | | | | | | | Piminodine | 1014 | | | | | |
| 272 | | | | | | | Phenazocine | 788 | | | | | |

TABLE XIV (*Continued*)

| Wave length (mμ) | Solvent 0.1 N HCl | | | | Solvent 0.1 N NaOH | | | | Solvent ethanol (50%) | | | | Wave length (mμ) |
|---|---|---|---|---|---|---|---|---|---|---|---|---|---|
| | Compound maximum | Molar extinction | Compound minimum | Molar extinction | Compound maximum | Molar extinction | Compound minimum | Molar extinction | Compound maximum | Molar extinction | Compound minimum | Molar extinction | |
| 274 | — | — | Dipipanone | 390 | — | — | — | — | Pholcodine | 1579 | — | — | 274 |
| — | — | — | Normethadone | 418 | — | — | — | — | — | — | — | — | — |
| 275 | — | — | — | — | — | — | — | — | — | — | — | — | 275 |
| 276 | — | — | — | — | — | — | Normethadone | 366 | Dipipanone | 293 | Normethadone | 303 | 276 |
| 277 | Phenazocine | 1982 | — | — | — | — | — | — | — | — | — | — | 277 |
| 278 | Levallorphan | 2452 | — | — | — | — | — | — | — | — | — | — | 278 |
| 279 | — | — | — | — | — | — | Dipipanone | 515 | — | — | — | — | 279 |
| 281 | — | — | — | — | — | — | — | — | Phenazocine | 2253 | — | — | 281 |
| 282 | — | — | — | — | — | — | — | — | Levallorphan | 2413 | — | — | 282 |
| — | — | — | — | — | — | — | — | — | — | — | — | — | — |
| 283 | Myrophine | 1690 | — | — | Myrophine | 1736 | — | — | Myrophine | 1630 | — | — | 283 |
| 284 | Pholcodine | 3270 | — | — | Pholcodine | 1602 | Nicomorphine | 1990 | — | — | — | — | 284 |
| — | — | — | — | — | — | — | — | — | — | — | — | — | — |
| 289 | — | — | — | — | Piminodine | 1523 | — | — | — | — | — | — | 289 |
| 292 | Dipipanone | 594 | — | — | — | — | Dipipanone | 556 | — | — | — | — | 292 |
| — | Normethadone | 598 | — | — | — | — | — | — | — | — | — | — | — |
| 293 | — | — | — | — | — | — | — | — | Piminodine | 1909 | — | — | 293 |
| 294 | — | — | — | — | — | — | Normethadone | 569 | Dipipanone | 448 | — | — | 294 |
| 295 | — | — | — | — | — | — | Nicomorphine | 2640 | Normethadone | 479 | — | — | 295 |
| 298 | — | — | — | — | — | — | Phenazocine | 3035 | — | — | — | — | 298 |
| 299 | — | — | — | — | — | — | Levallorphan | 3236 | — | — | — | — | 299 |
| 300 | — | — | — | — | — | — | — | — | — | — | — | — | 300 |

alcoholic solution of nicomorphine is spotted on the chromatogram and a drop of aqueous sodium hydroxide (0.1 *N*) is superimposed on the same spot prior to development.

There are four main facts which emerge from a study of the spectral changes produced in the acidic, basic, and neutral media:

(*i*) Phenyl groups which are dominant chromophores show little change;

(*ii*) Phenols undergo ionization to phenolates which reaction produces appreciable bathochromic shifts;

(*iii*) The aniline-anilinium tautomeric reaction in phenylaminochromophores causes noticeable phenyl structure changes;

(*iv*) Hydrolysis of esters produces ionic species which absorb differently than the acidic, or neutral molecule.

## 3. INFRARED SPECTRA

The general features of the infrared spectra of narcotics and the specific relationships of their functional groups to the IR bands are shown in Table XV, and discussed elsewhere (M5, B14).

## 4. X-RAY DIFFRACTION

Most of the weak lines ($I/I_1 \geq 3$) in the diffraction data in Table XVI are useful for checking the purity of the specimen. However, such weak lines do not appear on a negative exposed in the X-ray camera for shorter times. In the table the letters following the relative intensities of some of the lines are used to denote the reflection of sample condition in the crystallographic sense. The letter "d" refers to lines which are diffuse. They are probably caused by imperfections in the crystal lattice. Wide lines were marked "w." Lines whose relative intensities are set off by brackets are closely spaced, and are resolved by careful technique and use of the cobalt *k* source. A change in experimental conditions would probably result in the broadening of these lines into a single wide line with intermediate *d*-value.

The same order is used in the arrangement of the interplanar spacings and relative intensities of the twelve narcotics in Table XVII. No significant variations are observed in the patterns described in Table XVI or shown in Plate VII during the course of investigation.

Conventions regarding the two indexes Tables XVII and XVIII (H2), which are the numerical and innermost line indexes, are discussed by Barnes (B9) and Barnes and Sheppard (B10). In Table XVII the relative intensity of the innermost line of *dl*-dipipanone hydrochloride

TABLE XV

INFRARED IDENTIFICATION CHARACTERISTICS (M5)

| Fig. no. | Plate no. | Narcotic name | Common structural features | Functional group | IR band, wave numbers (cm$^{-1}$) |
|---|---|---|---|---|---|
| 1 | VIII | Piminodine | Methyl | —CH$_3$ | 1370–1380 (w)[a] |
| 3 | VIII | Propoxyphene | Methylene | —CH$_2$— | 1450 and 2900 |
| 4 | VIII | Levomoramide | Aromatic rings with substituents | (substituted aromatic ring structure) | 700 |
| 5 | IX | Normethadone | | | 750 |
| 6 | IX | Dipipanone | | | 1500–1600 |
| 8 | IX | Phenomorphan | Tertiary aliphatic base | >N— | 1325 |
| 12 | X | Nicomorphine | Pyridinium | (pyridine ring structure) | 700 |
| 1 | VIII | Piminodine | Carbon–oxygen ester | $-\overset{\displaystyle O}{\overset{\|}{C}}-OR$ | 1150 and 1250 |
| 2 | VIII | Etrhoheptazine | | | |
| 3 | VIII | Popoxyphene | | | |
| 11 | X | Myrophine | Carboxyl | COO— | 1700–1750 |
| 12 | X | Nicomorphine | | | |
| 4 | VIII | Levomoramide | Amide | CNO— | 1600–1650 |
| 5 | IX | Normethadone | Ketone | C=O | 1650–1750 |
| 6 | IX | Dipipanone | | | |

| No. | Group | Compound | Class | Structure | Band (cm⁻¹) |
|---|---|---|---|---|---|
| 7 | IX | Phenazocine | } Phenols | ⬡—OH | 3200–3400 |
| 8 | IX | Phenomorphan | | | |
| 9 | X | Levallorphan | | | |
| 10 | X | Pholcodine | } Ethers (furans) | (cyclic C–C–O structure) | 1070–1150 |
| 12 | X | Nicomorphine | | | |
| 11 | X | Myrophine | | | |
| 1 | VIII | Piminodine | Anilinium | ⬡—NH | 1325, 1600 |
| 1 | VIII | Piminodine | } Halide | [—C—NH₂]⁺X⁻ | 2400–2600 |
| 3 | VIII | Propoxyphene | | | |
| 5 | IX | Normethadone | | | |
| 6 | IX | Dipipanone | | | |
| 12 | X | Nicomorphine | | | |
| 2 | VIII | Ethoheptazine | Citrate | OH and H bonding | 2600–3000 (broad) |
| 9 | X | Levallorphan | Tartrate | OH and H bonding | 2600–3000 (broad) |

$^a$ w = weak intensity band.

monohydrate is less than 5 and therefore the *d* value of the third line
is listed. This entry is enclosed in square brackets.

TABLE XVI

Interplanar Spacings (*d*) and Relative Intensity ($I/I_1$) Values
of X-ray Diffraction Patterns of Twelve Narcotics (M5)

| $d$ (Å) | $I/I_1$ | $d$ (Å) | $I/I_1$ |
|---|---|---|---|
| 1. Piminodine Ethanesulfonate | | | |
| 16.4 | 5 | 2.89 | 20 |
| 12.2 | 5 | 2.83 | 1 |
| 11.1 | 55 | 2.76 | 15w[b] |
| 8.91 | 10 | 2.68 | 5w |
| 8.23 | 55 | 2.62 | 5w |
| 7.71 | 2 | 2.55 | 10 |
| 6.17 | 10 | 2.50 | 1 |
| 5.91 | 1 | 2.45 | 10 |
| 5.53 | 60 | 2.41 | 5 |
| 5.34 | 100 | 2.38 | 5 |
| 5.08 | 35 | 2.36 | 5 |
| 4.91 | 30 | 2.32 | 10 |
| 4.73 | 30 } | 2.27 | 4w |
| 4.65 | 20 } | 2.24 | 15 } |
| 4.49 | 3 | 2.23 | 2d } |
| 4.36 | 70 | 2.19 | 1 |
| 4.24 | 2 } | 2.16 | 3 |
| 4.20 | 5 } | 2.13 | 3 |
| 4.09 | 45 | 2.10 | 1 |
| 4.02 | 3d[a] | 2.07 | 5 |
| 3.91 | 30 | 2.01 | 2 |
| 3.83 | 30 | 1.97 | 3 |
| 3.69 | 80 | 1.93 | 5d |
| 3.46 | 25 | 1.87 | 2 |
| 3.38 | 35 | 1.85 | 1 |
| 3.29 | 35 | 1.83 | 5 |
| 3.22 | 3 | 1.79 | 1 |
| 3.15 | 10 | 1.78 | 2 |
| 3.04 | 20 | 1.76 | 2 |
| 2.96 | 20 | — | — |

[a] d stands for diffuse.
[b] w stands for wide.

TABLE XVI (*Continued*)

| $d$ (Å) | $I/I_1$ | $d$ (Å) | $I/I_1$ |
|---|---|---|---|
| | 2. Ethoheptazine Citrate | | |
| 20.8 | 50 | 3.03 | 15 |
| 11.5 | 25 | 2.94 | 3w |
| 8.51 | 80 | 2.86 | 20⎰ |
| 7.12 | 70w | 2.84 | 5⎱ |
| 6.71 | 40 | 2.76 | 2w |
| 6.35 | 1d | 2.69 | 1 |
| 6.08 | 5 | 2.63 | 35d |
| 5.89 | 40 | 2.55 | 15 |
| 5.71 | 35 | 2.50 | 2 |
| 5.37 | 30⎰ | 2.49 | 2 |
| 5.29 | 100⎱ | 2.43 | 2 |
| 5.11 | 10⎰ | 2.40 | 1 |
| 5.03 | 15⎱ | 2.36 | 2 |
| 4.87 | 40 | 2.32 | 1 |
| 4.71 | 5 | 2.29 | 2⎰ |
| 4.59 | 40 | 2.27 | 2⎱ |
| 4.41 | 35 | 2.23 | 3 |
| 4.26 | 35 | 2.20 | 2⎰ |
| 4.17 | 55 | 2.19 | 2⎱ |
| 4.07 | 30 | 2.15 | 1 |
| 3.96 | 35 | 2.09 | 3 |
| 3.81 | 5 | 2.04 | 2d |
| 3.71 | 5⎰ | 2.03 | 2d |
| 3.68 | 10⎱ | 2.00 | 2d |
| 3.59 | 10 | 1.98 | 2d |
| 3.47 | 10 | 1.93 | 3 |
| 3.38 | 65 | 1.91 | 1 |
| 3.28 | 2 | 1.88 | 2w |
| 3.23 | 20 | 1.84 | 1 |
| 3.14 | 2 | 1.82 | 1 |
| 3.08 | 1 | 1.79 | 2 |

TABLE XVI (*Continued*)

| d (Å) | I/I₁ | d (Å) | I/I₁ |
|---|---|---|---|
| | | | |

$$d\text{ (Å)} \qquad I/I_1 \qquad d\text{ (Å)} \qquad I/I_1$$

3. *d*-Propoxyphene Hydrochloride

| d (Å) | I/I₁ | d (Å) | I/I₁ |
|---|---|---|---|
| 9.40 | 10 | 2.85 | 20 |
| 8.75 | 45 | 2.82 | 5 |
| 8.13 | 1 | 2.77 | 5 |
| 7.84 | 1 | 2.71 | 15d |
| 7.38 | 40 | 2.62 | 15 |
| 6.89 | 1 | 2.56 | 1 |
| 6.57 | 1 | 2.52 | 30 |
| 6.40 | 10 | 2.46 | 15d |
| 6.07 | 45 ⎫ | 2.41 | 10 |
| 5.97 | 100 ⎭ | 2.36 | 5 |
| 5.81 | 2 | 2.33 | 5 |
| 5.66 | 10 | 2.30 | 2 |
| 5.42 | 10 | 2.26 | 3w |
| 5.22 | 3w | 2.23 | 15 |
| 5.05 | 40 | 2.19 | 1 |
| 4.85 | 1 | 2.16 | 5 |
| 4.69 | 3 | 2.14 | 10 |
| 4.52 | 35 | 2.12 | 1 |
| 4.37 | 35 | 2.10 | 2 |
| 4.26 | 15 | 2.08 | 2 |
| 4.17 | 25 | 2.06 | 1 |
| 4.07 | 100 ⎫ | 2.03 | 10 |
| 4.02 | 15 ⎭ | 2.00 | 3w |
| 3.87 | 25 | 1.97 | 3 |
| 3.82 | 2 | 1.95 | 3 |
| 3.74 | 40 | 1.93 | 2w |
| 3.66 | 5 ⎫ | 1.90 | 1 |
| 3.63 | 10 ⎭ | 1.88 | 2 |
| 3.57 | 1 | 1.85 | 2 |
| 3.50 | 10 ⎫ | 1.83 | 1 |
| 3.47 | 30 ⎭ | 1.81 | 5 |
| 3.39 | 10 | 1.79 | 5 |
| 3.33 | 10 | 1.77 | 1 |
| 3.28 | 10 | 1.75 | 2 |
| 3.21 | 30 | 1.71 | 2 |
| 3.17 | 10 | 1.70 | 1 |
| 3.10 | 15w | 1.68 | 2 |
| 3.02 | 10 ⎫ | 1.66 | 1 |
| 3.00 | 10 ⎭ | 1.64 | 2 |
| 2.91 | 30 | — | — |

TABLE XVI (*Continued*)

| d (Å) | I/I₁ | d (Å) | I/I₁ |
|-------|------|-------|------|

| d (Å) | $I/I_1$ | d (Å) | $I/I_1$ |
|-------|---------|-------|--------|
| | 4. Levomoramide (free base) | | |
| 10.2 | 35 | 2.78 | 1 |
| 9.23 | 15 | 2.73 | 5 |
| 8.57 | 80 | 2.64 | 35 |
| 8.07 | 1 | 2.58 | 3 |
| 7.67 | 30 | 2.53 | 2 |
| 7.33 | 50 | 2.48 | 2 |
| 7.04 | 65 | 2.43 | 20 |
| 6.66 | 60 | 2.38 | 3 |
| 6.42 | 1 | 2.34 | 20 |
| 6.12 | 65 | 2.30 | 1 |
| 5.85 | 60 | 2.28 | 1 |
| 5.52 | 2 } | 2.26 | 5 |
| 5.43 | 1 } | 2.24 | 3 |
| 5.17 | 40 | 2.21 | 1 |
| 4.97 | 70 | 2.19 | 15 |
| 4.83 | 1 | 2.16 | 5 |
| 4.69 | 40 | 2.11 | 5 |
| 4.59 | 100 | 2.08 | 5 |
| 4.50 | 45 | 2.04 | 5d |
| 4.37 | 45 } | 2.02 | 1 |
| 4.31 | 45 } | 1.99 | 1 |
| 4.17 | 5 | 1.97 | 8 |
| 4.05 | 70 | 1.95 | 1 |
| 3.93 | 65 | 1.92 | 1 |
| 3.81 | 40 | 1.90 | 5 |
| 3.72 | 40 | 1.88 | 1 |
| 3.64 | 15 | 1.86 | 4 |
| 3.52 | 15 | 1.85 | 3d |
| 3.43 | 65 | 1.81 | 4 |
| 3.31 | 3 | 1.80 | 1 |
| 3.22 | 10 } | 1.75 | 2 |
| 3.19 | 10 } | 1.72 | 2 } |
| 3.13 | 20 | 1.71 | 1 } |
| 3.06 | 15w | 1.65 | 2 |
| 2.99 | 1 | 1.64 | 1 |
| 2.92 | 5 } | 1.61 | 2 |
| 2.91 | 5 } | 1.58 | 2 |
| 2.85 | 20 | 1.56 | 1 |
| 2.82 | 15 | 1.54 | 1 |

TABLE XVI (*Continued*)

| d (Å) | I/I₁ | d (Å) | I/I₁ |
|-------|------|-------|------|

5. Normethadone Hydrochloride

| d (Å) | I/I₁ | d (Å) | I/I₁ |
|-------|------|-------|------|
| 12.3 | 20 | 2.58 | 10 |
| 8.40 | 2 | 2.54 | 10 |
| 8.04 | 60 | 2.50 | 4 |
| 7.69 | 50 | 2.46 | 4 |
| 7.24 | 85 | 2.39 | 8 |
| 6.77 | 2⎱ | 2.36 | 1 |
| 6.62 | 2⎰ | 2.32 | 5 |
| 6.26 | 10 | 2.28 | 10⎱ |
| 6.05 | 20 | 2.26 | 8⎰ |
| 5.68 | 5 | 2.21 | 3 |
| 5.47 | 2 | 2.17 | 8 |
| 5.27 | 5 | 2.13 | 5 |
| 5.03 | 2 | 2.09 | 3⎱ |
| 4.79 | 10⎱ | 2.08 | 3⎰ |
| 4.70 | 80⎰ | 2.05 | 5 |
| 4.55 | 20 | 2.03 | 3 |
| 4.36 | 100 | 1.99 | 2 |
| 4.21 | 20 | 1.98 | 2 |
| 4.11 | 25 | 1.95 | 1 |
| 4.01 | 25 | 1.93 | 2 |
| 3.89 | 20 | 1.91 | 2 |
| 3.76 | 20 | 1.88 | 5 |
| 3.66 | 20 | 1.85 | 2 |
| 3.63 | 3 | 1.84 | 2 |
| 3.45 | 10 | 1.80 | 5 |
| 3.34 | 10 | 1.79 | 1 |
| 3.21 | 25 | 1.75 | 2 |
| 3.15 | 2⎱ | 1.72 | 5 |
| 3.12 | 45⎰ | 1.70 | 1 |
| 3.04 | 45 | 1.67 | 1 |
| 2.97 | 20 | 1.66 | 3w |
| 2.89 | 5 | 1.61 | 1 |
| 2.87 | 25 | 1.60 | 2 |
| 2.75 | 1 | 1.59 | 1 |
| 2.73 | 5 | 1.56 | 2 |
| 2.69 | 10 | — | — |
| 2.65 | 10 | — | — |

TABLE XVI (*Continued*)

| $d$ (Å) | $I/I_1$ | $d$ (Å) | $I/I_1$ |
|---------|---------|---------|---------|
| 6. *dl*-Dipipanone Hydrochloride Monohydrate | | | |
| 15.0 | 2 | 2.40 | 15 |
| 8.93 | 1 | 2.35 | 1 |
| 8.09 | 80 | 2.32 | 3 |
| 7.32 | 20 | 2.29 | 15w |
| 6.99 | 1 | 2.25 | 1 |
| 6.70 | 2 | 2.22 | 3⎰ |
| 6.48 | 65 | 2.21 | 1⎱ |
| 6.25 | 55 | 2.16 | 10 |
| 5.30 | 60 | 2.14 | 2 |
| 5.17 | 30 | 2.11 | 10 |
| 5.02 | 75 | 2.07 | 8 |
| 4.79 | 60 | 2.05 | 5 |
| 4.34 | 60 | 2.02 | 8 |
| 4.24 | 35 | 2.01 | 3 |
| 4.14 | 35 | 1.97 | 10 |
| 4.02 | 100 | 1.95 | 2 |
| 3.90 | 5 | 1.93 | 4 |
| 3.80 | 20 | 1.90 | 10 |
| 3.68 | 55w | 1.88 | 2d |
| 3.58 | 5 | 1.85 | 5 |
| 3.52 | 20 | 1.83 | 2 |
| 3.46 | 15 | 1.81 | 3 |
| 3.34 | 15w | 1.79 | 2⎰ |
| 3.25 | 55 | 1.78 | 2⎱ |
| 3.16 | 25⎰ | 1.75 | 2 |
| 3.11 | 25⎱ | 1.72 | 2 |
| 3.05 | 5 | 1.70 | 2 |
| 2.98 | 35 | 1.66 | 2 |
| 2.90 | 55 | 1.63 | 1d |
| 2.82 | 2d | 1.60 | 2 |
| 2.80 | 20 | 1.58 | 1 |
| 2.76 | 5 | 1.57 | 1 |
| 2.71 | 20 | 1.53 | 2 |
| 2.64 | 10 | 1.52 | 1 |
| 2.60 | 10 | 1.480 | 1 |
| 2.56 | 10 | 1.461 | 1 |
| 2.52 | 2⎰ | 1.449 | 2 |
| 2.50 | 10⎱ | 1.422 | 1 |
| 2.47 | 5 | 1.410 | 2 |
| 2.44 | 10 | 1.373 | 2 |

TABLE XVI *(Continued)*

| $d$ (Å) | $I/I_1$ | $d$ (Å) | $I/I_1$ |
|---------|---------|---------|---------|

### 7. Phenazocine Hydrobromide

| $d$ (Å) | $I/I_1$ | $d$ (Å) | $I/I_1$ |
|---------|---------|---------|---------|
| 15.2 | 100 | 3.31 | 10 |
| 13.5 | 2 | 3.23 | 5⎱ |
| 10.6 | 2 | 3.20 | 30⎰ |
| 9.38 | 1 | 3.13 | 3 |
| 8.85 | 50 | 3.06 | 1 |
| 8.23 | 1 | 3.00 | 2 |
| 7.75 | 3 | 2.94 | 30 |
| 7.31 | 5 | 2.87 | 1 |
| 7.08 | 3 | 2.83 | 3⎱ |
| 6.75 | 1 | 2.81 | 3⎰ |
| 6.50 | 4 | 2.75 | 5 |
| 6.23 | 20 | 2.72 | 2 |
| 6.02 | 15 | 2.66 | 4 |
| 5.78 | 1 | 2.61 | 2⎱ |
| 5.51 | 25 | 2.59 | 2⎰ |
| 5.31 | 1 | 2.53 | 5 |
| 5.13 | 35 | 2.46 | 1⎱ |
| 4.93 | 30 | 2.44 | 2⎰ |
| 4.78 | 30 | 2.39 | 2w |
| 4.60 | 3 | 2.34 | 2 |
| 4.44 | 3 | 2.29 | 2 |
| 4.39 | 35 | 2.24 | 2 |
| 4.30 | 5 | 2.19 | 1 |
| 4.21 | 3 | 2.17 | 3 |
| 4.13 | 60 | 2.14 | 1 |
| 4.02 | 10 | 2.12 | 2 |
| 3.94 | 5 | 2.08 | 2 |
| 3.81 | 5 | 2.07 | 2 |
| 3.78 | 5 | 2.02 | 2 |
| 3.69 | 2 | 2.01 | 2 |
| 3.62 | 10 | 1.96 | 2 |
| 3.51 | 8 | 1.95 | 2 |
| 3.44 | 1 | 1.92 | 1 |
| 3.38 | 5 | — | — |

TABLE XVI (*Continued*)

| $d$ (Å) | $I/I_1$ | $d$ (Å) | $I/I_1$ |
|---|---|---|---|
| | | 8. *d*-Phenomorphan Hydrobromide | |
| 10.3 | 10 | 2.56 | 3⎫ |
| 9.38 | 75 | 2.53 | 5⎭ |
| 8.93 | 1 | 2.49 | 3 |
| 8.22 | 5 | 2.46 | 2d |
| 7.77 | 1 | 2.51 | 1 |
| 7.31 | 40 | 2.37 | 8d |
| 6.82 | 5 | 2.31 | 8 |
| 6.52 | 40 | 2.27 | 2 |
| 6.18 | 1w | 2.23 | 5 |
| 5.90 | 5⎫ | 2.20 | 3 |
| 5.81 | 5⎭ | 2.18 | 5 |
| 5.58 | 5 | 2.13 | 5 |
| 5.41 | 1 | 2.11 | 2 |
| 5.16 | 100 | 2.08 | 3 |
| 4.93 | 60 | 2.06 | 3⎫ |
| 4.74 | 1w | 2.05 | 2⎭ |
| 4.55 | 50 | 2.02 | 2⎫ |
| 4.40 | 70 | 2.01 | 3⎭ |
| 4.28 | 1 | 1.98 | 2 |
| 4.17 | 35 | 1.97 | 1 |
| 4.05 | 3 | 1.94 | 2 |
| 3.96 | 10 | 1.92 | 10 |
| 3.88 | 5 | 1.90 | 1 |
| 3.77 | 65 | 1.88 | 3 |
| 3.67 | 55 | 1.85 | 3d |
| 3.60 | 5 | 1.82 | 4 |
| 3.53 | 20 | 1.80 | 1 |
| 3.47 | 3 | 1.78 | 3 |
| 3.41 | 3 | 1.76 | 3 |
| 3.34 | 2 | 1.74 | 2 |
| 3.27 | 5 | 1.72 | 2 |
| 3.21 | 10 | 1.70 | 1w |
| 3.16 | 10 | 1.67 | 2w |
| 3.09 | 5 | 1.65 | 1 |
| 3.03 | 2⎫ | 1.64 | 1 |
| 3.01 | 2⎭ | 1.62 | 2 |
| 2.94 | 20 | 1.60 | 2 |
| 2.89 | 20 | 1.58 | 1 |
| 2.79 | 5 | 1.55 | 2 |
| 2.74 | 5 | 1.54 | 1 |
| 2.68 | 1⎫ | 1.52 | 2 |
| 2.67 | 3⎭ | — | — |
| 2.62 | 15 | — | — |

TABLE XVI (*Continued*)

| $d$ (Å) | $I/I_1$ | $d$ (Å) | $I/I_1$ |
|---|---|---|---|
| | 9. Levallorphan Tartrate | | |
| 9.50 | 50 | 2.53 | 40 |
| 7.34 | 35⎱ | 2.49 | 8 |
| 7.14 | 40⎰ | 2.46 | 8 |
| 6.70 | 75 | 2.42 | 2 |
| 6.36 | 1 | 2.38 | 1 |
| 6.30 | 15 | 2.35 | 5 |
| 5.93 | 1 | 2.30 | 45 |
| 5.72 | 100 | 2.27 | 2d |
| 5.51 | 80 | 2.23 | 25 |
| 5.29 | 2w | 2.18 | 15 |
| 5.08 | 20 | 2.14 | 2 |
| 4.92 | 1 | 2.10 | 1 |
| 4.74 | 40 | 2.09 | 1 |
| 4.58 | 15 | 2.04 | 20 |
| 4.43 | 30 | 2.01 | 1d |
| 4.35 | 40 | 2.00 | 10 |
| 4.20 | 50 | 1.98 | 8 |
| 4.04 | 70 | 1.96 | 8 |
| 3.92 | 2 | 1.93 | 1⎱ |
| 3.81 | 25 | 1.92 | 2⎰ |
| 3.69 | 30w | 1.90 | 5 |
| 3.55 | 70 | 1.86 | 3 |
| 3.46 | 1 | 1.84 | 2 |
| 3.38 | 35⎱ | 1.82 | 1 |
| 3.35 | 35⎰ | 1.81 | 1 |
| 3.25 | 2d | 1.79 | 25 |
| 3.21 | 3 | 1.76 | 5 |
| 3.16 | 3 | 1.74 | 1w |
| 3.09 | 2 | 1.72 | 1 |
| 3.04 | 10 | 1.71 | 1 |
| 2.99 | 5 | 1.69 | 3 |
| 2.93 | 5 | 1.67 | 2 |
| 2.85 | 30 | 1.65 | 1 |
| 2.79 | 35 | 1.62 | 2 |
| 2.72 | 2 | 1.60 | 1 |
| 2.64 | 1 | 1.58 | 3 |
| 2.60 | 5 | — | — |

TABLE XVI (*Continued*)

| $d$ (Å) | $I/I_1$ | $d$ (Å) | $I/I_1$ |
|---|---|---|---|
| | 10. Pholcodine Monohydrate (free base) | | |
| 7.59 | 100 | 2.49 | 10 |
| 6.71 | 35 | 2.39 | 35 |
| 6.25 | 40 | 2.36 | 5 |
| 6.00 | 20 | 2.33 | 10 |
| 5.82 | 1 | 2.28 | 15 |
| 5.55 | 100 | 2.24 | 5} |
| 5.37 | 25 | 2.23 | 10} |
| 5.27 | 100 | 2.17 | 35 |
| 4.71 | 25 | 2.15 | 2 |
| 4.64 | 80 | 2.13 | 1 |
| 4.48 | 40 | 2.10 | 5 |
| 4.33 | 40 | 2.08 | 5 |
| 4.23 | 1 | 2.05 | 10 |
| 4.12 | 35 | 2.02 | 8 |
| 3.96 | 35 | 2.01 | 2 |
| 3.87 | 1 | 1.98 | 10} |
| 3.79 | 80 | 1.97 | 5d} |
| 3.69 | 2} | 1.93 | 5 |
| 3.67 | 5} | 1.90 | 10w |
| 3.59 | 20 | 1.87 | 10 |
| 3.51 | 70 | 1.85 | 3 |
| 3.39 | 5d} | 1.83 | 3 |
| 3.36 | 25} | 1.80 | 5} |
| 3.31 | 10w | 1.79 | 5d} |
| 3.15 | 15 | 1.76 | 3 |
| 3.08 | 40 | 1.74 | 3w |
| 3.03 | 40 | 1.71 | 1 |
| 2.96 | 1 | 1.68 | 2 |
| 2.90 | 35 | 1.64 | 8 |
| 2.83 | 1 | 1.63 | 1 |
| 2.78 | 35 | 1.61 | 2 |
| 2.74 | 2 | 1.59 | 1 |
| 2.70 | 10 | 1.56 | 2} |
| 2.65 | 1 | 1.55 | 1} |
| 2.60 | 15 | 1.54 | 2 |
| 2.57 | 1 | 1.53 | 2 |
| 2.53 | 35 | — | — |

TABLE XVI (*Continued*)

| d (Å) | I/I₁ | d (Å) | I/I₁ |
|---|---|---|---|

| | 11. Myrophine (free base) | | |
|---|---|---|---|
| 14.4 | 65 | 2.97 | 2⎱ |
| 9.61 | 60 | 2.94 | 2⎰ |
| 8.96 | 1 | 2.88 | 5 |
| 8.82 | 1 | 2.83 | 1 |
| 8.30 | 85 | 2.79 | 2 |
| 7.69 | 15 | 2.72 | 1d |
| 7.22 | 15 | 2.66 | 1d |
| 6.83 | 1 | 2.61 | 4w |
| 6.57 | 35 | 2.55 | 4w |
| 6.27 | 3 | 2.50 | 3 |
| 5.97 | 40 | 2.46 | 1 |
| 5.74 | 3 ⎱ | 2.44 | 4 |
| 5.65 | 2d ⎰ | 2.39 | 5 |
| 5.31 | 25 | 2.34 | 3 |
| 5.01 | 100 | 2.29 | 1 |
| 4.87 | 3 | 2.27 | 10 |
| 4.72 | 40 | 2.24 | 5 |
| 4.58 | 1 | 2.21 | 1 |
| 4.44 | 20 | 2.19 | 2 |
| 4.30 | 3 | 2.15 | 3w |
| 4.16 | 35w | 2.11 | 2 |
| 4.02 | 30 | 2.09 | 2 |
| 3.92 | 30 | 2.06 | 3 |
| 3.83 | 3 | 2.01 | 4 |
| 3.74 | 10⎱ | 1.99 | 2 |
| 3.70 | 5⎰ | 1.96 | 5 |
| 3.58 | 20 | 1.92 | 2 |
| 3.49 | 10 | 1.90 | 1 |
| 3.43 | 3 | 1.87 | 2 |
| 3.36 | 2 | 1.84 | 1 |
| 3.29 | 3 | 1.80 | 2⎱ |
| 3.21 | 3 | 1.79 | 2⎰ |
| 3.13 | 3 | 1.74 | 2d |
| 3.03 | 5 | 1.70 | 1 |
| — | — | 1.68 | 1 |

TABLE XVI (*Continued*)

| $d$ (Å) | $I/I_1$ | $d$ (Å) | $I/I_1$ |
|---|---|---|---|
| 12. Nicomorphine Hydrochloride Dihydrate | | | |
| 15.6 | 95 | 2.80 | 15 |
| 11.2 | 10 | 2.75 | 1 |
| 10.3 | 1 | 2.71 | 8 |
| 9.43 | 90 | 2.67 | 2 |
| 8.72 | 1 | 2.62 | 3 |
| 7.84 | 3 | 2.58 | 2 |
| 7.30 | 1 | 2.54 | 5 |
| 7.00 | 1 | 2.48 | 3 |
| 6.56 | 25 | 2.42 | 4 } |
| 6.32 | 15 | 2.40 | 2d } |
| 5.97 | 85 } | 2.36 | 4 |
| 5.87 | 20 } | 2.33 | 1 |
| 5.61 | 10 | 2.28 | 1 |
| 5.41 | 1 | 2.26 | 4 |
| 5.20 | 20 | 2.23 | 1 |
| 4.98 | 1 | 2.17 | 4 } |
| 4.76 | 15 | 2.16 | 4 } |
| 4.52 | 80 | 2.12 | 2 |
| 4.34 | 100 | 2.09 | 1 |
| 4.16 | 10 | 2.06 | 3d |
| 4.04 | 1 | 2.03 | 1 |
| 3.92 | 15 | 2.00 | 3 |
| 3.82 | 1 | 1.97 | 4 |
| 3.66 | 35 | 1.95 | 1 |
| 3.58 | 5 | 1.93 | 1 |
| 3.48 | 45 | 1.90 | 4 |
| 3.39 | 20 | 1.88 | 1 |
| 3.33 | 5 | 1.83 | 2w |
| 3.26 | 20 | 1.77 | 2w |
| 3.18 | 10 | 1.73 | 2 } |
| 3.12 | 1 | 1.71 | 2 } |
| 3.07 | 5 | 1.69 | 1 |
| 3.01 | 3 | 1.66 | 2 |
| 2.95 | 10 | 1.65 | 1 |
| 2.88 | 3 | 1.63 | 2 |

[a] d stands for diffuse.
[b] w stands for wide.

TABLE XVII
INNERMOST LINE INDEX FOR TWELVE NARCOTIC
X-RAY DIFFRACTION PATTERNS (M5)

| $d$ (Å) | $I/I_1$ | Name | No. |
|---|---|---|---|
| 20.8 | 50 | Ethoheptazine citrate | 2 |
| 16.4 | 5 | Piminodine ethane sulfonate | 1 |
| 15.6 | 95 | Nicomorphine hydrochloride dihydrate | 12 |
| 15.2 | 100 | Phenazocine hydrobromide | 7 |
| 14.4 | 65 | Myrophine (free base) | 11 |
| 12.3 | 20 | Normethadone hydrochloride | 5 |
| 10.3 | 10 | $d$-Phenomorphan hydrobromide | 8 |
| 10.2 | 35 | Levomoramide (free base) | 4 |
| 9.50 | 50 | Levallorphan tartrate | 9 |
| 9.40 | 10 | $d$-Propoxyphene hydrochloride | 3 |
| [8.09 | 80 | $dl$-Dipipanone hydrochloride monohydrate | 6] |
| 7.59 | 100 | Pholcodine monohydrate (free base) | 10 |

5. PAPER CHROMATOGRAPHY

Table XIX gives the $R_f$ values of thirty-four narcotics and related bases in six paper chromatographic systems (G4). Four systems have strongly polar stationary phases and mobile phases of decreasing polarity (Nos. 1, 2, 3, and 6). The other two systems (Nos. 4 and 5) belong to the "reversed phase" category having a stronger polar mobile phase in contrast with the weakly polar stationary one. This set of solvents leads to a good distribution of $R_f$ values over the full range of the $R_f$ scale for the more important narcotics. Systems 1, 2, and 3 are most suitable for opiates, whereas nearly all opioids are found in the upper third of the $R_f$ scale. The latter narcotics are separable in systems 4 and 5. Most of the opiates in these systems travel as a group close to the front (system 4) or in the upper third (system 5). Tables XX, XXI, and XXII list the chromatographic observations on ninety-three, fifty-three, and thirty-three narcotics, alkaloids, antihistamines, and phenothiazines of toxicological importance. $R_f$ values, iodoplatinate spray reagent, color reactions, and the ultraviolet observations for about one hundred and ninety basic compounds are reported here, many for the first time (D2).

IV. Opium—Assay, Characteristics, Composition, and Origin

A. General

In 1948 the Economic and Social Council of the United Nations stated that "a major step in narcotic control would be made, when it became possible to trace the country of origin of illicit opium by physical and chemical methods." Since this beginning, the international research program on opium has made progress which is now worth reviewing and evaluating to see how close is the objective.

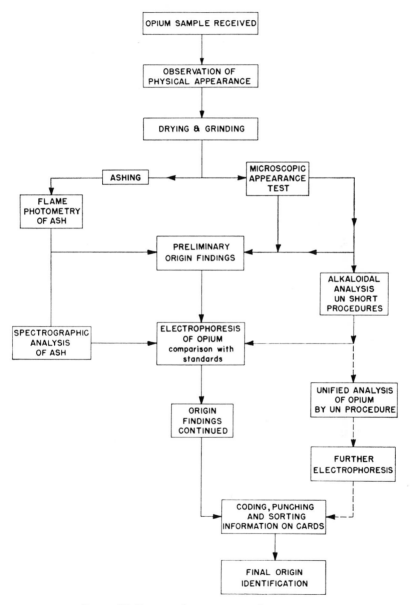

PLATE XI. Process of opium origin determination.

TABLE XVIII

NUMERICAL (HANAWALT) INDEX (M5)

| d-range | No. | d₁ (Å) | I | d₂ (Å) | I | d₃ (Å) | I | Substance | Ref |
|---|---|---|---|---|---|---|---|---|---|
| 15.9 to 14.0 | 84. | 14.4 | 100 | 5.01 | 85 | 8.30 | 65 | Myrophine (free base) | (11) |
| | | 15.6 | 100 | 4.34 | 90 | 9.43 | 95 | Nicomorphine hydrochloride dihydrate | (12) |
| | | 15.2 | 60 | 4.13 | 50 | 8.85 | 100 | Phenazocine hydrobromide | (7) |
| 9.49 to 9.00 | 79. | 9.38 | 100 | 5.16 | 70 | 4.40 | 75 | d-Phenomorphan hydrobromide | (8) |
| | | 9.43 | 100 | 4.34 | 95 | 15.6 | 90 | Nicomorphine hydrochloride dihydrate | (12) |
| 8.99 to 8.50 | 78. | 8.85 | 100 | 15.2 | 60 | 4.13 | 50 | Phenazocine hydrobromide | (7) |
| | | 8.75 | 100 | 5.97 | 100 | 4.07 | 45 | d-Propoxyphene hydrochloride | (3) |
| | | 8.51 | 100 | 5.29 | 70 | 7.12 | 80 | Ethoheptazine citrate | (2) |
| | | 8.57 | 100 | 4.59 | 70 | 4.97 | 80 | Levomoramide (free base) | (4) |
| 8.49 to 8.00 | 77. | 8.30 | 100 | 5.01 | 65 | 14.4 | 85 | Myrophine (free base) | (11) |
| | | 8.09 | 100 | 4.02 | 75 | 5.02 | 80 | dl-Dipipanone hydrochloride monohydrate | (6) |
| 7.99 to 7.50 | 76. | 7.59 | 100 | 5.55 | 100 | 5.27 | 100 | Pholcodine monohydrate (free base) | (10) |
| 7.49 to 7.00 | 75. | 7.12 | 100 | 5.29 | 80 | 8.51 | 70 | Ethoheptazine citrate | (2) |
| | | 7.24 | 100 | 4.36 | 80 | 4.70 | 85 | Normethadone hydrochloride | (5) |
| 6.99 to 6.50 | 74. | 6.70 | 100 | 5.72 | 80 | 5.51 | 75 | Levallorphan tartrate | (9) |
| 5.99 to 5.75 | 72. | 5.97 | 100 | 4.07 | 45 | 7.75 | 100 | d-Propoxyphene hydrochloride | (3) |
| 5.74 to 5.50 | 71. | 5.55 | 100 | 7.59 | 100 | 5.27 | 100 | Pholcodine (free base) (monohydrate) | (10) |

| | | | | | | | |
|---|---|---|---|---|---|---|---|
| 5.51 | 5.72 | 80 | 6.70 | 100 | 75 | Levallorphan tartrate | (9) |
| 5.72 | 5.51 | 100 | 6.70 | 80 | 75 | Levallorphan tartrate | (9) |
| | | | | 70. | 5.49 to 5.25 | | |
| 5.29 | 8.51 | 100 | 7.12 | 80 | 70 | Ethoheptazine citrate | (2) |
| 5.27 | 7.59 | 100 | 5.55 | 100 | 100 | Pholcodine monohydrate (free base) | (10) |
| 5.34 | 3.69 | 100 | 4.36 | 80 | 70 | Piminodine ethane sulfonate | (1) |
| | | | | 69. | 5.24 to 5.00 | | |
| 5.16 | 9.38 | 100 | 4.40 | 75 | 70 | d-Phenomorphan hydrobromide | (8) |
| 5.01 | 8.30 | 100 | 14.4 | 85 | 65 | Myrophine (free base) | (11) |
| 5.02 | 4.02 | 75 | 8.09 | 100 | 80 | dl-Dipipanone hydrochloride monohydrate | (6) |
| | | | | 68. | 4.99 to 4.90 | | |
| 4.97 | 4.59 | 70 | 8.57 | 100 | 80 | Levomoramide (free base) | (4) |
| | | | | 66. | 4.79 to 4.70 | | |
| 4.70 | 4.36 | 80 | 7.24 | 100 | 85 | Normethadone hydrochloride | (5) |
| | | | | 64. | 4.59 to 4.50 | | |
| 4.59 | 8.57 | 100 | 4.97 | 80 | 70 | Levomoramide (free base) | (4) |
| | | | | 63. | 4.49 to 4.40 | | |
| 4.40 | 5.16 | 70 | 9.38 | 100 | 75 | d-Phenomorphan hydrobromide | (8) |
| | | | | 62. | 4.39 to 4.30 | | |
| 4.34 | 15.6 | 100 | 9.43 | 95 | 90 | Nicomorphine hydrochloride dihydrate | (12) |
| 4.36 | 7.24 | 100 | 4.70 | 85 | 80 | Normethadone hydrochloride | (5) |
| 4.36 | 5.34 | 70 | 3.69 | 100 | 80 | Piminodine ethane sulfonate | (1) |
| | | | | 60. | 4.19 to 4.10 | | |
| 4.13 | 15.2 | 60 | 8.85 | 100 | 50 | Phenazocine hydrobromide | (7) |
| | | | | 59. | 4.09 to 4.00 | | |
| 4.02 | 8.09 | 100 | 5.02 | 80 | 75 | dl-Dipipanone hydrochloride monohydrate | (6) |
| 4.07 | 5.97 | 100 | 8.75 | 100 | 45 | d-Propoxyphene hydrochloride | (3) |
| | | | | 55. | 3.69 to 3.60 | | |
| 3.69 | 5.34 | 80 | 4.36 | 100 | 70 | Piminodine ethane sulfonate | (1) |

TABLE XIX

$R_f$ VALUES OF NARCOTICS IN SIX SOLVENT SYSTEMS (G4)

| No. | Name of narcotic | $R_f$ in system no. | | | | | |
|---|---|---|---|---|---|---|---|
| | | 1 | 2 | 3 | 4 | 5 | 6 |
| 1 | Oxymorphone | 0.21 | 0.10 | 0.06 | 0.93 | 0.80 | 0.08 |
| 2 | Morphine | 0.34 | 0.13 | 0.05 | 0.92 | 0.78 | 0.01 |
| 3 | Oxycodone | 0.34 | 0.22 | 0.16 | 0.92 | 0.81 | 0.16 |
| 4 | Hydrocodone | 0.46 | 0.26 | 0.23 | 0.95 | 0.81 | 0.08 |
| 5 | Codeine | 0.49 | 0.24 | 0.12 | 0.95 | 0.79 | 0.10 |
| 6 | Ethylmorphine | 0.66 | 0.45 | 0.33 | 0.94 | 0.77 | 0.18 |
| 7 | Diamorphine | 0.73 | 0.50 | 0.52 | 0.91 | 0.75 | 0.06 |
| 8 | Thebaine | 0.85 | 0.67 | 0.41 | 0.95 | 0.61 | 0.23 |
| 9 | Hydromorphone | 0.87 | 0.64 | 0.10 | 0.93 | 0.77 | 0.03 |
| 10 | Benzylmorphine | 0.94 | 0.84 | 0.62 | 0.97 | 0.34 | 0.30 |
| 11 | Myrophine | 0.98 | 0.98 | 1.00 | 0.01 | 0.01 | 0.97 |
| 12 | Cryptopine[a] | 0.56 | 0.34 | 0.53 | 0.00 | 0.55 | 0.10 [0.00][b] |
| 13 | Narceine[a] | 0.80 | 0.75 | 0.62 | 0.82 | 0.78 | 0.00 |
| 14 | Papaverine[a] | 0.88 | 0.78 | 0.64 | 0.98 | 0.02 | 0.04 |
| 15 | Narcotine[a] | 0.88 | 0.78 | 0.72 | s[b] | 0.02 | 0.10[L][b] |
| 16 | Cocaine | 0.83 | 0.67 | 0.56 | 0.60[L][b] | 0.71 | 0.67 |
| 17 | Pyrahexyl | 1.00 | 1.00 | 1.00 | 0.01 | 0.00 | 1.00 |
| 18 | Anileridine | 0.76 | 0.40 | 0.54 | 0.56 | 0.35 | 0.40 |
| 19 | Pethidine | 0.91 | 0.77 | 0.63 | 0.95 | 0.60 | 0.78 |
| 20 | Alphaprodine | 0.91 | 0.81 | 0.77 | 0.51 | 0.62 | 0.77 |
| 21 | Alphameprodine | 0.94 | 0.90 | 0.84 | 0.85 | 0.33 | 0.84 |
| 22 | Ethoheptazine[a] | 0.92 | 0.82 | 0.66 | 0.87 | 0.70 | 0.80 |
| 23 | Normethadone | 0.97 | 0.95 | 0.90 | 0.11 | 0.30 | 0.87 |
| 24 | *l*-Dipipanone | 0.99 | 0.98 | 0.91 | 0.00 | 0.07 | 0.98 |
| 25 | Phenadoxone | 0.99 | 0.98 | 0.90 | 0.02 | 0.00 | 0.98 |
| 26 | Methadone | 1.00 | 0.96 | 0.88 | 0.15 | 0.27 | 0.94 |
| 27 | *l*-Isomethadone | 1.00 | 0.96 | 0.90 | 0.02 | 0.19 | 0.93 |
| 28 | Alphaacetylmethadol | 1.00 | 1.00 | 0.96 | 0.06 | 0.05 | 0.97 |
| 29 | Propoxyphene | 0.97 | 0.94 | 0.93 | 0.22 | 0.11 | 0.94 |
| 30 | Diethylthiambutene | 0.90 | 0.89 | 0.90 | 0.08 | 0.10 | 1.00 |
| 31 | Levomoramide | 0.97 | 0.95 | 0.87 | 0.0– 0.5s[b] | 0.02 | 0.6s[b] |
| 32 | Levallorphan | 0.95 | 0.92 | 0.66 | 0.88 | 0.60 | 0.58 |
| 33 | *dl*-Methorphan | 0.99 | 0.92 | 0.78 | 0.47[L][b] | 0.36 | 0.91 |
| 34 | Phenazocine | 0.95 | 0.92 | 0.91 | 0.67 | 0.07 | 0.82 |

[a] Not narcotic under international law.
[b] See list of abbreviations at end of Table XXII.

Fulton (F21, F22, F23) in 1948 showed that chemical and physical determination of origin of opium was possible. In one paper he reported the first practical origin determination on a seizure from 373 lb of opium found on the ship M. V. Manoran, in Vancouver B.C., 9 October 1947 (U.S. No. 64451). The following data were determined: percentages of codeine, morphine, narcotine, papaverine, thebaine, cryptopine, fats, chloroform solubles, ash, and moisture. The porphyroxine-meconidine (PM) Lovibond color was obtained along with the general physical and microscopic appearance. After comparison with the same values on known samples Fulton concluded that the origin was Indian. It was on the basis of these findings that a research program under the auspices of the U.N. was inaugurated. Laboratory facilities were loaned by the Government of the U.S.A. to the U.N. in the Alcohol Tax Unit Laboratory in the City of New York in 1948. Samples are being supplied from many countries and various legal and illegal growing areas (S14, S15, S16, S17). Governments with laboratories and scientific personnel were asked to participate and more than sixty are now taking part.

In 1954 a U.N. laboratory was set up in Geneva, at the Palais des Nations. It is equipped for routine chemical analysis, paper chromatography, paper electrophoresis, and spectrographic and spectrophotometric analysis (P15). A U.N. document series entitled "The Assay, Characteristics, Composition and Origin of Opium" is provided in which the reports contributed by the participating scientists are being published. The earlier ones (June 23, 1947 to October 19, 1950) are to be found in the Narcotic Commission series E/CN7/ . . . ; those since January 25, 1951 are published in the special opium series, ST/SOA/SER.K/. . . . Reports of two international committees of experts on opium under the chairmanship of Jermstad in 1954 (C8) and of Farmilo in 1958 (C9) give detailed accounts of the progress made until that time. A report for analytical chemists in 1958 (A1a) and a review by Pfeifer (P10a) in 1960 describe the work on opium. Since 1948 about 120 papers have been published; the next few paragraphs give a summary of these results.

### B. Methods

A summary of a process for the origin determination is illustrated in Plate XI. Data about the sample history and appearance are recorded on a punched card, Plate XII.

After a sample is taken for moisture determination in its original state, the sample is air-dried, ground, and sieved to obtain a 25- to 40-mesh powder. One milligram is used for a microscopic appearance test (F21, F22, A1, F39, B27, R6); 2–10 gm are ashed for spectrochemical analysis (B4a, B11, F11, P12, P13). The opium ash color varies, and has been discussed in relation to types of opium (F21, P2, J2). Potassium, calcium, sodium, and phosphate, major constituents in the ash, have been correlated with sample provenance (B11, F11). Recent preliminary

TABLE XX

CHROMATOGRAPHIC OBSERVATIONS FOR NARCOTICS AND RELATED COMPOUNDS FOR IsoBUOH:ACOH:H₂O (10:1:2.4) ON SULFATE- (SO₄) AND PHOSPHATE- (PO₄) TREATED PAPERS[a] (D2)

| Compound | $R_f$ values | | Iodoplatinate color | | UV observations | | | |
|---|---|---|---|---|---|---|---|---|
| | | | | | SO₄ | | PO₄ | |
| | SO₄ | PO₄ | SO₄ | PO₄ | 3660 Å | 2537 Å | 3660 Å | 2537 Å |
| Acetoketobemidone | 0.71 | 0.80 | B(V) | V | — | — | — | — |
| Acetyldihydrocodeine | 0.53 | 0.72 | B(V) | B | — | A$^L$ | — | A$^L$ |
| α-Acetylmethadol[b] | 1.00 | 1.00 | RV | V | — | — | — | — |
| β-Acetylmethadol[b] | 1.00 | 1.00 | RV | V | — | — | — | — |
| Acetylmorphenol | 0.93 | 0.94 | — | — | — | V$^L$ | — | V$^L$ |
| Allylprodine (alperidine) | 0.88 | 0.93 | RV | V | — | — | — | — |
| Anileridine | 0.40 | 0.76 | V | V | G | A | GY | A |
| Apomorphine | 0.44 | 0.68 | V | V → B | A | BG | A(GYB) | BG |
| Benzylmorphine | 0.84 | 0.94 | V | V | G | A$^L$ | A$^L$ | A |
| Cocaine | 0.67 | 0.83 | V | V | A$^L$ | A | A | A |
| Codeine | 0.24 | 0.49 | BV | BV | A$^L$ | A | A$^L$ | A |
| Codeinone | 0.78 | 0.91 | V | V | VG(V) | (A)VG | Y$^L$A | Y$^L$A |
| Cotarnine | 0.63 | 0.80 | RV | RV | Or | Or | Or = 0.5 | Or = 0.5 |
| Cryptopine | 0.34 | 0.56 | V | V | Ol | Ol | Or | Or |
| Desomorphine | 0.43 | 0.65 | B(V) | B | B | B | B | B |
| Diacetylmorphine | 0.50 | 0.73 | B | V | — | — | — | — |
| Diacetylmorphol | 0.94 | 0.95 | — | — | — | V$^L$ | — | B$^{VL}$ |
| Diethylthiambutene | 0.90 | 0.89 | RV | V | A$^L$ | A | A$^L$ | A |
| Dihydrocodeine | 0.33 | 0.56 | BV | BV | A$^L$ | A | A$^L$ | A |
| Dihydromorphine | 0.14 | 0.30 | B | B | — | A | A$^L$ | A$^L$ |
| Dimethylthiambutene | 0.87 | 0.88 | RV | V | — | A | A | A |

| | | | | | | | | |
|---|---|---|---|---|---|---|---|---|
| Dioxaphetylbutyrate | 0.92 | 0.95 | RV | V | — | — | — | — |
| Dioxyline | 0.87 | 0.96 | Br$^{VL}$ | Br$^{VL}$ | Y | Y | Y | Y |
| dl-Dipipanone | 0.97 | 0.98 | RV | V | BY | A$^L$ | BV | A$^L$ |
| l-Dipipanone | 0.98 | 0.99 | RV | V | BY | A$^L$ | BY | A$^L$ |
| Ethoheptazine | 0.82 | 0.92 | V | V | — | — | — | B |
| Ethylmethyl thiambutene | 0.89 | 0.90 | RV | V | — | A | A | A |
| Ethylmorphine | 0.45 | 0.66 | BV | V | A$^L$ | A | A$^L$ | A |
| Ethylnarceine | 0.94 | 0.98 | V | V$^L$ | — | A | — | A |
| Ethylpethidine | 0.86 | 1.00 | V$^L$ | V | A$^L$ | A | A$^L$ | — |
| Hydrocodone | 0.26 | 0.46 | BV | VB | A$^L$ | A | A$^L$ | A |
| Hydromorphone | 0.64 | 0.87 | B(V) | VB | A$^L$ | A | A$^L$ | A |
| Hydroxypethidine (bemidone) | 0.70 | 0.79 | V | V | BY | A$^L$ | BY | — |
| dl-Isodipipidone (pipidone) | 0.97 | 0.97 | RV | V | — | — | — | A |
| d-Isomethadone | 0.96 | 1.00 | RV | V | — | — | — | — |
| l-Isomethadone | 0.96 | 1.00 | RV | V | — | — | — | — |
| Ketobemidone | 0.58 | 0.80 | B(V) | VB | — | A$^{VL}$ | — | A$^L$ |
| Levallorphan | 0.86 | 0.94 | V | V | — | — | — | — |
| Meconic acid | 0.10 | 0.04 | NC | NC | B | B | B | B |
| α-Meprodine$^b$ | 0.90 | 0.94 | V | BV | — | — | B | — |
| α-d-Methadol$^b$ | 0.94 | 1.00 | RV | V | — | — | — | — |
| β-d-Methadol$^b$ | 0.94 | 1.00 | RV | V | — | — | — | — |
| Methadone | 0.96 | 1.00 | V | V | — | A | — | A |
| Methazocine | 0.61 | 0.77 | B | BV | — | — | — | A |
| d-Methorphan$^b$ | 0.92 | 0.99 | V(B) | BV | — | — | — | — |
| l-Methorphan$^b$ | 0.92 | 0.99 | V(B) | BV | — | — | — | — |
| dl-Methorphan$^b$ | 0.92 | 0.98 | V(B) | BV | — | — | — | — |
| l-2-Methoxy-N-methylmorphinan | 0.91 | 0.96 | V(B) | V | — | — | — | — |
| Methyldesorphine | 0.53 | 0.78 | B | B | — | — | G | B |
| Methyldihydromorphine | 0.21 | 0.42 | VGy | BV | — | — | B | A$^L$ |
| Methyl ketobemidone | 0.33 | 0.65 | V | BV | — | A$^L$ | — | A |
| Methylmorphenol | 0.98 | 0.96 | NC | NC | A$^L$ | A | — | V$^L$ |

TABLE XX (*Continued*)

| Compound | $R_f$ values | | Iodoplatinate color | | UV observations | | | |
|---|---|---|---|---|---|---|---|---|
| | | | | | SO₄ | | PO₄ | |
| | SO₄ | PO₄ | SO₄ | PO₄ | 3660 Å | 2537 Å | 3660 Å | 2537 Å |
| Metopon | 0.20 | 0.46 | V | B | — | A | — | — |
| O⁶-Monoacetylmorphine | 0.32 | 0.56 | V | V | — | $A^L$ | — | — |
| d-Moramide$^b$ | 0.95 | 0.96 | RV | RV | — | $A^L$ | — | $A^L$ |
| l-Moramide$^b$ | 0.95 | 0.97 | RV | RV | — | $A^L$ | — | $A^L$ |
| Morpheridine | 0.43 | 0.71 | B | B | — | — | — | — |
| Morphine | 0.13 | 0.34 | B | B | $A^L$ | A | G, $A^L$ | G, A |
| Morphine-N-oxide | 0.18 | 0.33 | $R^L$ | — | $A^L$ | A | A | A |
| Morphothebaine | 0.32 | 0.58 | V | V | $V^L$ | B($A^L$) | $V^L$ | B, $A^L$ |
| Myrophine | 0.98 | 0.98 | B, L | $B^P$, T | — | $A^L$ | — | $A^L$ |
| Nalorphine (allylnormorphine) | 0.24 | 0.48 | VB | BV | $A^L$ | A | $A^L$ | A |
| Narceine | 0.75 | 0.80 | V(Br) | BV | $A^L$ | A | $A^L$ | A |
| l-α-Narcotine (noscapine) | 0.78 | 0.88 | V(Br) | V | B | B | BG | A |
| Norlevorphanol | 0.78 | 0.88 | V | B | $A^L$ | A | — | A |
| Normethadone | 0.95 | 0.97 | V | VB | — | — | — | — |
| Normorphine | 0.13 | 0.31 | B | — | $A^L$ | A | — | — |
| Opianic acid | 0.92 | 0.82 | NC | NC | $VV^L$ | A | — | A |
| d-Orphan$^b$ | 0.77 | 0.92 | V | V | — | — | — | — |
| dl-Orphan$^b$ | 0.78 | 0.93 | V | V | — | — | — | — |
| l-Orphan$^b$ | 0.77 | 0.92 | V | V | — | — | — | — |
| Oxycodone | 0.22 | 0.34 | V | $V^L$ | $A^L$ | A | $A^L$ | A |
| Oxymorphone | 0.10 | 0.21 | V | V | B | $A^L$ | B | A |
| Papaverine | 0.78 | 0.88 | V | V | YG | YG | YG | Y |
| Pethidine | 0.77 | 0.91 | V | V | — | — | — | — |
| Phenadoxone | 0.98 | 0.99 | B(RV) | $RV^L$ | — | — | — | — |

| | | | | | | | | |
|---|---|---|---|---|---|---|---|---|
| Phenazocine | 0.92 | 0.95 | RV | V | — | A^L | — | A^L |
| d-Phenomorphan | 0.97 | 0.96 | RV | VB | A | — | A | — |
| l-Phenomorphan | 0.97 | 0.95 | RV | BV | A | — | A | — |
| Pholcodine | 0.03 | 0.08 | BV | V | — | — | — | A |
| Piminodine (anoprodine) | 0.86 | 0.95 | V | VB | G(A) | G(A) | — | A |
| α-Prodine^b | 0.81 | 0.91 | V(B) | V | — | — | — | — |
| β-Prodine^b | 0.81 | 0.91 | V | V | — | — | — | — |
| Proheptazine | 0.84 | 0.93 | V(B) | BV | — | — | G^D | — |
| d-Propoxyphene | 0.94 | 0.97 | RV | B | A | A | — | A |
| Propylketobemidone | 0.77 | 0.81 | V(W) | V | — | — | — | — |
| Pseudomorphine | 0.03 | 0.09 | BV | V | B | B | — | B |
| Sinomenine | 0.40 | 0.58 | V(Br) | V | A | A | A | A |
| Thebacon | 0.16 | 0.32 | BrV | V^L | A^L | A | A^L | A |
| Thebaine | 0.67 | 0.85 | V | RV | A^L | A | A^L | A |
| Thebenine | 0.58 | 0.78 | RV, T | V | V | A^L | A(Br) | A |
| Xanthaline | 0.98 | 0.98 | BrV, T | BrV, T | A | A | A(Y) | A |

^a See list of abbreviations after Table XXII.
^b International names: alpha and beta acetylmethadol; alpha meprodine; alpha and beta methadol; dextro-, levo-, and racemethorphan; dextro- and levomoramide; dextrorphan, racemorphan, and levorphanol; alphaprodine and betaprodine.

TABLE XXI

CHROMATOGRAPHIC OBSERVATIONS FOR ALKALOIDS AND RELATED BASES FOR IsoBUOH:ACOH/:H₂O (10:1:2.4) ON SULFATE- (SO₄) AND PHOSPHATE- (PO₄) TREATED PAPERS[a] (D2)

| Compound | $R_f$ values SO₄ | $R_f$ values PO₄ | Iodo platinate color SO₄ | Iodo platinate color PO₄ | UV observations SO₄ 3660 Å | UV observations SO₄ 2537 Å | UV observations PO₄ 3660 Å | UV observations PO₄ 2537 Å |
|---|---|---|---|---|---|---|---|---|
| Aconotine | 0.94 | 0.97 | R | R | — | A^L | — | A^L |
| Ajamaline | 0.86 | 0.93 | V | V | NC^VL | — | NC | A |
| Amphetamine sulfate | 0.53 | 0.71 | B, DOS | B, DOS | NC | — | B(G) | — |
| Apomorphine | 0.44 | 0.66 | RV | BV | A | A | — | A |
| Aspidospermine | 0.88 | 0.85 | RV | V | — | — | — | — |
| Atropine sulfate | 0.53 | 0.72 | RV | BV | — | — | Y^VB | — |
| Berberine chloride | 0.53 | 0.67 | Or(Br) | OI(Br), T | Y | BY | V | — |
| Boldine | 0.36 | 0.57 | R | RV | V | — | — | A |
| Brucine | 0.40 | 0.54 | B | B | — | A | — | — |
| Cadaverine HCl | 0.06 | 0.12 | G^L | BG^L | — | — | — | A |
| Caffeine | 0.85 | 0.86 | — | — | — | A | — | — |
| Cevadine | 0.96 | 0.97 | R | R | — | A | — | — |
| Cinchonine HCl | 0.36 | 0.83 | B | B | BV | — | V | — |
|  | 0.42 |  |  |  |  |  |  |  |
| Colchicine | 0.98 | 0.98 | R | B^L | OI^L(Br) | — | OI(Br) | A |
| Cupreine | 0.26 | 0.73 | B | B, TMS | BV^L | — | B^LOr(V) | — |
|  | 0.31 |  |  |  |  |  |  |  |
| Dihydroergocristine | 0.94 | 0.91 | V | V, T | B^VL | — | B^L, T | — |
| Emetine | 0.45 | 0.97 | V | V | B | — | B^L | — |
| l-Ephedrine | 0.38 | 0.63 | R^L(NC) | BV^L(NC) | — | A | — | A^L |
| Ergocristine | 0.94 | 0.92 | V | V | BV | — | V^L, T | — |
| Ergometrine | 0.34 | 0.53 | V | V | — | — | V^L | — |
| Ergometrinine | 0.52 | 0.62 | V | V | V^L | — | B | — |
| Ergonovine maleate | 0.29 | 0.56 | — | — | B, YG, T | — | B | — |
| Ergotamine | 0.92 | 0.89 | V | V | B^VB | — | BV, T | — |

| Compound | Rf | Rf | | | | | | |
|---|---|---|---|---|---|---|---|---|
| Ergotamine tartrate | 0.93 | 0.97 | — | — | BV, T | — | BL, T | — |
| Ergotaminine | 0.93 | 0.84 | V | V | — | A | BV, T | — |
| Eserine | 0.51 | 0.72 | BV | BV | GB | — | V | A |
| Eupaverine | 0.82 | 0.95 | B | RV | — | A | — | — |
| Homatropine HBr | 0.33 | 0.56 | BV | BV | B$^b$ | — | B$^{Lb}$ | A |
| Hordenine | 0.17 | 0.41 | BVL | B | — | A | — | A |
| Hydrastinine | 0.22 | 0.36 | B | BV(Br) | B$^b$ | A | B$^b$ | A |
| Lobeline | 0.78 | 0.90 | RV | EXWS | — | — | — | — |
| | 0.91 | 0.96 | BVL | R(V), HDOS | NC | — | NC | A |
| Methamphetamine HCl | 0.61 | 0.73 | B(R), HDOS | VB, BV | — | A$^{VL}$ | A | A |
| Methylphenidate HCl | 0.76 | 0.88 | V(B) | B | — | — | — | — |
| Nicotine | 0.00 | 0.23 | B | B(Br) | — | — | A | A |
| Phenothiazine | 0.98 | 0.98 | BVD | B$^P$(Gy)BWGH | — | — | — | — |
| Pilocarpine | 0.15 | 0.29 | B(G$^L$) | BV | G$^{VL}$ | A$^L$ | G$^L$ | A$^L$ |
| Procaine HCl | 0.35 | 0.59 | BV(Gy), T | BV | — | A | — | A |
| Psicaine | 0.92 | 0.96 | V | B(G) | — | — | — | — |
| Putrescine dihydrochloride | 0.06 | 0.12 | G$^L$ | V | — | — | — | — |
| Quinidine | 0.40 | 0.86 | RV | V | B$^{VB}$ | — | B$^{VB}$ | A |
| Quinine bismuthiodide | 0.39 | 0.86 | RV | V | B$^{VB}$ | — | B$^{VB}$ | — |
| Quinine bisulfate | 0.12 | — | BV | B$^{VB}$ | B$^{VB}$ | — | A | A |
| Raubasine | 0.41 | 0.84 | BV | V | GB | — | G$^{VL}$ | — |
| Reserpine | 0.91 | 0.95 | BV, TTF | — | G | — | G | — |
| Scopolamine HCl | 0.95 | 0.94 | B | B | — | — | — | — |
| Scopoline | 0.28 | 0.49 | R$^L$(B) | V$^L$(B) | — | — | — | — |
| Serpentine | 0.05 | 0.11 | BV | V | B$^{VB}$, T | — | B$^{VB}$ | — |
| Sparteine sulfate | 0.82 | 0.90 | B | B$^P$ | — | — | — | A |
| | 0.04 | 0.13 | | | | | | |
| | 0.29 | — | | | | | | |
| Strychnine | 0.54 | 0.70 | BV | B | B | A | A$^L$ | A |
| Trigonelline | 0.08 | 0.12 | B$^{VL}$ | B$^L$ | — | A | — | A |
| Tropacocaine HCl | 0.71 | 0.84 | B$^{VD}$ | BV | — | A | — | — |
| Veratridine | 0.94 | 0.97 | RV | RV | — | A$^L$ | — | A$^L$ |
| α-Yohimbine | 0.70 | 0.82 | R$^L$, FOS | V$^L$ | NC | — | G$^L$ | — |

$^a$ See list of abbreviations after Table XXII.

$^b$ Extra spots—no color with iodoplatinate.

TABLE XXII

CHROMATOGRAPHIC OBSERVATIONS FOR THIRTY-THREE ANTIHISTAMINES AND PHENOTHIAZINES FOR
ISOBUTANOL:ACETIC ACID:WATER ON SULFATE- AND PHOSPHATE-TREATED PAPERS[a] (D2)

| Compound | Rf values SO4 | Rf values PO4 | Iodoplatinate color SO4 | Iodoplatinate color PO4 | UV SO4 3660 Å | UV SO4 2537 Å | UV PO4 3660 Å | UV PO4 2537 Å |
|---|---|---|---|---|---|---|---|---|
| Antazoline phosphate | 0.88 | 0.94 | BV | VR | A$^L$ | A | A$^L$ | A |
| Anthallan | 0.80 | 0.91 | NC, T | NC[2] | (A)G$^L$ | A$^L$ | A(G)$^L$ | A$^L$ |
| Bromodiphenhydramine HCl | 0.92 | 0.95 | V, VR | V(VR) | — | — | — | — |
| Carbinoxamine maleate | 0.61 | 0.84 | BV | B | — | A | — | A |
| Chlorcyclizine HCl | 0.94 | 0.95 | B | BV(V) | V$^B$ | A | — | A$^L$ |
| Chlorothen citrate | 0.68 | 0.92 | B[2] | V | — | — | — | A |
| Chlorpheniramine maleate | 0.52 | 0.87 | B[L] | V | — | A$^L$ | — | A$^L$ |
| Cyclizine mono-HCl[b] (M)[c] | 0.85 | 0.94 | B$^D$ | B | BrR | RP | BrR | RP |
| Diethazine HCl[b] (P)[d,e] | 0.93 | 0.95 | V | BV | — | — | — | — |
| Dimenhydrinate HCl[b] (M)[c] | 0.89 | 0.94 | BV | V(VR)[2] | — | — | — | — |
| Diphenhydramine HCl | 0.90 | 0.94 | BV | V(VR) | — | — | — | — |
| Diphenylpyraline HCl | 0.91 | 0.81 | V | V | — | A | — | A |
| Doxylamine succinate | 0.29 | 0.56 | B$^D$[2, T] | BV[2, T] | RV(A) | RV(A) | RV | RV |
| Ethopropazine HCl[b] (P)[d] | 0.94 | 0.94 | RV, (BV) | V | Y$^L$A | A$^L$ | GY | A$^L$ |
| Isothipendyl HCl | 0.84 | 0.90 | VB$^D$ | BV$^D$ | — | — | — | — |
| Methafurylene fumarate[e] | 0.15 | 0.70 | B, [2] | B[2] | A$^L$ | — | A(G)$^L$ | — |
| Methaphenilene HCl | 0.86 | 0.92 | V | V | BV$^L$ | — | V | — |
| Methapyrilene fumarate | 0.36 | 0.75 | B[2] | B[2] | — | A | — | A |
| Parabromdylamine maleate[e] | 0.62 | 0.87 | B$^D$T | B$^D$[2] | YG | — | YG | — |
| Phenindamine tartrate | 0.91 | 0.95 | VR | VR | — | A | — | A |
| Pheniramine maleate | 0.19 | 0.72 | B[L] | BV | — | A | — | — |
| Phenyltoloxamine dihydrogen citrate | 0.92 | 0.94 | BV | V | — | A | — | A |
| Promethazine HCl | 0.90 | 0.93 | VR | BV | BrR | A$^L$RV | BrR | RV$^L$ |
| Pyrathiazine HCl | 0.92 | 0.94 | BV | V | Br$^L$ | R | Br$^L$ | R |

| Compound | | | | | | | | |
|---|---|---|---|---|---|---|---|---|
| Pyrilamine maleate | 0.34 | 0.79 | BP[L] | BP | B | — | B | — |
| Pyrrobutamine phosphate | 0.94 | 0.95 | BR | RV | — | A | — | A |
| Thenalidene HCl[e] | 0.76 | 0.81 | B[2] | V | $A^L$ | A | A | A |
| Thenyldiamine HCl | 0.27 | 0.71 | B[2, L] | BV[2] | V | — | V | — |
|  | 0.16 | 0.71 | B[L, NR] | — | V | — | — | — |
| Thonzylamine HCl | 0.72 | 0.86 | BV | BV(V) | $A^L$ | A | $A^L$ | A |
| Trihexyphenidyl[b] (P)[d] | 0.94 | 0.96 | VR | VR | — | — | — | — |
| Tripelennamine HCl | 0.39 | 0.76 | B[L] | BV | BV | — | V | — |
| Triprolidine HCl[e] | 0.69 | 0.91 | BP | B(BV) | $AV^L$ | AV | — | $A^{LV}$ |
| Zolamine HCl | 0.61 | 0.85 | BP[2] | B(BV)[2] | — | A | — | A |

[a] See list of abbreviations below.
[b] Not usual antihistamine.
[c] M = Motion sickness remedy.
[d] P = Parasympatholytic.
[e] Name not approved.

### Abbreviations

| | | | | |
|---|---|---|---|---|
| A | absorbance | | Or | orange |
| B | blue | | R | red |
| BWGH | blue with grey halo | | s | streaking |
| D | (superscript) dark | | T | tailing |
| DOS | color develops on standing | | TMS | tailing main spot |
| EXWS | extra spot when sprayed | | TTF | tailing to front |
| FOS | fading on standing | | V | violet |
| G | green | | vB | (superscript) very bright |
| Gy | grey | | vD | (superscript) very dark |
| HDOS | halo develops on standing | | vL | (superscript) very light |
| [L] | elongated spot | | W | white |
| L (superscript) | light | | Y | yellow |
| NC | no color reaction or indefinite fluoresence if listed under UV observations | | [0.00] | some material remains at start |
| | | | ( ) | color or absorbance of center of spot |
| NR | not resolved | | [2] | two extra spots |
| Ol | olive | | | |

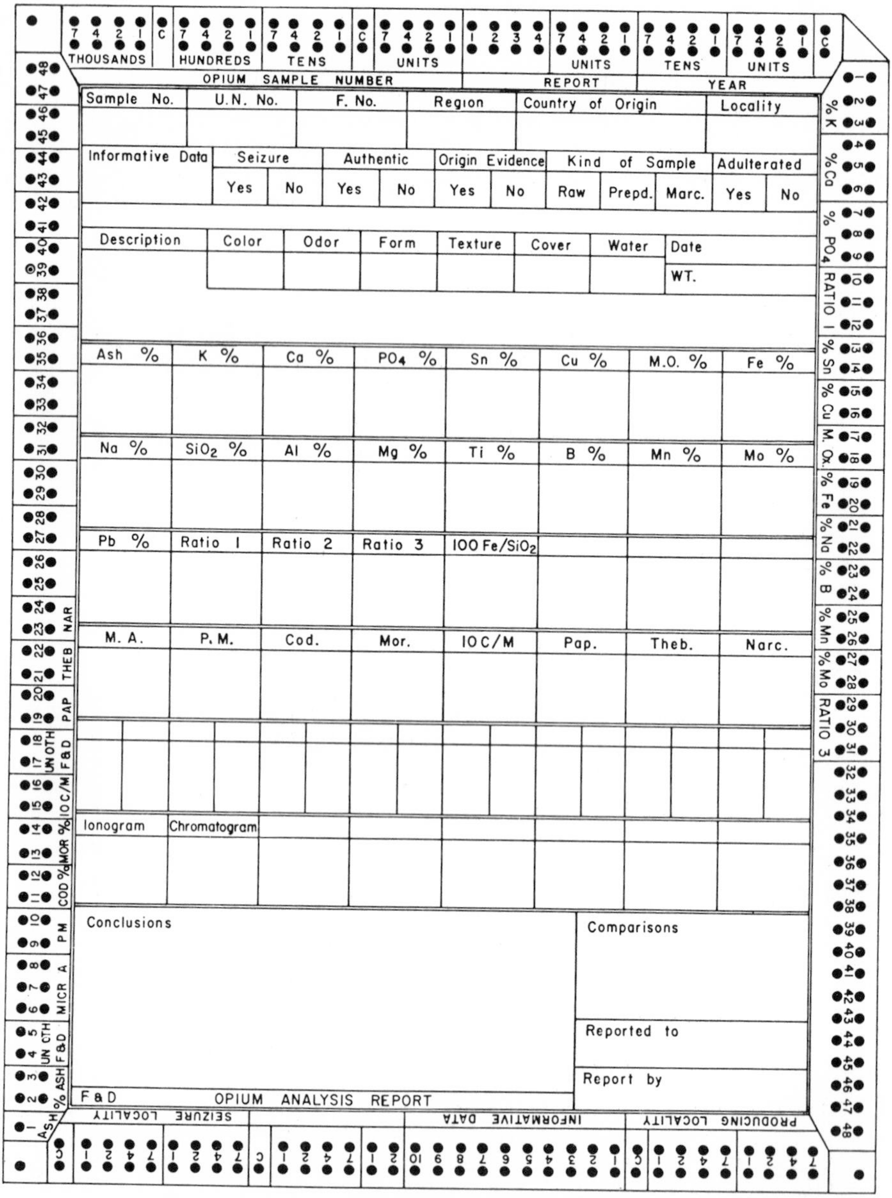

OPIUM SAMPLE NUMBER      REPORT

| Sample No. | U.N. No. | F. No. | Region | Country of Origin | Locality |
|---|---|---|---|---|---|

| Informative Data | Seizure | | Authentic | | Origin Evidence | | Kind of Sample | | | Adulterated | |
|---|---|---|---|---|---|---|---|---|---|---|---|
| | Yes | No | Yes | No | Yes | No | Raw | Prepd. | Marc. | Yes | No |

| Description | Color | Odor | Form | Texture | Cover | Water | Date |
|---|---|---|---|---|---|---|---|
| | | | | | | | WT. |

| Ash % | K % | Ca % | PO4 % | Sn % | Cu % | M.O. % | Fe % |
|---|---|---|---|---|---|---|---|

| Na % | SiO2 % | Al % | Mg % | Ti % | B % | Mn % | Mo % |
|---|---|---|---|---|---|---|---|

| Pb % | Ratio 1 | Ratio 2 | Ratio 3 | 100 Fe/SiO2 | | | |
|---|---|---|---|---|---|---|---|

| M. A. | P. M. | Cod. | Mor. | 10 C/M | Pap. | Theb. | Narc. |
|---|---|---|---|---|---|---|---|

| Ionogram | Chromatogram |
|---|---|

| Conclusions | | Comparisons |
|---|---|---|
| | | Reported to |
| | | Report by |

F & D      OPIUM ANALYSIS REPORT

PLATE XII. Punched card for opium analysis reports and origin determinations.

work on the neutron activation analysis method for raw opium promises to yield a still further sensitive method to detect and assay minor metallic elements (L1a, P9). The amino acids (J0, M14), meconic acid (N2,

N3, N4, F36, A10, M13, W9a), sulfuric acid, and total acids of raw opium have also been studied and show typical variations (M13, M14). The ultraviolet examination of opium extracts, which is an economical, rapid, and simple method developed by Grlić (G9, G10, G11, G16, B22, P21b), has been applied by others (A9, B4, B15, B16, K19, B26, R5, M6, A4). It is a popular method for opium origin determination.

There is a natural similarity between the UV spectra of opium extracts, but the judicious choice of ratios of certain absorbances at given absorption wavelengths yields a measure of what are assumed to be responses of given constituents. For example, Grlić states that the ratio $E_{250}/E_{270}$ is inversely related to the ratio of the thebaine and papaverine content, while a high ratio of $E_{280}/E_{290}$ indicates a low amount of meconic acid in the sample. The quotient $E_{300}/E_{310}$ is directly proportional to thebaine and papaverine content, but is influenced as well by other factors. The various workers have selected other sets of ratios to compare.

Still another qualitative method based on color reactions has been developed by Braenden *et al.* (B18, B28, B22, B23, B24, B25, B29, B30) and applied to a large number of opium samples by others (B3, B6, B6a, P14, R6). Braenden claims that four color tests with aqueous ferric sulfate, acidic iodic acid, dilute hydrochloric acid, and a modified formaldehyde sulfuric acid reaction, when applied to an acetic acid extract of opium, yield color intensities which, when measured, may be correlated to the origin of the sample. Several hundred samples have been investigated with the procedure and application of various colorimeters for the measurement of color intensities has ben made (P21a). The color of a buffered aqueous extract has been used to estimate the production year of the opium (G17, G18, G18a, G18b, P9a).

*Quantitative methods for assay of the opium alkaloids.* Reports are published on assays of: morphine (A14, F36, A6, P6, V2, A7, W9, A10, B1, P22, B34, B36, F26, K9, K10, F29, A2, F40, R6); codeine (F23, F25, F39, F40, A14, F36, P6, P8, A7a, R6); thebaine (F22, F31, A11, R6); papaverine (L3, F31, R6); narcotine (L3, N2, N3, N4, F36, M13, R6); and porphyroxine-meconidine (F21, F22, F24, F6, F38, F19, F7, F20, F39, F11, G4a, G4b, R6). Morphine, the most important commercial alkaloid in opium, is of course the one most extensively studied. The minor phenolic alkaloids are separated and assayed as a group (F22, F28, F40, F35). In the process of working out the above assays of the individual compounds several authors—Liang (L7, L8), Fulton (F34, F35), Asahina (A8), and Farmilo *et al.* (B7, G4a)—propose unified procedures by which the major and the minor alkaloids may be determined in sequence (F35) or simultaneously (B7, G4a).

Studies of the composition of opium to obtain criteria for origin determination have been published (F21, F27, F28, F30, C1, F41, F42, F11, M2, F37, F2, K18, K2, K3, B19, B20). Pruner (P21, P23, P24) has investigated the influence of molds on the stability of morphine and the effect of the addition of extracts of *Papaver orientale* on the assay of opium for origin determinations.

Analytical data from opium is presented in a number of different ways for use in establishing discriminatory criteria: by tabulation (F39, F42, F11), by frequency distribution charts, or by histograms (F6) to indicate the mean, median, and range of each value (F27). Distributions about a median value are given (B11) for ash components. Scatter diagrams which correlate two values and show a third in a color code are used (F2). Other examples of this type of plotting are given in references (F33) and (F41). A statistical treatment of data was carried out by Dunnet (F2) to maximize variations in nine values and reduce them to two numbers for plotting. A still more attractive method of correlating many values for comparison with those of a given sample consists of the use of edge-punched cards of which a detailed description is published for use in opium origin determinations (B12). Paper chromatographic studies of opium of various types have been made (P3, F13, P4, P5, P7, A5, A6, A7a, R6). A statistical study of variance of $R_f$ values for morphine, codeine, thebaine, and papaverine/narcotine in the isoBuOH: AcOH:$H_2O$ (10:1:2.4) system has been published (F12). Paper electrophoresis of raw opium extracts was carried out and its application to origin determinations is discussed (F14). A qualitative infrared method was first studied (J2a) and quantitative methods developed by Bakre *et al.* (B7) and Genest and Farmilo (G4a). An extraction apparatus for alkaloids is described (B21). Gas chromatographic methods for the semiquantitative analysis of alkaloids (E1) and a quantitative determination of the fatty acids of opium fat (M5a) for use in determination of origin of opium have been described.

## C. Reliability of Origin Determinations

The question of certainty of the results of physical-chemical methods for origin determination has been extensively discussed by the Commission members and the scientists participating in the program (F17). Five trials to determine the certainty of the physicochemical methods of origin determination have been carried out in various laboratories (F28, F4, F2, K19, N4a, M2a, K18). Opium samples of which the origin was known to the Narcotic Laboratory of the United Nations, and unknown to Farmilo and Bartlet, were submitted for origin determination on three occasions (F32, F2, F4). A total of eighty-nine samples were assayed as follows: ash, macro- and microscopic appearance, codeine, porphyroxine-meconidine, papaverine, narcotine, thebaine, morphine, and paper chromatography. Punched card–sorting of the data was used in the latter trials (F4, F2).

The tests of reliability of opium origin determinations have been applied to seizures from the international illicit traffic. In the trials fifteen samples of this type were examined as unknowns, and checked with the findings of the U.N. laboratory. In thirteen cases the same country was designated in both laboratories. In two cases the same region was designated. In 1955 results of examination of eight samples were published (F3) at the request of the Government of the U.S.A. Four samples were Indian, two Turkish, one Mexican, and the eighth was a new type of Mediterranean origin. In 1958, Krishnan (K18) published alkaloidal data on thirty samples of opium seized by the Indian authorities, but did not indicate his conclusions as to the origin of the samples. Bakre and Karaata in our laboratory obtained the composition of the ash of these samples on ash prepared in India. Krishnan provided the alkaloidal and other data on the samples. Farmilo and Bartlet carried out the origin determinations using the punched card data. Results of a comparison of findings of Krishnan with those of Farmilo, Bartlet, Bakre, and Karaata are shown in Table XXIII. These may be summarized as follows: sixteen were of Indian origin, nine were of Iranian origin, one was probably Pakistan opium, and three samples which were alleged to have come from Nepal by police evidence yielded inconclusive results and their origin remains unknown. One sample was impossible to identify because of adulteration.

Tests of reliability of the color reaction and UV method on twenty samples selected by Nicholls from the UN collection in Geneva were carried out by Secretariat chemists. Although the color tests and UV methods were both applied to the unknowns, they were said to be identified as to "origin" mainly by the UV method alone. The UV method developed by Grlić et al. (G9) was assessed by Kuśević (K19) in a trial carried out on sixty unknowns supplied by the UN Narcotic Laboratory. These findings are summarized along with other "scores" in Table XXIV.

A still further collaborative determination of origins on ten unknowns recommended by the committee of experts (C9) was carried out by Macleod et al. (M2a). The analytical data on each of the ten samples was processed through the punch cards and origin determinations made by Martin (M5c) in cooperation with Farmilo and Bartlet.

In Table XXIV the samples are divided into three main types: first, samples which have been contributed by governments and are authenticated representative types from the country of origin; second, seizures of

TABLE XXIII

COMPARISON OF OPIUM ORIGIN DETERMINATIONS BY DIFFERENT METHODS

| Sample | Circumstantial evidence | Alkaloid data (K18) | Total data | Comparison samples | Remarks |
|---|---|---|---|---|---|
| 1 | Iran | Iran | Iran | UN50, UN85 | Many comparison samples |
| 2 | India | Probably India | Probably India | 43385 | Not completely typical |
| 3 | Iran | Iran | Iran | L of N III, Fars (old) | Ca higher than usual for Iran |
| 4 | Iran | Iran | Iran | UN48 | Ca higher than usual for Iran |
| 5 | Iran | Probably Iran | Iran | UN47 | UN47 virtually same composition |
| 6 | Iran | Iran | Iran | UN121 | Many comparison samples |
| 7 | Nepal | Possibly Indian | Unknown | UN163 | These samples are probably from |
| 8 | Nepal | Far East or China | Unknown | UN163 } | the same source, possibly Nepal |
| 9 | Nepal | Probably India | Unknown | UN163 | or India |
| 10 | — | Probably India | Probably India | UN163 | Not typical |
| 11 | — | Probably India | India | 63913 | Typical |
| 12 | — | Probably India | Probably India | 43385 | Not typical |
| 13 | — | Probably India | Probably India | 63913, UN34 | Many comparison samples for alkaloid data |
| 14 | India | India | India | 63913, UN34 | Typical |
| 15 | India | India | India | 43385 | Ash not typical |
| 16 | India | India | India | UN185 | Many comparison samples |
| 17 | India | India | India | 63913, In No. 10 | Many comparison samples |
| 18 | India | India | India | 63913, In No. 10 | Many comparison samples |
| 19 | — | Probably India | Possibly India | UN34 | Not typical |
| 20 | — | Difficult to place | Possibly India | 63913 | Low narcotine and thebaine |
| 21 | — | Impossible to identify because of adulteration | | | |
| 22 | Iran | Probably Iran | Iran | UN74 | Alkaloid composition typical |
| 23 | — | Possibly Himachal, Pradesh, India | Possibly Himachal, Pradesh, India | UN61 | Papaverine extremely high (5.7%) |
| 24 | — | Iran | Iran | UN50 | Typical |

| | | | | |
|---|---|---|---|---|
| 25 | Pakistan, Iran | India or Pakistan | India or Pakistan | (K18) | Papaverine high |
| 26 | Probably India | Probably India | India | 63913 | Typical |
| 27 | Pakistan | Possibly Pakistan | Possibly Pakistan | UN100 | Insufficient data on Pakistani samples for complete identification |
| 28 | Iran | Iran | Iran | UN51 | Alkaloid data corrected for adulteration is typical of Iranian opium |
| 29 | India | Probably India | India | UN59 | Typical |
| 30 | — | Probably Iran | Iran | UN50 | Not entirely typical |

TABLE XXIV

"Scores" on Determinations of Opium Origin of "Unknowns"

| Answer | Sample types | Government contributed authenticated, method[a] | | | Seizures illicit traffic, method[a] | | New, method[a] | Totals cumulative |
|---|---|---|---|---|---|---|---|---|
| | | 1 | 2 | 3 | 1 | 4 | 1 | |
| 1 | (a) correct country | 54 | 29 | — | — | — | — | — |
| | (b) definite locality within country | — | 13 | — | — | — | — | — |
| | Total type 1 | 54 | 42 | 19 | 13 | 25 | [9][b] | 162 |
| 2 | (a) correct geographic region | 6 | 6 | — | — | — | — | — |
| | (b) alternative country | — | 12 | — | — | — | — | — |
| | Total type 2 | 6 | 18 | 1 | 2 | 1 | 0 | 28 |
| 3 | (a) inconclusive | 0 | 0 | 0 | 0 | 3 | [3][b] | — |
| | (b) not identifiable | 0 | 0 | 0 | 0 | 1 | 0 | — |
| | (c) incorrect | 2 | 0 | 0 | 0 | 0 | 0 | — |
| | Total type 3 | 2 | 0 | 0 | 0 | 4 | [3][b] | 9 |
| Grand totals | | 62 | 60 | 20 | 15 | 30 | 12 | 199 |

[a] Methods: (1) ash, alkaloidal, and other methods (F28, F4, F2); (2) UV method (B16A, K19); (3) color tests and UV method (N4a); (4) alkaloidal, ash, and other methods compared with circumstantial (police) evidence (K18).

[b] No origin named.

opium from the illicit traffic, which are sometimes accompanied by circumstantial evidence of country of origin; third, the new types, which are opiums not previously examined by the chemists carrying out the tests. The kind of origin determinations which are reported are shown in the rows labeled "answers" 1, 2, and 3. The first kind of answer is the one which specifies the correct country of origin, and in some cases either the type, e.g., Turkey (soft) or Turkey (medicinal), or the province, India (Uttar Pradesh), etc. The second type of origin answer is the one which describes a broad geographical area, e.g., Mediterranean type; in this class are included some opiums which are closely similar in characteristics, e.g., certain Turkish soft and Indian opiums. In these cases the answer can only be given as an alternative with the one showing the predominate character stated first, i.e., Turkey soft or India. In the third group of origin determinations are included the answers which are inconclusive, where the type is not well defined, or where the comparisons come from more than two countries. There are some opiums which are not identifiable as a result of heavy adulteration. The incorrect answers are those in which samples have been determined to have come from one origin and are known to have come from a different origin. Incorrect answers cannot be stated in the case of seizure examinations, so that a different method of assessment is employed. The seizure samples were studied independently by two laboratories and the final conclusions compared. In the case of matching answers the determinations of origin are assumed to be "correct." In the trials, no mismatches were obtained. The new samples are recognized as not being from countries for which samples were previously examined, and this is recorded as a correct answer; no definite origin is named but the sample is recognized as a new type.

The number of correct results of origin determinations for 142 authenticated samples is 140. Ninety-eight per cent of the determinations of origin by combined physical-chemical methods of analysis are right in three separate trials. For seizures, agreement on the same country of origin is found in 90% of cases between analysts from separate laboratories in three countries on two independent trials.

The United Nations Commission on Narcotic Drugs is not unanimous in its acceptance of the origin determinations (C6, I1) in spite of the fact that the majority opinion of twenty-three experts is that "opium origin research has developed to the point where origin can be determined with reasonable accuracy, and . . . the methods are ready for practical application" (F18). The result has been the passage of a resolution which requires the United Nations Laboratory to carry out opium origin determinations on seizure samples provided by governments, and to report the results in confidence to the government making the seizure and to the country of origin named. The origin results on seizures cannot be known and no mandatory public discussion of origin findings is required. It is difficult, therefore, to evaluate the effect that the determination of origin of seized opium has had in helping to combat illicit traffic. Public debate of the origin findings must be allowed before the enforcement value of the methods can be measured.

## V. Cannabis (Marihuana)

### A. General

In 1955 the Commission on Narcotic Drugs requested a review of the identification tests for active principles in cannabis (F14a); this is cited in the Commission report (C7). Certain microscopic, botanical, UV, IR, paper chromatographic, and electrophoretic methods and color tests are recommended for collaborative study by interested scientists

(F14b). Some familiar cannabis color tests—alkaline Beam's, Ghamrawy's, Duquenois'—were studied by Grlić (G12, G13). The study confirmed the value of the Beam and Duquenois–Moustapha–Negm reactions, while limiting the usefulness of the Ghamrawy test, which reacts positively with a number of plant extracts. Further color test results (Gibbs', Blackie's) on fifty-two cannabis samples from various origins— Greece, Sweden, Brazil, Morocco, Cardiff, Germany, Switzerland, Canada, Eygpt—are given by Farmilo (F14c). A modified Duquenois' test for marihuana (B31, B32) was applied to thirty-nine substances, mostly volatile oils of aromatic plants. It is found that the positive reacting substances like carvacrol, citral, citronellal, citronellol, farnesol, geraniol, juglone, and resorcinol gave colors (blue-red-violet) which were insoluble in chloroform. Hops extracted with petrol ether yield a residue, which with Duquenois' gives a green color changing to blue-green on standing. The extraction with chloroform produces a yellow chloroformsoluble substance and a green acid layer. The modified Duquenois' is advantageous in testing for marihuana.

Grlić (G15) investigates a reaction of hydrogen peroxide–sulfuric acid with cannabinol compounds. Cannabidiol, tetrahydrocannabinol, and cannabinol yield a pink to blood red, a violet, and a green changing rapidly to a green-brown, respectively. Cannabidiol acid acetate reacts orange to pink. The colors vary with concentration of the reactants. Forty-nine cannabis samples from eleven countries are analyzed. The colors range from pink (samples from temperate regions) to brown or green-brown (samples from tropical regions).

## B. Methods

### 1. Preparation of Extracts of Cannabinols

Cannabis material (1 gm or less) is extracted in the cold with successive portions of methanol, until the methanol residue fails to give a positive Duquenois' test. The filtered methanol solution is placed in a dry ice–acetone freezing mixture and the cold-precipitated waxy material is filtered at −80°C. The solution is evaporated at room temperature in a draft of air and the residue taken up in a minimum amount of benzene and filtered through a bed of Florisil (60/100 mesh) to absorb the pigments. Benzene is passed through the filter pad in successive small portions until the clear, colorless filtrate gives a negative Duquenois' test. The benzene is transferred to a clean, dry, weighed dish, and evaporated to dryness, desiccated, and weighed. The residue weight represents the major cannabinols. Th appropriate volume of solvent (e.g., 1 or 2 ml ethanol is often suitable) may be added and the elegant solution used for paper chromatography, ultraviolet and infrared spectrophotometry, and color tests. The solutions turn red on standing.

## 2. Paper Chromatography (D4, F9)

Cyclohexane is shaken with an excess of dimethylformamide. The upper layer is used as the mobile phase for descending paper chromatography. Whatman No. 1 paper (54 × 23.5 cm) is spotted with the benzene extracts. Volumes corresponding to 200 μg of residue are used. The chromatographic chamber is presaturated with lower layer (dimethylformamide saturated with cyclohexane) and the same solution used to impregnate the prepared paper prior to development. It is equilibrated 1 hour, the solvent added to the troughs in the chamber, and developed for 5–6 hours in a draftless quiet room. The developed papers are removed, the front marked immediately with red ball-point ink, and dried at room temperature in a hood. The paper is examined under ultraviolet light at 2537 and 3660 Å, and the absorbing and fluorescing areas marked. For a rapid ascending procedure (1–3 hours) rectangular jars (10 × 10 × 5 inches) and paper (8 × 8¾ inches) are recommended. No equilibration is necessary.

The following spray reagents are recommended:

*a. Diazo.* A solution of *p*-nitraniline (0.3% in HCl 8%, 25 ml) is mixed with sodium nitrite (5% in $H_2O$, 1.5 ml) at the time required. The reagent is stable for 4 days, and may be revived by addition of a few crystals of solid sodium nitrite.

*b. Indophenol.* 2,6-Dibromo-*p*-benzoquinone-4-chlorimine (0.3 gm) is shaken with methanol (25 ml) and the supernatant solution used. The reagent is unstable, and should be freshly prepared before spraying.

*c. Beam.* A solution of ethanolic potassium hydroxide (5%) is used.

*d. Duquenois.* A solution of vanillin (0.8 gm) and acetaldehyde (1 ml) in ethanol (40 ml) is sprayed on the chromatogram. The paper is then sprayed with concentrated hydrochloric acid. Other modifications of this test are available (G12, F14c). The vanillin aldehyde solution is unstable and should be made only when ready for use.

Combinations of the above reagents have been recommended by Korte and Sieper (K17) for use in marihuana identification for court cases.

## 3. Ultraviolet Spectrophotometry

The ethanol solution (Section V,B,1) (0.1 ml) was diluted in a volumetric flask with ethanol (10 ml); 2 ml of each of 0.2 N HCl and 0.2 N NaOH are added to 2-ml portions of the ethanol solution. The spectra are obtained. In the case of the examination of hashish extracts, or tropical and Mediterranean types of cannabis, dilution of the solutions will be required. After the spectra of the cannabinols are obtained against ethanol, 0.1 N ethanolic HCl, and 0.1 N ethanolic NaOH as blanks, it is then useful to obtain differential spectra of the acidic cannabinols against the alkaline cannabinols.

The phenolic properties of cannabinols are discussed by several authors (F14a, F14b, F15, S13, S8, G13, F14c) who investigated the spectral assay of cannabinols. The shifts observed in the acid-base differential spectra may be due to cannabinol and tetrahydrocannabinol acids as well as the phenolic homologs. The characteristic bands for hashish are: maxima (245, 327 m$\mu$), minima (235, 270 m$\mu$), inflections (295, 305 m$\mu$). The differential curves for hops and tobacco extracts alone and mixed with marihuana show distinct differences from those of marihuana. Similar comparisons for extracts of catnip, origanum, tobacco, tea, ragweed, peppermint, hops, rosemary, savory, sage, geranium, fig, buckthorn, tarragon, and eucalyptus are made by Scaringelli (S8). He found that differential spectra obtained in acid and base solutions could be distinguished from those of marihuana.

4. Gas-Liquid Phase Partition Chromatography (F9)

Recent work in this laboratory with a gas chromatographic apparatus equipped with a beta ray ionization detector has been carried out under the following conditions:

A methyl-silicone gum rubber (3% SE-30) on Chromosorb W column packing is activated by heating at 225° for 12 hours in the argon gas stream in the chromatographic column oven, and then at 325° for 24 hours without the gas flow. A 20- or 30-inch column is used, at 174–190°, for the assay of the samples. The argon carrier gas flow rate is 100 ml/minute. Typical sample sizes are: steam-distilled oils, 0.5 $\mu$l; light petroleum (30–60°) extracts of fresh and dry green leaf and flowering tops, 40 $\mu$g; hashish extracts with methanol, 3 $\mu$g; with light petroleum, 10 $\mu$g; police seizures from northern countries involving green plant parts found in reefers, 10–40 $\mu$g depending on the quality of the product. Standards of cannabidiol, cannabinol, and tetrahydrocannabinol give good chromatograms at 0.5–1 $\mu$g.

The gas chromatography retention values (RT values) for cannabidiol, tetrahydrocannabinol, and cannabinol are 9.3, 13.5, and 18.3 minutes at 174°/30 inches and 109 ml/minute. On standing the cannabidiol standard develops a new material which gives a peak at 8.5 minutes. The material is found in an extract from Canadian hemp. Pyrahexyl has an RT value of 23.5 minutes for the main band at 180°/30 inches and 100 ml/minute. The relative retention time values (RRT values) for tetrahydrocannabinol in terms of cannabidiol are 1.83, 1.58, and 1.42 for Pyrahexyl®, natural tetrahydrocannabinol, and synthetic tetrahydrocannabinol, respectively. When using light petroleum or methanol extracts of cannabis it is recommended that RRT values relative to cannabinol be used for identification purposes, i.e., 0.595 and 0.80 for cannabidiol and tetrahydrocannabinol, respectively.

## C. Origin of Cannabis Constituents

A theoretical scheme for the biogenesis of cannabinols is discussed (F14c,d). The relationship between chemical constituents and the geographical origin of cannabis is seen, and the following generalizations emerge:

(*i*) The amounts of constituents of oil and resin vary with the main geographical areas and climatic factors (G14, S13, F14d);

(*ii*) Temperature and maturity (S13, G14) affect the amounts present;

(*iii*) The sex of the plant (F15) does not alter the kind of constituent present, but influences the amount;

(*iv*) Parts of the plant (M5b) show variations in the amount of constituents. The roots and seeds contain no cannabinols;

(*v*) The antibiotic and marihuana activity of cannabis depend on the cannabidiol acid and tetrahydrocannabinol content which vary with geographic origin (R0).

ACKNOWLEDGMENTS

We wish to thank G. Machata, Institut für Gerichtliche Medizin der Universität, and Springer Verlag, Wien, for permission to copy and use the information in Plate I; H. Rapoport and Leong Way, University of California, for information on the metabolism of narcotics; J. Cochin for chromatographic data; and H. J. Anslinger for the report on neutron activation analysis of opium.

Our co-workers T. W. McConnell Davis and Ruth Lane have kindly supplied the data on paper chromatography of narcotics, alkaloids, and antihistamines and the information on the assay of marihuana. M. Osadchuk suggested the use of the short jars for rapid screening of marihuana samples. L. Martin and R. Cloutier contributed the UV, IR, and X-ray data of twelve narcotics.

The illustrations were made by G. Morris, and the photographs were produced by the Biological Photo Laboratory of this Department. Miss Valerie Hash, our typist, prepared the manuscript for publication.

REFERENCES

(A1) Akcasu, A. U. N. Document, ST/SOA/SER.K/2 (June 11, 1951).
(A1a) Anonymous *Anal. Chem.* **30**, No. 8, 19A (1958).
(A2) Asahina, H. U. N. Document, ST/SOA/SER.K/15 (March 11, 1953).
(A3) Asahina, H. *Bull. Narcotics U. N. Dept. Social Affairs* **9** (4), 17 (1957).
(A4) Asahina, H. U. N. Document, ST/SOA/SER.K/113 (October 6, 1961).

# 286 Charles G. Farmilo and Klaus Genest

(A5) Asahina, H., and Ōno, M. U. N. Document, ST/SOA/SER.K/39 (June 30, 1955).

(A6) Asahina, H., and Ōno, M. U. N. Document, ST/SOA/SER.K/40 (August 25, 1955).

(A7) Asahina, H., and Ōno, M. U. N. Document, ST/SOA/SER.K/45 (February 19, 1957).

(A7a) Asahina, H., and Ōno, M. U. N. Document, ST/SOA/SER.K/46 (February 19, 1957).

(A8) Asahina, H., and Ōno, M. U. N. Document, ST/SOA/SER.K/50 (October 1, 1957).

(A9) Asahina, H., and Ōno, M. U. N. Document, ST/SOA/SER.K/73 (June 20, 1958).

(A10) Asahina, H., and Ōno, M. U. N. Document, ST/SOA/SER.K/90 (October 22, 1959).

(A11) Asahina, H., and Ōno, M. U. N. Document, ST/SOA/SER.K/91 (October 30, 1959).

(A12) Asahina, H., and Ōno, M. *Eisei Shikensho Hokoku* **78**, 39 (1960); *Chem. Abstr.* **55**, 25159 (1961).

(A13) Asahina, H., and Mizumachi, S. *Eisei Shikensho Hokoku* **76**, 113 (1958); *Chem. Abstr.* **53**, 16465 (1959).

(A14) Asahina, H., and Shiuchi, Y. U. N. Document, ST/SOA/SER.K/32 (August 30, 1954).

(A15) Asahina, H., and Shiuchi, Y. *Eisei Shikensho Hokoku* **76**, 65 (1958); *Chem. Abstr.* **53**, 16465 (1959).

(A16) Asahina, H., and Shiuchi, Y. *Eisei Shikensho Hokoku* **76**, 115 (1958); *Chem. Abstr.* **53**, 16463 (1959).

(A17) Attisso, M. *Therapie* **14**, 650 (1959).

(A18) Attisso, M. *Montpellier Med.* **55**, 380 (1959).

(A19) Axelrod, J., and Inscoe, J. K. *Proc. Soc. Exptl. Biol. Med.* **103**, 675 (1960).

(B1) Baerheim-Svendsen, A. U. N. Document, ST/SOA/SER.K/92 (November 3, 1959).

(B2) Baerheim-Svendsen, A., and Bergane, K. *Bull. Narcotics U. N. Dept. Social Affairs* **10** (4), 17 (1958).

(B3) Baggesgaard-Rasmussen, H. U. N. Document, ST/SOA/SER.K/72 (May 12, 1958).

(B4) Baggesgaard-Rasmussen, H. U. N. Document, ST/SOA/SER.K/84 (October 21, 1959).

(B4a) Baggesgaard-Rasmussen, H. U. N. Document, ST/SOA/SER.K/86 (March 31, 1959).

(B5) Baggesgaard-Rasmussen, H., and Reimers, F. *Arch. Pharm.* **273**, 129 (1935).

(B6) Baggesgaard-Rasmussen, H., Eichsted-Nielsen, B., and Folting, K. U. N. Document, ST/SOA/SER.K/76 (January 7, 1959).

(B6a) Baggesgaard-Rasmussen, H., Eichsted-Nielsen, B. E., and Folting, K. U. N. Document, ST/SOA/SER.K/80 (January 7, 1959).

(B7) Bakre, V. J., Karaata, Z., Bartlet, J. C., and Farmilo, C. G. U. N. Document, ST/SOA/SER.K/79 (December 1, 1958).

(B8) Balatre, P. H., Traisnel, M., and Delcambre, J. P. *Ann. Pharm. Franc.* **19**, 171 (1961).

(B9) Barnes, W. H. *Bull. Narcotics U. N. Dept. Social Affairs* **6** (1), 20 (1954).

(B10) Barnes, W. H., and Sheppard, H. *Bull. Narcotics U. N. Dept. Social Affairs* 6 (2), 27 (1954).

(B11) Bartlet, J. C., and Farmilo, C. G. U. N. Document, ST/SOA/SER.K/30 (July 12, 1954).

(B12) Bartlet, J. C., Farmilo, C. G., and Taker, G. U. N. Document, ST/SOA/SER.K/56 (November 19, 1957).

(B13) Bäumler, J., and Rippstein, S. *Pharm. Acta Helv.* 36, 382 (1961).

(B14) Bellamy, L. J. "Infrared Spectra of Complex Molecules," 2nd ed., p. 102. Methuen, New York, 1958.

(B15) Bićan-Fišter, T. U. N. Document, ST/SOA/SER.K/88 (May 20, 1959).

(B16) Bićan-Fišter, T. U. N. Document, ST/SOA/SER.K/93 (December 11, 1959).

(B16a) Bićan-Fišter, T. U. N. Document, ST/SOA/SER.K/94 (February 12, 1960).

(B17) Borke, M. L., and Kirch, E. R. *J. Am. Pharm. Assoc.* 42, 627 (1953).

(B18) Braenden, O. J., and Lumsden, E. S. U. N. Document, ST/SOA/SER.K/65 (January 20, 1958).

(B19) Braenden, O. J., and Lumsden, E. S. U. N. Document, ST/SOA/SER.K/69 (March 31, 1958).

(B20) Braenden, O. J., Lumsden, E. S., and Inoue, I. U. N. Document, ST/SOA/SER.K/71 (July 9, 1958).

(B21) Braenden, O. J., and Lumsden, E. S. U. N. Document, ST/SOA/SER.K/74 (July 11, 1958).

(B22) Braenden, O. J., and Grlić, L. U. N. Document, ST/SOA/SER.K/87 (April 6, 1959).

(B23) Braenden, O. J., Lumsden, E. S., and Inoue, I. U. N. Document, ST/SOA/SER.K/81 (January 22, 1959).

(B24) Braenden, O. J., Grlić, L., Lumsden, E. S., and Inoue, I. U. N. Document, ST/SOA/SER.K/85 (February 18, 1959).

(B25) Braenden, O. J., Grlić, L., Lumsden, E. S., and Inoue, I. U. N. Document, ST/SOA/SER.K/99 (March 15, 1960).

(B26) Braenden, O. J., Grlić, L., Lumsden, E. S., and Inoue, I. U. N. Document, ST/SOA/SER.K/100 (March 15, 1960).

(B27) Braenden, O. J., Grlić, L., Ibañez, M. L., Ramanathan, V. S., and Gnadinger, E. U. N. Document, ST/SOA/SER.K/104 (November 3, 1960).

(B28) Braenden, O. J., and Ramanathan, V. S. U. N. Document, ST/SOA/SER.K/105 (November 30, 1960).

(B29) Braenden, O. J., Lumsden, E. S., Inoue, I., and Ibañez, M. L. U. N. Document, ST/SOA/SER.K/115 (November 16, 1961).

(B30) Braenden, O. J., Lumsden, E. S., Inoue, I., and Ibañez, M. L. U. N. Document, ST/SOA/SER.K/116 (December 19, 1961).

(B31) Braenden, O. J. U. N. Document, ST/SOA/SER.S/3 (November 28, 1960).

(B32) Braenden, O. J., and Grlić, L. U. N. Document, ST/SOA/SER.S/5 (November 30, 1961).

(B33) Brandt, R., Ehrlich-Rogozinsky, S., and Cheronis, N. D. *Microchem. J.* 5, 215 (1961).

(B34) Bruchhausen von, F. U. N. Document, ST/SOA/SER.K/29 (May 26, 1954).

(B35) Büchi, J., Huber, R., and Schumacher, H. *Bull. Narcotics U. N. Dept. Social Affairs* 12 (2), 25 (1960).

(B36) Büchi, J., and Huber, R. *Pharm. Acta Helv.* 36, 119 (1961).

(B37) Büchi, J., and Huber, R. *Pharm. Acta Helv.* **36**, 571 (1961).
(C1) Chari, T. S. T., Parthasarthy, C., Rajagopalan, N., and Subramanian, K. S. U. N. Document, ST/SOA/SER.K/25 (March 10, 1954).
(C2) Cheronis, N. D., and Entrikin, J. B. "Semimicro Qualitative Organic Analysis," 2nd ed. Wiley (Interscience), New York, 1957.
(C3) Chih-Yung Ch'ên *Yao Hsueh Hsueh Pao* **5**, 249 (1957); *Chem. Abstr.* **55**, 23929 (1961).
(C4) Clarke, E. G. C. *Nature* **184**, 451 (1959).
(C5) Cochin, J., and Daly, J. *Experientia* **18**, 294 (1962).
(C6) Commission on Narcotic Drugs, U. N. Document, E/CN7/278 (March 22, 1954).
(C7) Commission on Narotic Drugs, U. N. Document, E/CN7/315 (April 23–May 18, 1956).
(C8) Commission on Narcotic Drugs, U. N. Document, E/CN7/LI31/add. 36 (May 17, 1956).
(C9) Commission on Narcotic Drugs, U. N. Document, E/CN7/338 (February 20, 1958).
(D1) Dal Cortivo, L. A., Willumsen, C. H., Weinberg, S. B., and Matusiak, W. *Anal. Chem.* **33**, 1218 (1961).
(D2) Davis, T. W. McConnell, Genest, K., Lane, R., and Farmilo, C. G. (Organic Chemistry and Narcotic Section.) Unpublished results.
(D2a) Davis, T. W. McConnell, and Farmilo, C. G. *Abstr. 141st Meeting Am. Chem. Soc.* p. 11B (March, 1962); *Anal. Chem.* **35**, 751 (1963).
(D3) Demoen, P. J. A. W. *J. Pharm. Sci.* **50**, 79 (1961).
(D4) De Ropp, R. S. *J. Am. Pharm. Assoc.* **49**, 756 (1960).
(E1) Eddy, N. B., Fales, H. M., Haahti, E., Highet, P. F., Horning, E. C., May, E. L., and Wildman, W. C. U. N. Document, ST/SOA/SER.K/114 (October 6, 1961).
(E2) Eisenman, A. J., Fraser, H. F., Sloan, J., and Isbell, H. *J. Pharmacol. Exptl. Therap.* **124**, 305 (1958).
(E3) Eisleb, O. *Chem. Ber.* **74**, 1433 (1941); U. S. Patent 2,167,351 (July, 1939).
(E4) Elizabeth II. Statutes of Govt. of Canada, Chapter 35. Schedule, Control of Narcotic Drugs Act, p. 220. Queen's Printer, Ottawa, 1960.
(E5) Elliott, H. W., and Elison, C. *J. Pharmacol. Exptl. Therap.* **131**, 31 (1961).
(E6) Erdös, E. G., Foldes, F. F., Baart, N., Zsigmond, E. K., and Zwartz, J. A. *Biochem. Pharmacol.* **2**, 97 (1959).
(F1) Farmilo, C. G. *Bull. Narcotics U. N. Dept. Social Affairs* **6** (3), 18 (1954).
(F2) Farmilo, C. G., and Bartlet, J. C. U. N. Document, ST/SOA/SER.K/55 (November 26, 1957).
(F3) Farmilo, C. G., and Bartlet, J. C. U. N. Document, E/CN7/301 (April 22, 1955).
(F4) Farmilo, C. G., and Bartlet, J. C. U. N. Document, ST/SOA/SER.K/36 (April 20, 1955).
(F5) Farmilo, C. G., and Genest, K. *In* "Toxicology: Mechanisms and Analytical Methods" (C. P. Stewart and A. Stolman, eds.), Vol. II, Chapter 7. Academic Press, New York, 1961.
(F6) Farmilo, C. G., and Kennett, P. M. L. U. N. Document, E/CN7/207 (October 19, 1950).
(F7) Farmilo, C. G., and Kennett, P. M. L. U. N. Document, ST/SOA/SER.K/14 (January 26, 1953).

(F8) Farmilo, C. G., and Levi, L. *Bull. Narcotics U. N. Dept. Social Affairs* **5** (4), 20 (1953).

(F9) Farmilo, C. G., and Davis, T. W. McConnell *J. Pharm. Pharmacol.* **13**, 767 (1961).

(F10) Farmilo, C. G., Oestreicher, P. M. L., and Levi, L. *Bull. Narcotics U. N. Dept. Social Affairs* **6** (1), 7 (1954).

(F11) Farmilo, C. G., Bartlet, J., Oestreicher, P., and Almond, A. U. N. Document, ST/SOA/SER.K/47 (February 19, 1957).

(F12) Farmilo, C. G., Genest, K., Davis, T. W. McConnell, and Airth, J. M. U. N. Document, ST/SOA/SER.K/110 (April 11, 1961).

(F13) Farmilo, C. G., Genest, K., Clair, E. G. C., Nadeau, G., Sobolewski, G., and Fiset, L. U. N. Document, ST/SOA/SER.K/58 (November 29, 1957).

(F14) Farmilo, C. G., McKinley, W. P., Bartlet, J. C., Oestreicher, P. M., and Almond, A. U. N. Document, ST/SOA/SER.K/61 (December 20, 1957).

(F14a) Farmilo, C. G. U. N. Document, E/CN7/304 (June 15, 1955).

(F14b) Farmilo, C. G., and Genest, K. U. N. Document, E/CN7/373 (April 15, 1959).

(F14c) Farmilo, C. G. U. N. Document, ST/SOA/SER.S/4 (April 27, 1961).

(F14d) Farmilo, C. G., and Davis, T. W. McConnell *Proc. 3rd Intern. Meeting Forensic Immunol., Pathol. Med., Toxicol, London, 1963,* Part VII, Paper No. 6, 35 pp.

(F15) Farmilo, C. G., Davis, T. W. McConnell, Vandenheuvel, F. A., and Lane, R. U. N. Document, ST/SOA/SER.S/7 (April, 1962).

(F16) Fisher Scientific Company. Technical Data Sheet, TD 119, 1/60. New York (1960).

(F17) Foldes, F. F., Erdös, E. G., Baart, N., Zwartz, J., and Zsigmond, E. K. *Arch. Intern. Pharmacodyn.* **120**, 286 (1959).

(F18) Fuchs, L., Ullrich, W., Farmilo, C. G., Oestreicher, P. M., McKinley, W. P., Bartlet, J. C., Krishnan, P. S. Witte, A. H., Jermstadt, A., Acba, S., Nicholls, J. R., Small, L. F., Macleod, L. N., Liang, C. K., and Nordal, A. U. N. Document E/CN7/312, and add. 1 (March 22, 1956).

(F19) Fuchs, L., and Ullrich, W. U. N. Document, ST/SOA/SER.K/10 (September 25, 1952).

(F20) Fuchs, L., and Ullrich, W. U. N. Document, ST/SOA/SER.K/19 (September 1, 1953).

(F21) Fulton, C. C. U. N. Document, E/CN7/117, Add. 2 (May 19, 1947).

(F22) Fulton, C. C. U. N. Document, E/CN7/117, Annex A (June 23, 1947).

(F23) Fulton, C. C. U. N. Document, E/CN7/117, Add. 1 (September 22, 1948).

(F24) Fulton, C. C. U. N. Document, E/CN7/195 (March 26, 1950).

(F25) Fulton, C. C. U. N. Document, E/CN7/202 (September 18, 1950).

(F26) Fulton, C. C. U. N. Document, ST/SOA/SER.K/1 (January 25, 1951).

(F27) Fulton, C. C. U. N. Document, ST/SOA/SER.K/8 (February 11, 1952).

(F28) Fulton, C. C. U. N. Document, ST/SOA/SER.K/9 (June 9, 1952).

(F29) Fulton, C. C. U. N. Document, ST/SOA/SER.K/12 (October 14, 1952).

(F30) Fulton, C. C. U. N. Document, ST/SOA/SER.K/13 (January 12, 1953).

(F31) Fulton, C. C. U. N. Document, ST/SOA/SER.K/17 (March 25, 1953).

(F32) Fulton, C. C. U. N. Document, ST/SOA/SER.K/28 (April 29, 1954).

(F33) Fulton, C. C. U. N. Document, ST/SOA/SER.K/31 (October 15, 1954) and add. 1.

(F34) Fulton, C. C. U. N. Document, ST/SOA/SER.K/33 (September 14, 1954).

(F35) Fulton, C. C. U. N. Document, ST/SOA/SER.K/34 (September 14, 1954).

(F36) Fulton, C. C. U. N. Document, ST/SOA/SER.K/35 (August 25, 1955).
(F37) Fulton, C. C. U. N. Document, ST/SOA/SER.K/53 (October 22, 1957).
(F38) Fulton, C. C., and Engleke, B. U. N. Document, ST/SOA/SER.K/4 (September 11, 1951).
(F39) Fulton, C. C., and Engleke, B. U. N. Document, ST/SOA/SER.K/21 (September 24, 1953).
(F40) Fulton, C. C., and Engleke, B. U. N. Document, ST/SOA/SER.K/22 (December 29, 1953).
(F41) Fulton, C. C., and Engleke, B. U. N. Document, ST/SOA/SER.K/38 (August 25, 1955).
(F42) Fulton, C. C., and Engleke, B. U. N. Document, ST/SOA/SER.K/41 (April 5, 1956).
(G1) Gautier, J. A., Renault, J., and Rabiant, J. Ann. Pharm. Franc. 17, 401 (1959).
(G2) Genest, K., and Farmilo, C. G. Bull. Narcotics U. N. Dept. Social Affairs 11 (4), 20 (1959).
(G3) Genest, K., and Farmilo, C. G. Bull. Narcotics U. N. Dept. Social Affairs 12 (1), 15 (1960).
(G4) Genest, K., and Farmilo, C. G. J. Chromatog. 6, 343 (1961).
(G4a) Genest, K., and Farmilo, C. G. U. N. Document, ST/SOA/SER.K/119 (April, 1962).
(G4b) Genest, K., and Farmilo, C. G. Am. Chem. Soc. Abstr. 141st Meeting p. 11B, (March, 1962); Anal. Chem. 34, 1464 (1962).
(G5) Ghielmetti, G., and Mela, C. Boll. Chim. Farm. 99, 452 (1960).
(G6) Gillam, A. E., and Stern, E. S. "Introduction to Electronic Absorption Spectroscopy," p. 134. Arnold, London, 1958.
(G7) Glasstone, S. "Text-Book of Physical Chemistry," p. 982. Van Nostrand, Princeton, New Jersey, 1940.
(G8) Goldbaum, L., and Kazyak, L. Anal. Chem. 28, 1289 (1956).
(G9) Grlić, L. U. N. Document, ST/SOA/SER.K/54 (December 13, 1957); Acta Pharm. Jugoslav. 7, 199 (1957).
(G10) Grlić, L. U. N. Document, ST/SOA/SER.K/75 (August 22, 1958); Acta Pharm. Jugoslav. 9, 103 (1959).
(G11) Grlić, L., and Petričić, J. U. N. Document, ST/SOA/SER.K/48 (July 4, 1957); Farm. Glasnik 12, 487 (1956).
(G12) Grlić, L. U. N. Document, ST/SOA/SER.S/1 (March 15, 1960).
(G13) Grlić, L. U. N. Document, ST/SOA/SER.S/2 (April 29, 1960).
(G14) Grlić, L., and Andrec, A. Experientia 17, 325 (1961).
(G15) Grlić, L. J. Pharm. Pharmacol. 13, 637 (1961).
(G16) Grlić, L. J. Pharm. Belg. 14, 45 (1959).
(G17) Grlić, L., and Petričić, J. Experientia 15, 319 (1959).
(G18) Grlić, L. U. N. Document, ST/SOA/SER.K/117 (February 27, 1962).
(G18a) Grlić, L. J. Criminal Law Criminol. Police Sci. 52, 229 (1961).
(G18b) Grlić, L. J. Forensic Sci. Soc. 2, 62 (1961).
(G19) Grossmann, V., and Chaloupka, Z. Arch. Exptl. Pathol. Pharmakol. 236, 14 (1959).
(G20) Grossmann, V., and Kvetina, J. Arch. Exptl. Pathol. Pharmakol. 238, 107 (1960).
(H1) Halbach, H. World Health Mag. 15 (1), 22 (1962). (Published by World Health Organization, Palais des Nations, Geneva, Switzerland.)
(H2) Hanawalt, J. D., Rinn, H. W., and Frevel, L. K. Ind. Eng. Chem. Anal. Ed. 10, 457 (1938).

(H3) Henderson, L. J., and Hasselbach, K. A. Cited *in* "Biochemistry" (E. S. West and W. R. Todd, eds.), p. 53. Macmillan, New York, 1955.

(H4) Herken, H., Neubert, D., and Timmler, R. *Arch. Exptl. Pathol. Pharmakol.* **237**, 319 (1959).

(H5) Hilf, R., Castano, F. F., and Lightbourn, G. A. *J. Lab. Clin. Med.* **54**, 634 (1959).

(H6) Hubley, C. E., and Levi, L. *Bull. Narcotics U. N. Dept. Social Affairs* **7** (1), 20 (1955).

(H7) Huebner, I. *Nature* **167**, 119 (1951).

(I1) Incekara, F., and Karaata, Z. U. N. Document, ST/SOA/SER.K/57 (November 27, 1957).

(I2) Isbell, H. *Trans. Studies Coll. Physicians Phila.* **24** (1), 1 (1956).

(I3) Isbell, H. *Brit. J. Addic.* **57**, (1), 17 (1961).

(I4) Izmailov, N. A., and Schraiber, M. S. *Farmatsija* (*Sofia*) (3), 1 (1938). Cited in ref. (W11).

(I5) Izmailov, N. A., Franke, A. K., and Simon, I. S. *Med. Prom. SSSR* **13** (11), 36 (1959); *Chem. Abstr.* **55**, 15838 (1961).

(J0) Jabbar, A., and Brochmann-Hanssen, E. U. N. Document, ST/SOA/SER.K/102 (August 3, 1960).

(J1) Jambor, B., and Bajusz, E. *Pharmazie* **14**, 447 (1959).

(J2) Jermstad, A., and Waaler, T. U. N. Document, ST/SOA/SER.K/23 (April 23, 1954).

(J2a) Jermstad, A., and Lothe, J. U. N. Document, ST/SOA/SER.K/24 (May 5, 1954).

(J3) Johnson, C. A., and Lloyd, C. J. *J. Pharm. Pharmacol.* **10**, (Suppl.) 60T (1958).

(K1) Kalinowski, K., and Zwierchowski, Z. *Acta Polon. Pharm.* **16**, 377 (1959); *Chem. Abstr.* **54**, 7978 (1960).

(K2) Karaata, Z., and Incekara, F. U. N. Document, ST/SOA/SER.K/62 (January 2, 1958).

(K3) Karaata, Z. U. N. Document, ST/SOA/SER.K/66 (January 23, 1958).

(K4) Kaye, S., and Goldbaum, L. R. Toxicology. *In* "Legal Medicine" (R. B. H. Gradwohl, ed.), Chapter 24. Mosby, St. Louis, Missouri, 1954.

(K5) Kazyak, L. *J. Forensic Sci.* **4**, 264 (1959).

(K6) Kingston, C. R., and Kirk, P. L. *Anal. Chem.* **33**, 1794 (1961).

(K7) Kirchner, J. G., Miller, J. M., and Kellner, G. I. *Anal. Chem.* **23**, 420 (1951).

(K8) Kleinschmidt, G. *Pharmazie* **15**, 663 (1960).

(K9) Knaffl-Lenz, E. U. N. Document, ST/SOA/SER.K/3 (August 1, 1951).

(K10) Knaffl-Lenz, E. U. N. Document, ST/SOA/SER.K/11 (October 2, 1952).

(K11) Kolankiewicz, J., and Nikonorow, M. *Acta Polon. Pharm.* **16**, 115 (1959); *Chem. Abstr.* **53**, 18319 (1959).

(K11a) Kolšek, J., Matićić, M., and Repić, R. *Arch. Pharm.* **295**, 151 (1962).

(K12) Kolthoff, I. M. *Biochem. Z.* **762**, 289 (1925).

(K13) Kopp, E., Kotilla, E., and Csedo, K. *Pharmazie* **14**, 263 (1959).

(K14) Kori, S., and Kono, M. *Yakugaku Zasshi* **80**, 728 (1961).

(K15) Kori, S., and Kono, M. *Yakugaku Zasshi* **81**, 776 (1961); *Chem. Abstr.* **55**, 26368 (1961).

(K16) Korte, F., and Sieper, H. *Ann. Chem.* **630**, 71 (1960); *Tetrahedron* **10**, 153 (1960).

(K17) Korte, F., and Sieper, H. *Angew. Chem.* **72**, 210 (1960).

(K18) Krishnan, P. S. U. N. Document, ST/SOA/SER.K/59 (December 10, 1957).

(K19) Kuśević, V. U. N. Document, ST/SOA/SER.K/95 (February 22, 1960).

(K20) Kvetina, J. *Czesk. Fysiol.* **7**, 357 (1958).
(K21) Kvetina, J. *Radiobiol. Radiotherap.* **1**, 268 (1960).
(L1) Latshaw, W. E., and MacDonnell, D. R. *J. Pharm. Sci.* **50**, 792 (1961).
(L1a) Leddicotte, G. W., Emery, J. F., and Bate, L. C. U. S. A.E.C. Oak Ridge National Laboratory 62-2-71 (February, 1962).
(L2) Lee, H. M., Scott, E. G., and Pohland, A. *J. Pharmacol. Exptl. Therap.* **125**, 14 (1959).
(L3) Lee, K.-T., and Farmilo, C. G. U. N. Document, ST/SOA/SER.K/49 (July 17, 1957).
(L4) Lerner, M. *Anal. Chem.* **32**, 198 (1960).
(L5) Levi, L., Oestreicher, P. M., and Farmilo, C. G. *Bull. Narcotics U. N. Dept. Social Affairs* **5** (1), 15 (1953).
(L6) Levi, L., Hubley, C. E., and Hinge, R. A. *Bull. Narcotics U. N. Dept. Social Affairs* **7** (1), 42 (1955).
(L7) Liang, C. K. U. N. Document, ST/SOA/SER.K/18 (April 30, 1953).
(L8) Liang, C. K. U. N. Document, ST/SOA/SER.K/26 (April 29, 1954).
(L9) Lloyd, H. A., Fales, H. M., Highet, P. F., Van Den Heuvel, W. J. A., and Wildman, W. C. *J. Am. Chem. Soc.* **82**, 3791 (1960).
(M1) Machata, G. *Mikrochim. Acta* p. 79 (1960).
(M2) Macleod, L. N. U. N. Document, ST/SOA/SER.K/52 (October 17, 1957).
(M2a) Macleod, L. N., Martin, L., and Roberts, G. Private communication to C. Farmilo (February 11, 1960).
(M3) Makisumi, S., Kotoku, S., Ota, H., Ishihera, F., Hino, M., and Nishi, K. *Yonago Acta Med.* **3**, 126 (1958).
(M4) Mannering, G. J., and Takemori, A. E. *J. Pharmacol. Exptl. Therap.* **127**, 187 (1959).
(M5) Martin, L., Genest, K., Cloutier, J. A. R., and Farmilo, C. G. *Bull. Narcotics U. N. Dept. Social Affairs* **15** (3–4), 17 (1963).
(M5a) Martin, L., Davis, T. W. McConnell, Lane, R., and Farmilo, C. G. *Proc. Can. Soc. Forsenic Sci., 9th Meeting, Toronto, October, 1961.*
(M5b) Martin, L., Smith, D. M., and Farmilo, C. G. *Nature* **191**, 774 (1961).
(M5c) Martin, L. Research Report No. 3, p. 4 (May, 1960). Food and Drug Directorate, Ottawa, Canada.
(M6) May, E. L., Eddy, N. B., and Ager, J. H. U. N. Document, ST/SOA/SER.K/111 (October 6, 1961).
(M7) Mellett, L. B., and Woods, L. A. *Proc. Soc. Exptl. Biol. Med.* **106**, 221 (1961).
(M8) Meloun, B. Private communication to I. M. Hais. *In* "Handbuch der Papierchromatographie" (I. M. Hais and K. Macek, eds.). 1st ed., p. 179. Fischer, Jena, Germany, 1958.
(M9) Micheel, I., and Leifels, W. *Mikrochim. Acta* p. 444 (1961).
(M10) Milos, C. *J. Pharm. Sci.* **50**, 837 (1961).
(M11) Milthers, K. *Acta Pharmacol. Toxicol.* **15**, 21 (1958).
(M12) Miram, R., and Pfeifer, S. *Sci. Pharm.* **26**, 22 (1958).
(M13) Miyamoto, S., and Brochmann-Hanssen, E. U. N. Document, ST/SOA/SER.K/106 (January 23, 1961).
(M14) Miyamoto, S., and Brochmann-Hanssen, E. U. N. Document, ST/SOA/SER.K/109 (March 30, 1961).
(M15) Morgan, P. J. *Analyst* **84**, 418 (1959).
(M16) Morgan, P. J. *Analyst* **86**, 631 (1961).

(N1) Nakamura, G. R. *J. Forensic Sci.* **5**, 259 (1960).
(N2) Nicholls, J. R., and Kellett, E. G. U. N. Document, ST/SOA/SER.K/5 (September 24, 1951).
(N3) Nicholls, J. R., and Kellett, E. G. U. N. Document, ST/SOA/SER.K/6 (September 24, 1951).
(N4) Nicholls, J. R., and Kellett, E. G. U. N. Document, ST/SOA/SER.K/7 (September 24, 1951).
(N4a) Nicholls, J. R., and Eddy, N. B. U. N. Document, ST/SOA/SER.K/97 (February 19, 1960).
(N5) Niyogi, S. K., Tompsett, S. L., and Stewart, C. P. *Clin. Chem. Acta* **6**, 739 (1961).
(N6) Niyogi, S. K., Tompsett, S. L., and Stewart, C. P. *Clin. Chim. Acta* **6**, 741 (1961).
(N7) Nürnberg, E. *Arch. Pharm.* **292**, 617 (1959).
(O1) Oestreicher, P. M., Farmilo, C. G., and Levi, L. *Bull. Narcotics U. N. Dept. Social Affairs* **6** (3), 42 (1954).
(P1) Paerregaard, P. *Acta Pharmacol. Toxicol.* **14**, 53 (1957).
(P2) Panopoulos, G., and Vassiliou, A. U. N. Document, ST/SOA/SER.K/16 (March 24, 1953).
(P3) Panopoulos, G., and Vassiliou, A. U. N. Document, ST/SOA/SER.K/27 (April 29, 1954).
(P4) Panopoulos, G., and Vassiliou, A. U. N. Document, ST/SOA/SER.K/37 (April 4, 1955).
(P5) Panopoulos, G., and Vassiliou, A. U. N. Document, ST/SOA/SER.K/42 (April 18, 1956).
(P6) Panopoulos, G., and Vassiliou, A. U. N. Document, ST/SOA/SER.K/43 (May 8, 1956).
(P7) Panopoulos, G., and Vassiliou, A. U. N. Document, ST/SOA/SER.K/51 (October 7, 1957).
(P8) Parthasarathy, C., and Rajagopalan, N. U. N. Document, ST/SOA/SER.K/20 (July 20, 1953).
(P9) Perkons, N., and Jervis, R. E. "Activation Analysis of Raw Opium." Unpublished results, private communication.
(P9a) Petričić, J., and Grlić, L. U. N. Document, ST/SOA/SER.K/78 (October 16, 1958).
(P10) Pfeifer, S., and Weiss, F. *Pharmazie* **15**, 349 (1960).
(P10a) Pfeifer, S. *Pharmazie* **15**, 320 (1960).
(P11) "Pharmacopoeia of the United States of America," 14th revision, pp. 734, 795. Mack Publ. Co., Easton, Pennsylvania, 1950.
(P12) Pinta, M. U. N. Document, ST/SOA/SER.K/63 (December 23, 1957).
(P13) Pinta, M. U. N. Document, ST/SOA/SER.K/68 (March 31, 1958).
(P14) Pinta, M. U. N. Document, ST/SOA/SER.K/77 (October 14, 1958).
(P15) Pinta, M. U. N. Document, ST/SOA/SER.K/96 (February 18, 1960).
(P16) Pinxteren van, J. A. C., and Verloop, M. E. *Pharm. Weekblad* **96**, 545 (1961); *Chem. Abstr.* **55**, 26371 (1961).
(P17) Porter, C. C. *J. Pharmacol. Exptl. Therap.* **120**, 447 (1957).
(P18) Pride, R. R. A., and Stern, E. S. *J. Pharm. Pharmacol.* **4**, 59 (1954).
(P19) Pro, M. J. *J. Assoc. Offic. Agr. Chemists* **42**, 177 (1959).
(P20) Pro, M. J. *J. Assoc. Offic. Agr. Chemists* **42**, 458 (1959).
(P21) Pruner, G. U. N. Document, ST/SOA/SER.K/108 (March 20, 1961).

(P21a) Pruner, G. U. N. Document, ST/SOA/SER.K/83 (March 9, 1959).
(P21b) Pruner, G. U. N. Document, ST/SOA/SER.K/98 (March 15, 1960).
(P22) Pruner, G. U. N. Document, ST/SOA/SER.K/101 (April 12, 1960).
(P23) Pruner, G. U. N. Document, ST/SOA/SER.K/112 (June 14, 1961).
(P24) Pruner, G., and Dentice di Accadia, F. U. N. Document, ST/SOA/SER.K/107 (March 20, 1961).
(R0) Radošević, A., Kupinić, M., and Grlić, L. U. N. Document, ST/SOA/SER.S/6 (January 25, 1962).
(R1) Rapoport, H., Look, M., Binks, R., Sauermann, W., and Keumg, W. Private communication from H. Rapoport (Dept. of Chemistry, University of California, Berkeley, California) to C. Farmilo (January 25, 1962).
(R2) Revitch, E., and Weiss, G. *Diseases Nervous System* **20**, 317 (1959).
(R3) Rösler, Ch., Pfeifer, S., and Weiss, F. *Pharm. Zentralhalle* **99**, 349 (1960).
(R4) Roux, A., and Roux-Matignon, J. *Ann. Pharm. Franc.* **18**, 135 (1960).
(R5) Ruiz-Gizon, J. U. N. Document, ST/SOA/SER.K/103 (October 18, 1960).
(R6) Ruzhentseva, A. K., Merlis, V. M., Lyamina, G. G., and Bagreyeva, M. R. U. N. Document, ST/SOA/SER.K/89 (June 25, 1959).
(S1) Sakurai, H. *Yakugaku Zasshi* **81**, 155 (1961).
(S2) Sakurai, H. *Yakugaku Zasshi* **81**, 865 (1961).
(S3) Sakurai, H. *Yakugaku Zasshi* **81**, 869 (1961).
(S4) Sakurai, H., and Umeda, M. *Yakugaku Zasshi* **80**, 736 (1961).
(S5) Sakurai, H., and Umeda, M. *Yakugaku Zasshi* **81**, 1027 (1961); *Chem. Abstr.* **55**, 26367 (1961).
(S6) Sanchez, C. A. *Anales Fac. Farm. Bio-Quim. Univ. Nacl. Mayor San Marcos* (*Lima*) **8**, 82 (1957); *Chem. Abstr.* **53**, 22466 (1959).
(S7) Saunders, L., and Srivastava, R. S. *J. Pharm. Pharmacol.* **3**, 78 (1951).
(S8) Scaringelli, F. *J. Assoc. Offic. Agr. Chemists* **44**, 296 (1961).
(S9) Schaumann, O. *Arch. Exptl. Pathol. Pharmakol.* **239**, 311 (1960).
(S10) Schaumann, O. *Arch. Exptl. Pathol. Pharmakol.* **239**, 321 (1960).
(S11) Schaumann, O. *Oesterr. Apotheker Ztg.* **44**, 249 (1960).
(S12) Schmidlin-Mészáros, J., and Hartmann, H. *Arch. Toxicol.* **18**, 259 (1960).
(S13) Schultz, O. E., and Haffner, G. *Arch. Pharm.* **293**, 1 (1960).
(S13a) Schultz, O. E., and Mohrmann, H. L. *Arch. Pharm.* **295**, 66 (1962).
(S14) Secretariat, U. N. Document, ST/SOA/SER.K/60 (January 3, 1958).
(S15) Secretariat, U. N. Document, ST/SOA/SER.K/70 (March 31, 1958).
(S16) Secretariat, U. N. Document, ST/SOA/SER.K/82, Add. 1 (March 14, 1961).
(S17) Secretariat, U. N. Document, ST/SOA/SER.K/82, Add. 2 (March 14, 1961).
(S18) Sjöström, E., and Randell, A. *J. Am. Pharm. Assoc.* **48**, 445 (1959).
(S19) Spengler, G. A. *Helv. Med. Acta* **25**, 430 (1958).
(S20) Stahl, E. *Chemiker Ztg.* **82**, 323 (1958).
(S21) Stahl, E. *Angew. Chem.* **73**, 646 (1961).
(S22) Stainier, C., and Gloesener, E. *Farmaco* (*Pavia*) *Ed. Prat.* **15**, 721 (1960); *Chem. Abstr.* **55**, 18011 (1961).
(S23) Stermitz, F. R., and Rapoport, H. *Nature* **189**, 310 (1961).
(S24) Street, H. V. *J. Pharm. Pharmacol.* **14**, 56 (1962).
(S25) Sung, hen-Yu, and Way, E. L. *J. Pharmacol. Exptl. Therap.* **110**, 260 (1954).
(S26) Swanson, H. E. "Table for Conversion of X-ray Diffraction Angles to Interplanar Spacings," Appl. Math. Ser. 10. National Bureau of Standards, Washington, D. C., 1950.

(T1) Takemori, A. E. Univ. Microfilms, L.C. Card No. Mic 58-1935; *Dissertation Abstr.* 18, 2165 (1958); *Chem. Abstr.* 52, 16619 (1958).
(T2) Takemori, A. E., and Mannering, G. J. *Pharmacol. Exptl. Therap.* 123, 171 (1958).
(T3) Teichert, K., Mutschler, E., and Rochelmeyer, H. *Deut. Apotheker-Ztg.* 100, 283, 477 (1960) from ref. (S17).
(T4) Teijgeler, C. A. *Pharm. Weekblad* 94, 201 (1959).
(T5) Ternikova, R. M. *Sudebno-Med. Ekspertiza Min. Zdravookhr. SSSR* 1 (2), 27 (1958); *Chem. Abstr.* 54, 13235 (1960).
(T6) Ternikova, R. M. *Aptechn. Delo* 6 (2), 38 (1957); *Chem. Abstr.* 52, 5751 (1958).
(U1) United Nations Documents, Permanent Central Opium Board. Reports to the Economic and Social Council on the Work of the Board. Document Series No. E/OB/6 (November, 1950); *ibid.* E/OB/16 (November, 1960; released January 9, 1961).
(U2) Same as ref. (U1), Annex B to Statistical forms, 5th ed. (December, 1960).
(U3) United Nations Document, Permanent Central Opium Board. Report to the Economic and Social Council on the Work of the Board in 1961, Series E/OB/17.
(V1) Vacek, J., and Tyrolova, L. *Mitt. Deut. Pharm. Ges.* 28, 176 [in *Arch. Pharm.* 291] (1958).
(V2) Vaille, C. U. N. Document, ST/SOA/SER.K/44 (December 12, 1956).
(V3) Vidic, E. *Arzneimittel-Forsch.* 11, 408 (1961).
(V4) Vidic, E. *Arch. Toxicol.* 19, 254 (1961).
(W1) Wachsmuth, H., and Van Koeckhoven, L. *J. Pharm. Belg.* 14, 215 (1959).
(W2) Waldi, D., Schnackerz, K., and Munter, F. *J. Chromatog.* 6, 61 (1961).
(W3) Walkenstein, S. S., MacMullen, J. A., Knebel, C., and Seifter, J. *J. Am. Pharm. Assoc.* 47, 20 (1958).
(W4) Way, E. L., and Adler, T. K. *Pharmacol. Revs.* 12, 383 (1960).
(W5) Way, E. L., Kemp, J. W., Young, J. M., and Grassetti, D. R. *J. Pharmacol. Exptl. Therap.* 129, 144 (1960).
(W6) Weijlard, J., Orahovats, P. D., Sullivan, A. P., Purdue, G., Health, F. K., and Pfister, K. *J. Am. Chem. Soc.* 78, 2342 (1956).
(W7) Williams, L. A., Brusock, Y. M., and Zak, B. *Anal. Chem.* 32, 1883 (1960).
(W8) Willner, K. *Arch. Toxicol.* 17, 347 (1959).
(W9) Witte, A. H. U. N. Document, ST/SOA/SER.K/67 (March 31, 1958).
(W9a) Witte, A. H. U. N. Document, ST/SOA/SER.K/64 (February 21, 1958).
(W10) Wolf, S. *Naturwissenschaften* 46, 649 (1959).
(W11) Wollish, E. G., Schmall, M., and Hawryshyn, M. *Anal. Chem.* 33, 1138 (1961).
(Y1) Yu, Yun-Hsiang *Yao Hsueh Hsueh Pao* 6, (2), 101 (1958); *Chem. Abstr.* 53, 11765 (1959).

# Toxicity of Air Pollutants

by Milton Feldstein

*Bay Area Air Pollution Control District, San Francisco, California*

## I. Introduction

The emission of dusts, gases, vapors, and mists from industrial operations, combustion sources, and the general activities of man forms the basis for man-made air pollution. The intensity and frequency of air pollution incidents are closely associated with meteorological and topographical phenomena. The effects of pollutants on human health are functions of concentration, exposure time, the nature of the pollutant, and the presence of possible potentiating materials.

A review of some of these factors would be helpful in considering the specific toxicity of air pollutants. The term air pollution itself is much too general to afford an intelligible background to the study of the toxicity of air pollutants. There are many kinds of air pollution, each relating to the nature of the pollutants emitted, and to the reaction or interaction of such pollutants in the atmosphere. Generally speaking, however, air pollution may be divided into two broad classes, based upon certain observations and measurements as shown in Table I.

TABLE I
CHARACTERISTICS OF "LONDON" AND "LOS ANGELES" AIR POLLUTION MIXTURES

| Characteristics | London or East Coast metropolitan areas | Los Angeles or West Coast metropolitan areas |
|---|---|---|
| Major characteristic components | Sulfur compounds, particulate matter, carbon monoxide | Ozone, nitrogen oxides, carbon monoxide, particulate matter, hydrocarbons |
| Industrial sources | Various | Various |
| Rubbish burning sources | Major | Minor |
| Combustion fuel sources | Coal and petroleum | Petroleum |
| Effect on reagents | Reducing | Oxidizing |
| Effect on man | Lung and throat irritation | Eye irritation |
| Visibility reduction | Severe | Moderate to severe |
| Maximum occurrence | | |
| Months | December, January | August, September |
| Time of day | Early morning | Midday |
| Temperature | 30–40°F | 75–90°F |
| Relative humidity | 85% | Less than 75% |
| Wind speed | 0 | Less than 5 mph |

"Reducing" type air pollution has often been referred to as "London" type or "industrial" type, or even "classical" air pollution. As seen from the table, its predominating features are the presence of sulfur dioxide, industrial dusts, and soot from coal-burning operations. Much has been written about this kind of air pollution (M1, M2, M3, T1).

Another type of air pollution has received attention in recent years. This type is referred to as "oxidizing" air pollution, resulting from photochemical processes which occur in the atmosphere. Recent studies have shown that nitrogen dioxide and hydrocarbons are the key elements in the formation of photochemical air pollution. The process involves the absorption of radiant energy by $NO_2$ to form NO and atomic oxygen.

Reaction between atomic oxygen and molecular oxygen results in the formation of ozone, the principal oxidizing agent of photochemical smog. Further reactions involve ozone and reactive hydrocarbons (olefins) to produce many products, the nature of which is not as yet fully known (H1, H2).

However, it is generally accepted that the products of these reactions give rise to many of the effects associated with photochemical air pollution. The principal effects include eye irritation, vegetation damage, and visibility reduction (F1, L1, M4, R1, S1). To further complicate the picture, it seems reasonable to assume that under the proper conditions both "classical" and "photochemical" air pollution may coexist.

It is the purpose of this chapter to discuss some of the factors associated with photochemical smog, and to point out the possible effects on health of exposure to the mixture of chemicals which are present.

## II. Photochemical Smog

### A. Meteorological Factors

Studies of air pollution on the west coast of the United States have implicated several factors of meteorological origin which are generally associated with intense episodes. These factors tend to limit the movement of air so that rapid accumulation of the reactants in the photochemical process can occur. The major factors involved are reduced wind speeds and the presence of a layer of warm air blanketing an area (W1). Under these conditions pollutants emitted into the atmosphere are not dissipated by dilution or by being blown away, and gradually build up to concentrations necessary for photochemical reaction. These conditions generally occur during periods of intense heat and low relative humidity.

### B. Topographic Factors

Coupled with stagnation of the air mass and presence of an inversion lid is the topographic structure of many areas of the west coast. Features generally include mountain barriers creating huge bowls within which the accumulated pollutants tend to stagnate. The net effect of this combination of low wind speeds, inversion layer, high temperature, and natural bowl is to create a huge chemical reaction cell in which the photochemical processes may occur.

### C. Radiant Energy

The prime mover under the conditions outlined above is the energy derived from the sun which initiates the atmospheric reactions resulting in smog. The intensity of sunlight and the general absence of cloud cover and ultraviolet absorbing layers tend to make the area under discussion ideally suited for maximal intensities of energy in the 3000 Å range to reach the surface of the earth.

## D. Pollutants

Many varieties of chemical substances are emitted to the atmosphere by the activities of man. A catalogue of every species of substance would occupy many pages of text. Of particular interest in the formation of photochemical smog are nitrogen oxides and hydrocarbons (H1, H2).

Nitrogen dioxide and nitric oxide are formed during high temperature combustion of organic substances in the presence of air. Such operations or processes as incineration, open dump burning, power plants, auto exhaust, and gas- and oil-fired heating units all give rise to quantities of nitrogen oxides. During smoggy periods values for $NO_2$ as high as 1.5 ppm have been measured in Los Angeles (S2).

Hydrocarbons are derived primarily from the incomplete combustion of organic substances in incineration, open dump burning, and auto exhaust. Other sources include petroleum processing and solvent and gasoline evaporation. Much evidence has accumulated indicating that the most reactive hydrocarbons taking part in the photochemical process are the olefins (H3, S3). Olefins react more rapidly than do the paraffins and most of the oxygenates or aromatics.

## E. Photochemical Reactions

The photochemically catalyzed reactions which take place in the atmosphere are extremely complex. The principal reactants include nitrogen oxides, hydrocarbons, and oxygenated hydrocarbons. For a full discussion of the reactions and reaction rates the reader is referred to Leighton's work (L2).

A simplified summary of the processes involved indicates that nitrogen dioxide and olefins when irradiated by sunlight produce ozone, organic peroxides, and compounds which cause eye irritation, vegetation damage, and reduced visibility. The photodissociation of nitrogen dioxide to nitric oxide and atomic oxygen appears to be the most important primary photochemical reaction:

$$NO_2 + h\nu \rightarrow NO + O \tag{1}$$

Atomic oxygen in the presence of a catalyzing surface (denoted by M) may react with molecular $O_2$ to form ozone:

$$O + O_2 + M \rightarrow O_3 + M \tag{2}$$

Ozone reacts very rapidly with NO to form $NO_2$:

$$O_3 + NO \rightarrow NO_2 + O_2 \tag{3}$$

This provides an additional source of $NO_2$ for the formation of $O_3$ (Eqs. 1 and 2) since the concentration of NO in the atmosphere at the start of the photochemical cycle is greater than the concentration of $NO_2$. Ozone can also react with olefins:

$$O_3 + \;\diagdown\!\!C\!\!=\!\!C\!\!\diagup \to R, \overset{.}{R}O, \overset{.}{R}CO, ROH, ROOH, RCOOH, \text{polymers} \qquad (4)$$

Thus the ozone concentration measured in the atmosphere is the net result of two processes:

($a$) A light-catalyzed reaction leading to the formation of ozone (Eq. 2);

($b$) A light-independent reaction leading to the removal of ozone (Eqs. 3 and 4).

If one considers the wide variety of reactive organic compounds which are emitted to the atmosphere daily and which are capable of reacting with ozone or of becoming photolyzed or of reacting with the free radicals formed during the photochemical process, the nature of the reaction products formed would be complex indeed.

## F. Factors Affecting the Intensity of Photochemical Smog

The severity of a smog episode is related to the factors which have previously been discussed. At the risk of oversimplification, the intensity of a smog attack might be pictured as:

$$S = f\left(P \times E \times T \times \frac{1}{W} \times \frac{1}{I}\right)$$

where

$S$ = intensity of smog,

$P$ = concentration of reactive pollutants (hydrocarbons, nitrogen oxides),

$E$ = intensity of radiant energy of proper wavelength,

$T$ = temperature,

$W$ = wind speed,

$I$ = inversion height.

Thus, when the hydrocarbons and nitrogen oxides are present in sufficient concentration, when the irradiating energy is sufficiently intense, when the temperature is sufficiently high, when the wind speeds are low, and when the inversion level is close to the ground, a maximum smog effect will be obtained. This implies that eye irritation, visibility reduction, and vegetation damage will be at maximum levels. As each factor is varied, the intensity of the reaction is varied accordingly. For example, if all of the factors outlined above were present, except that the inversion level were at 3000 ft, the smog intensity would be reduced because the greater mixing volume would permit reduction of the concentration of reactive pollutants to the point at which no reaction or lesser reaction would occur. Alternatively, if the wind speed were to increase to 10–20 miles an hour, it would have a similar effect. If all other factors were present, but a heavy cloud cover substantially reduced the intensity of ultraviolet radiation reaching the surface of the earth, a similar diminution of the severity of the smog reaction would occur.

It is not inconceivable that quantitative measurements of all of the factors involved may soon be achieved so that a quantitative relationship between them may be established.

## III. Effects of Photochemical Smog

### A. Eye Irritation

Research into the nature of photochemical reactions occurring in the atmosphere had as its stimulus the eye-smarting and vegetation-damaging effects of Los Angeles smog. The exact chemical nature of the specific eye irritants found in the outside air during smoggy periods has not as yet been determined (R1). Recent work on the irradiation of synthetic mixtures of hydrocarbons and nitrogen oxides and the irradiation of dilute auto exhaust has implicated three specific eye irritants: formaldehyde, acrolein, and peroxyacetylnitrate (PAN) (S4, S5). These substances have been isolated and identified in smoggy air, but it is doubtful if the concentrations found can account for the degree of eye irritation noted during smoggy periods. Considering the complexity of the reaction mixture in the atmosphere, it is likely that other materials are formed which are eye-irritating, or that aerosols play some potentiating role in eye irritation.

Certainly, as analytical techniques become more refined and more sensitive, the number and nature of specific eye irritants will become better understood. Present studies on the role of particulate material as concentrating and transmitting agents of irritants to the eye may unravel one of the causes of intense eye irritation so common to photochemical smog mixtures.

### B. Vegetation Damage

Early studies on the effect of air pollution on vegetation centered around smoke and fumes from industrial processes, particularly from chemical manufacture, smelting, and the combustion of coal. In 1944 a new type of vegetation damage was observed in the Los Angeles area, and since that time has spread to most of the coastal areas of western

United States. The symptoms of this new type of plant injury consisted of silvering, bronzing, glazing, and necrosis of the lower leaf surface. The injuries generally occurred during episodes of intense air pollution associated with eye irritation and visibility reduction. Susceptible crops include leafy vegetable and forage crops, ornamentals, grapes, tomato, cereal, and cotton.

Recent studies (D1) have disclosed at least two classes of phytotoxicants which are formed in photochemical smog. The first of these is ozone which produces a mottling or bleaching of the upper surfaces of plant leaves. The second may well consist of a number of specific agents. The exact nature of these materials is not as yet known. The effects seem to include glazing or bronzing of the undersurface of the leaf.

Effects of photochemical smog damage have been duplicated in laboratory experiments. Studies with irradiated mixtures of olefins and $NO_2$ indicate that there may be a number of specific phytotoxicants, each having more or less effect on different species and ages of plants (S6).

## C. Visibility Reduction

One of the most readily discernible effects of air pollution is the reduction of visibility due to the presence of aerosols in the atmosphere. Smog aerosols are predominantly in the 0.3–1.0 $\mu$ size range (G1). As this size range is practically not subject to fallout by gravity, and also coincides with the optically visible wavelengths of light, such particles are the most effective light scatterers, and cause strong visibility reduction (M3, R2). Of additional interest is the fact that particles of this size range are most effectively deposited in the pulmonary spaces. Larger particles are trapped along the upper respiratory tract, whereas smaller particles are not caught because of low settling velocity and insufficient residence time in the lungs.

While the predominating concern with aerosols from an air pollution point of view relates to their visibility-reducing characteristics, of interest to the toxicologist are the size and rate of deposition of particles in the lungs, and surfaces of particles acting as condensation nuclei for absorption, concentration, and reaction of gases.

In general, there are two primary sources of the particles which are found in the atmosphere during heavy episodes of air pollution. The first of these are particles emitted as such directly to the atmosphere from various sources. These are emitted in a wide variety of chemical species and particle sizes. The second source consists of particles which are formed in the atmosphere as a result of the photochemical process (G1).

Much less is known about this aspect of aerosol formation. Recent work has indicated that these particles may result from the condensation of reaction products of the hydrocarbon–nitrogen dioxide–sunlight reaction on nucleating surfaces present in the atmosphere from other sources (G1). The final size of these aerosol particles is dependent on the size of the nucleating particles, their concentration, and the concentration of reaction products. Evidence has accumulated that they are predominantly in the 0.3–1.0 $\mu$ size range.

Much speculation concerning the role of $SO_2$ in aerosol formation has occurred over the past few years. Early studies (G2) indicated that the photochemical conversion of $SO_2$ to $SO_3$ in concentrations around 1 ppm in the atmosphere was only about 0.1%/hour. This conversion to aerosol did not contribute significantly to visibility reduction. Subsequent work (C1) indicated that the conversion rate may be substantially increased in the presence of catalytic dusts such as $MnSO_4$ and $FeSO_4$. However, the concentrations of catalyst required seemed much greater than has been encountered in the ambient atmosphere. Most recent studies have shown that, in the presence of hydrocarbons, nitrogen oxides, and radiant energy of the intensity and wavelength equivalent to that reaching the surface of the earth, the presence of $SO_2$ greatly enhances the formation of aerosol and may indeed be a significant source of visibility reduction (J1, R3). The sulfur-containing aerosol resulting from this mixture has tentatively been identified as $H_2SO_4$.

While the discussion above has divided classes of aerosols on the basis of preformed or emitted particulates and atmospherically generated particulates, it is not intended to imply that this differentiation characterizes specific visibility reduction in specfic areas. Indeed, it has been suggested (L3) that combinations of both kinds of particulates are present in classical and West Coast types of air pollution. The major source of aerosols causing visibility restriction during episodes of photochemical smog is from the photochemical process.

## IV. Toxicity of Air Pollutants

### A. Introduction

Comparisons are sometimes made between exposure to occupational pollutants and exposure to substances which are present in the ambient air during periods of air pollution. Many of the materials are the same in both cases. There are, however, some decided differences, in concentration, time of exposure, and in the type of population being exposed:

(1) Occupational exposures usually occur with some single substance, or at most only a few, in contrast with exposure to a wide variety of substances during air pollution episodes;

(2) Occupational exposures occur generally with adult, male popula-

tions in good health, contrasted with exposure of the very young, the aged, and the chronically ill populations exposed to periods of air pollution.

(3) Occupational exposures generally occur for an 8-hour period during perhaps 5 days a week, contrasted with continuing exposure to greater or lesser concentrations of air pollutants.

Consideration of these major differences in exposure to air pollutants and occupational pollutants leads to the conclusion that threshold limits or maximum allowable concentrations (MAC) for occupational exposures are not applicable to the general population exposed to air pollution. An MAC for exposure to community levels of air pollution should consider the differences in age, condition of health, concentration and time of exposure, and potentiating effects of groups of pollutants present at one time (S2).

## B. Carbon Monoxide

Carbon monoxide as a community air pollutant is emitted to the atmosphere from most combustion operations where incomplete combustion of organic matter occurs (Table II). Sources include incineration,

TABLE II
TONNAGES OF VARIOUS POLLUTANTS EMITTED TO THE
ATMOSPHERE PER DAY IN LOS ANGELES[a]

| Substance | Tons emitted per day |
|---|---|
| Carbon monoxide | 9950 |
| Sulfur oxides | 585 |
| Nitrogen oxides | 695 |
| Hydrocarbons | 1990 |
| Aerosols | 125 |

[a] Air Pollution Control District, Engineering Division, Los Angeles, 1961.

internal combustion engines, and the burning of various fuels for the production of heat and power. Community levels as high as 70–90 ppm (Table III) have been measured in the atmosphere for short periods of time (S2). Longer exposures during episodes of high air pollution may average 15–30 ppm.

Because of the cumulative action associated with exposure to carbon monoxide it is possible that the most serious effects may be noted in persons with chronic heart and lung conditions, that is, persons who may be acutely responsive to interference with oxygen transport. Recent studies (G3) have shown that exposures to 30 ppm for 4–6 hours may result in blood carboxyhemoglobin levels as high as 8%. At such levels,

*Milton Feldstein*

TABLE III
COMPARISON OF INDUSTRIAL THRESHOLD LIMITS (MAC)[a]
AND AIR POLLUTION VALUES[b]

| Substance | MAC | Maximum air pollution value | Average air pollution value |
|---|---|---|---|
| | (ppm) | (ppm) | (ppm) |
| Carbon monoxide | 100 | 72 | 26 |
| Nitrogen dioxide | 5 | 0.65 | 0.10 |
| Nitric oxide | — | 2.08 | 0.50 |
| Ozone | 0.1 | 0.90 | 0.25 |
| Sulfur dioxide | 5 | 3.16[c] | 0.10[d] |
| Hydrogen fluoride | 3 | 0.08[c] | 0.002[d] |
| Hydrogen sulfide | 20 | 0.9[c] | 0.002[d] |
| | (mg/m³) | (mg/m³) | |
| Sulfuric acid | 1.0 | 0.02[e] | |
| Beryllium | 0.002 | 0.00011[f] | |
| Lead | 0.2 | 0.042[c] | |

[a] Threshold Limit Values for 1960, ACGIH. *A.M.A. Arch. Environ. Health* **1**. 140 (1960).
[b] Los Angeles Air Pollution Control District Repts. (unnumbered).
[c] From reference (S14).
[d] From Cholak, J. *A.M.A. Arch. Ind. Hyg. Occup. Med.* **10**, 203 (1954).
[e] Estimated.
[f] From reference (S13).

detectable effects of carbon monoxide on visual sensitivity may occur (H4). Further research will be required to determine the permanence of such effects.

It should be pointed out that residual carbon monoxide hemoglobin concentrations as high as 8% may occur in heavy smokers. An additional 5–8% from exposure to community air pollution may pose added risks to health.

## C. Ozone

It has long been known that ozone is formed in the upper atmosphere by interreaction of molecular oxygen and ultraviolet radiation of 2000 Å. The greatest concentration of ozone occurs at distances of 10–20 miles above the surface of the earth (B1). However, the major source of ozone encountered at the surface of the earth is derived as a by-product of the photochemical cycle involving reactive hydrocarbons, nitrogen oxides, and ultraviolet radiation (H1, H2). Ozone levels in Los Angeles as high as 0.9 ppm have been measured, while ordinary levels during periods of smog may reach as high as 0.2–0.3 ppm for extended periods of time.

Short exposures to ozone in the range of a few ppm result chiefly in action on the lung tissue. Ozone acts as an oxidizing irritant, producing pulmonary edema and hemorrhage (S7). It is interesting to note that the MAC for ozone for occupational exposures is 0.1 ppm for 8 hours. This concentration has been exceeded in community levels of air pollution in the Los Angeles area on innumerable occasions.

Specific effects of long term exposure to community air pollution levels of ozone have not as yet been made clear. Experimental work with animals has revealed that there are other factors which may affect toxicity due to exposure to ozone (S8). Animals exposed to low levels of ozone develop a tolerance to the pulmonary effects of subsequent exposure (M5). Vitamin C and other reducing agents lessen the acute response (M5). In addition, it has been shown that oil mists protect animals in subsequent exposure to lethal ozone concentrations (W2). On the other hand, certain substances have been shown to have a potentiating effect on the acute toxicity of ozone in experimental animals (S9).

The mode of action of ozone has been likened to the action of ionizing radiation on biological systems (B2). It is apparent that much more information on the effects of long term exposures to community air pollution levels of ozone is needed. Additional information concerning the potentiating and inhibiting agents present in smog on the chronic effects of ozone is also needed.

### D. Nitrogen Oxides (Nitric Oxide and Nitrogen Dioxide)

Nitrogen dioxide is the primary reactant in the photochemical smog process because of its dissociation into nitric oxide and atomic oxygen under the influence of ultraviolet radiation. The majority of nitrogen oxides emitted to the atmosphere are formed during combustion processes of all kinds. Fixation of nitrogen and oxidation of nitrogen-containing organic matter occur during incineration, combustion of fuel in the internal combustion engine, and combustion of fuel for the production of heat and power. Community levels of nitrogen oxides as high as 0.65 ppm for $NO_2$ and 2.08 ppm for NO have been reported (Table III) in the Los Angeles area.

The toxicity of relatively high concentrations of $NO_2$ are fairly well known (S10), with acute pulmonary edema as the major finding. In animal exposures nitric oxide is about one-fifth as toxic as $NO_2$, with the major toxicity probably due to the conversion of NO to $NO_2$. Nitric oxide has an unusually high affinity for hemoglobin, but nitric oxide hemoglobin has not been observed in exposures at community air pollution levels. Studies of animals exposed to $NO_2$ at levels of 1 ppm produced no detectable changes in the lungs after 1 year of exposure (S11).

Further work needs to be done on the effects of inhibiting and potentiating substances present in photochemical smog mixtures on the chronic toxicity of $NO_2$. In addition, the possibility of tolerance development to intermittent exposures of low concentrations of $NO_2$ needs further study.

## E. Lead

The acute and chronic toxicity of exposure to lead is well documented (E1). Levels which may lead to chronic effects in exposed workers have been adopted; the MAC has been set at 200 $\mu g/m^3$ of air. The National Air Sampling Network (A1) of the United States Public Health Service has reported the average national value of lead in the air as 1.4 $\mu g/m^3$. Values ranged from 0.1 $\mu g$ in rural areas to about 3.5 $\mu g/m^3$ in populated areas. Community sources of atmospheric lead include emissions from foundries, automobile exhaust, and the smelting and refining of lead ores and products.

Of major concern in discussing the toxicity of lead present in the atmosphere is the particle size distribution of the material. Experiments on animals exposed to lead sesquioxide showed that absorption was about 35–50% when the particle size was in the neighborhood of 0.01–0.05 $\mu$, and about 50–60% when the particle size approached 0.75 $\mu$ in diameter (K1).

An index of exposure to community levels of lead can be estimated by comparison of urine and blood lead levels in exposed and control groups. Recent studies have shown that persons living in urban areas and persons with occupational exposure to auto exhaust tend to have higher levels than persons living in rural areas (H5) (Table IV). Blood lead levels of greater than 80 $\mu g/100$ gm of blood indicate incipient lead intoxication (K2).

TABLE IV
BLOOD LEAD LEVELS IN VARIOUS POPULATIONS[a]

|        | Urban | Rural | Exposed to auto exhaust |
|--------|-------|-------|-------------------------|
| Male   | 21    | 16    | 30                      |
| Female | 16    | 11    | —                       |

[a] Micrograms/100 gm.

In addition to the atmospheric burden of lead must be the consideration of other sources of daily exposure to lead such as cigarette smoking, food and beverage intake, and occupational exposures. The daily intake of atmospheric lead may in some cases provide the necessary additional lead to result in increased lead storage and chronic toxicity in selected individuals. Community studies at present being conducted may provide further insight into the role of atmospheric lead in chronic lead toxicity.

## F. Sulfur Oxides

Sulfur oxides are emitted to the atmosphere from such operations as the combustion of sulfur-containing fuels, refining of petroleum, and certain chemical- and insecticide-manufacturing processes. Atmospheric levels vary quite widely, tending to be higher in areas where high sulfur fuels are used for heat or power production. Ambient levels as high as 3.6 ppm have been measured in Chicago. In the severe London air pollution incident during December 5–9, 1952, values around 1–1.3 ppm were recorded. The average atmospheric values in natural gas and low sulfur fuel burning areas rarely exceed 0.05–0.10 ppm except in the vicinity of large sources of $SO_2$.

Sulfur trioxide is apparently much more toxic than $SO_2$ (G4). The MAC for occupational exposures to $SO_3$ is 1 mg/m$^3$ as $H_2SO_4$, and for $SO_2$ is 5 ppm (or 13 mg/m$^3$). Data on ambient levels for $H_2SO_4$ is very sparse; average values around 0.02–0.04 mg/m$^3$ have been assumed (S2). Exposures of 0.12 mg/m$^3$ of $H_2SO_4$ have been shown to have no effect on human subjects. Levels of 0.25 mg/m$^3$ may have effects on persons who are ill or who have chronic respiratory disease (S2). An additional factor which must be considered in discussing the toxicity of $H_2SO_4$ is particle size. Optimum size for maximum effect appears to be around 1 $\mu$ or slightly less. Very little is known about the particle size distribution of $H_2SO_4$ in the atmosphere.

Physiological response to low concentrations of both $SO_2$ and $SO_3$ is similar and involves bronchial constriction, and hence increased airway resistance (S2). The response with $SO_3$ is some four to twenty times greater in experimental animals than with $SO_2$ on an equimolar basis.

There are reports that concentrations of $SO_2$ as low as 1 ppm may produce measurable physiological response in man (A2). Contrary findings have also been reported (L4). It is generally agreed, however, that between 1 and 5 ppm most human subjects will show a detectable response to $SO_2$. Persons suffering from chronic bronchitis showed aggravated symptoms when exposed to community levels of $SO_2$ and soot (L5).

It should be pointed out that the presence of inert aerosols may potentiate the bronchial restricting action of $SO_2$ (A3, A4, D2). The action of such aerosols is dependent on the chemical nature, the particle size, and the concentration of the aerosol. Because of the diversity of particle size, chemical composition, and concentration of aerosols present in air pollution mixtures, the assessment of chronic exposure to $SO_2$ in the presence of these aerosols must await full evaluation of these factors. An additional factor which must be considered in discussing chronic exposure to $SO_2$ is the acute response which may occur in sensitive individuals (S12).

The possibility of atmospheric conversion of $SO_2$ to $SO_3$ is of interest to the toxicologist because of the greater toxicity of $SO_3$, and because the conversion could result in the formation of sulfur-containing aerosols which might possibly potentiate other pollutants, provide condensation nuclei for reaction in the atmosphere, and generally contribute to visibility reduction. Early work indicated relatively low photochemical conversion of $SO_2$ to $SO_3$, on the order of 0.1%/hour at concentrations of 1 ppm (G2). Additional studies indicated that the conversion may be much more rapid in the presence of such catalysts as $MnSO_4$ or $FeSO_4$ (C1). Recently the rate of production of a visibility-reducing aerosol from $SO_2$ was shown to be greatly increased in the presence of nitrogen oxides and olefinic hydrocarbons (R3).

It should be pointed out that $SO_2$ is toxic to vegetation at levels which do not apparently affect humans. Impaired yield and interference with photosynthesis may occur with alfalfa and buckwheat after 7-hour exposures of 0.4 ppm (B3, Z1).

### G. Fluoride

Major concern with fluoride levels in the atmosphere has been with the effect on vegetation and on cattle foraging on such vegetation. The literature is fairly comprehensive in this field (A5, N1, P1, M3, R4). Sources of fluoride include the manufacture of aluminum, clay bricks, phosphate chemicals, fertilizers, and steel. Reported ambient air levels of HF in areas of high air pollution average around 0.002 ppm, with much higher concentrations around heavily emitting sources. The National Air Sampling Network of the United States Public Health Service showed from 0.1 to 0.4 $\mu$g of fluoride per $m^3$ of air in urban areas. The maximum concentration reported was 1.64 $\mu g/m^3$ (A1).

Health effects from human exposure to these levels have not been reported in literature.

### H. Beryllium

Beryllium is a highly specialized air pollutant, emitted to the atmosphere from sources specifically involved in the processing or fabrication of the metal or its compounds. Close control on both in-plant and emission levels is generally maintained because of the toxic effects of the metal. The MAC for beryllium has been set at 0.002 $mg/m^3$. Maximum air pollution level measured was 0.003 mg/m³ (A1). Average levels within three-quarters of a mile distance from a specific source were 0.0001 mg/m³ (S13). Most known cases of beryllium poisoning occur among persons working with the metal or living close to sources of the material (K3, V1).

## I. Hydrogen Sulfide

Hydrogen sulfide is produced in the coking of coal and in petroleum-refining operations. It is also present in emissions from kraft paper pulping process, smelters, and the production of natural gas. Local non-industrial sources include sewer outfalls and decaying organic matter. Its presence in the atmosphere is manifested by its odor, discoloration of paints, and tarnishing of brass. The MAC for $H_2S$ has been set at 20 ppm. Levels as high as 0.9 ppm have been measured in the atmosphere (S14). Minimum detectable concentration by odor may be around 0.002 ppm.

The toxicity of $H_2S$ in large concentrations is well documented (H6). Levels this high are unlikely to be encountered in community air pollution episodes, except in cases of discharge of large quantities by accident. Toxic effects may be manifested by levels above the odor threshold by particularly sensitive persons.

The air pollution problem resulting from its presence is associated primarily with its nauseating odor.

## J. Carcinogens

Polynuclear hydrocarbons are produced from the incomplete burning of fuels, waste materials, or other combustible materials. Greater concentrations of these materials are produced during the combustion of coal than of other fuels. Atmospheric concentrations are generally three to twenty times higher in winter months than during the warmer seasons (S15).

One of the polynuclear hydrocarbons, 3,4-benzpyrene, has been shown to cause cancer in experimental animals. This substance is also present in cigarette smoke. Recent studies by the United States Public Health Service (S15) have indicated that levels of 3,4-benzpyrene as high as 61 μg/m³ of air have been measured in certain American cities. The range of values found in ninety-four urban American sites was 0.11–61 μg/m³ of air. The range in twenty-eight nonurban sites was 0.01–1.9 μg/m³ of air. Samples analyzed from London air showed values as high as 366 μg/m³ of air.

A number of researchers now hold the view that there is no tolerable dose of a carcinogen. Skin tumors have been produced in animals by as little as 0.4 μg of benzpyrene. Numerous observations indicate that carcinogens have a cumulative effect over a period of years. With the rate of lung cancer increasing rapidly, most studies have shown that the rate is higher in cities than in rural areas (D3, E2, M6, S16). Part of the reason, at least, is ascribed to carcinogens present in the air.

## K. Particulates

Specific particulates or aerosols including lead, beryllium, sulfuric acid, and carcinogens have been discussed earlier. These are only four of a wide variety of suspended liquid and solid droplets which are present in the atmosphere over urban areas. Factors which determine the potential toxicity of this vast number of substances include:

(a) the particle size distribution;
(b) the chemical nature;
(c) the quantity of each substance present in the atmosphere;
(d) the length of time during which individuals are exposed;
(e) the potentiating effects which one or more substances may have on others (see discussion in Section IV,F).

Table V shows the weight and analyses of particulate matter collected

TABLE V

PARTICULATE ANALYSES FROM SELECTED CITIES[a]

| Analysis | San Francisco | Los Angeles | New York | Detroit | Cincinnati |
|---|---|---|---|---|---|
| Total loading | 104 | 265 | 244 | 344[b] | 176 |
| Organic matter | 19.4 | 57.3[b] | 37.7 | 50.9 | 31.4 |
| Mn | 0.11 | 0.15 | 0.07 | 0.74[b] | 0.24[b] |
| Pb | 2.4[b] | 5.2 | 2.8 | 2.9 | 1.6 |
| Sn | 0.02 | 0.02 | 0.08 | 0.06 | 0.03[b] |
| Fe | 2.4 | 4.7 | 5.2 | 8.3[b] | 4.5 |
| V | 0.002 | 0.002 | 0.322[b] | 0.025 | 0.09[b] |
| Cu | 0.07 | 0.13 | 0.30 | 0.57 | 0.18 |
| Be | 0.0001 | 0.0001 | 0.0003 | 0.0004 | 0.0002 |
| Ti | 0.04 | 0.30 | 0.41[b] | 0.28 | 0.06 |
| As | 0.01 | 0.02 | 0.05 | 0.04 | 0.02[b] |
| F$^-$ | 0.37[b] | 0.38[b] | 0.21 | 0.04 | 0.21 |
| SO$_4{}^{2-}$ | 1.8 | 14.4 | 14.8 | 7.5 | 5.6[b] |
| NO$_3{}^{2-}$ | 3.4 | 14.4[b] | 0.8 | 1.2 | 1.0 |

[a] Average values in micrograms per cubic meter.
[b] Represents maximum value rather than average.

from the atmosphere over various cities as reported by the United States Public Health Service (A1). This represents a partial analysis of a few selected substances. In addition, very little concerning the nature of the organic fraction is known, as is very little concerning the particle size distribution of the large number of species of aerosols present in the atmosphere. Until more information concerning these factors is accumulated, the contribution of aerosols to health effects of air pollution must remain in the conjectural stage.

## L. Photochemical Smog

The question has often been asked, particularly by residents of the Los Angeles area, as to what the health effects of exposure to photochemical smog might be. The first effect noted, and one which is persistently present during severe episodes of photochemical smog, is eye irritation. Several substances have been shown to be present in smog mixtures which have eye-irritating effects. These include formaldehyde, acrolein, and peroxyacetyl nitrate. However, the concentrations present during smog episodes are insufficient to account for the degree of eye irritation experienced. The influence of particulate matter in enhancing the eye-irritating effect is at present being studied. In spite of the widespread incidence of eye irritation in areas experiencing photochemical smog, no evidence has accumulated concerning permanent eye injury.

Mortality and morbidity studies (G5) following severe episodes of smog have failed to produce conclusive evidence concerning the lethal or toxic nature of the mixture. Other studies have shown statistically significant correlation between attacks of asthma and oxidant index on particular days (S17).

Reports that lung function of patients with severe emphysema (M7) is affected by smog have increased concern about the chronic disease potential of this type of air pollution. These factors have led to the statement that photochemical air pollution poses a serious threat to the health of individuals (G5). It seems reasonable to assume that specific etiological factors will be unraveled as a result of research currently under way in this field. At the present time it is difficult to state whether the serious threat to the health of individuals is the result of exposure to the complex mixture known as photochemical smog or due to one or more of the specific components of photochemical smog discussed in Sections IV,B–K, above.

### REFERENCES

(A1) Air Pollution Measurements of the National Air Sampling Network. *Public Health Serv. Publ.* **637** (1958).
(A2) Amdur, M. O., Melvin, W. W., Jr., and Drinker, P. *Lancet* ii, 758 (1953).
(A3) Amdur, M. O. *Am. Ind. Hyg. Assoc. Quart.* **18**, 149 (1957).
(A4) Amdur, M. O. *Publ. Health Repts.* (*U.S.*) **69**, 503 (1954).

(A5) Agate, J. M. "Industrial Fluorosis." *Med. Res. Council Memo.* 22 (1949).

(B1) Blacet, F. E. *Ind. Eng. Chem.* 44, 1339 (1952).

(B2) Brinkman, R., and Lamberts, H. B. *Nature* 181, 1202 (1958).

(B3) Brandt, C. S. *In* "Air Pollution Handbook" (P. L. Magill, F. R. Holden, and C. Ackley, eds.), Chapter 8. McGraw-Hill, New York, 1956.

(C1) Coughanour, D. R. "Oxidation of Sulfur Dioxide in Fog Droplets." Ph.D. Thesis, University of Illinois, Urbana, Illinois, 1956.

(D1) Darley, E. F., Stephens, E. R., Middleton, J. T., and Houst, P. L. *Intern. J. Air Pollution* 1, 155 (1959).

(D2) Dautrebande, L., Shaver, J., and Capp, R. *Arch. Internal Med.* 85, 17 (1951).

(D3) Dean, G. *Brit. Med. J.* ii, 852 (1959).

(E1) Elkins, H. B. "The Chemistry of Industrial Toxicology." Wiley, New York, 1951.

(E2) Eastcott, D. F., and Lond, M. B. *Lancet* i, 37 (1956).

(F1) Ford, H. W. Tech. Rept. No. X, Project C-1388. Stanford Research Inst., Menlo Park, California, 1955.

(G1) Goetz, A. "Visibility Restriction by Photochemical Aerosol Formation." Presented at Air Pollution Research Conference, University of Southern California, Los Angeles, 1961.

(G2) Gerhardt, E. R., and Johnstone, H. F. *Ind. Eng. Chem.* 47, 972 (1955).

(G3) Goldsmith, J. R., and Rogers, L. H. *Public Health Repts. (U.S.)* 74, 6 (1959).

(G4) Greenwald, I. *A.M.A. Arch. Ind. Hyg. Occupational Med.* 10, 455 (1954).

(G5) Goldsmith, J. R., and Breslow, L. *J. Air Pollution Control Assoc.* 9, 129 (1959).

(H1) Haagen-Smit, A. J. *Ind. Eng. Chem.* 44, 1342 (1952).

(H2) Haagen-Smit, A. J., Bradley, C. E., and Fox, M. M. *Ind. Eng. Chem.* 45, 2086 (1953).

(H3) Haagen-Smit, A. J., and Fox, M. M. *Ind. Eng. Chem.* 48, 1484 (1956).

(H4) Halperin, M. H., McFarland, R. A., Niven, J. I., and Roughton, F. J. W. *J. Physiol. (London)* 146, 583 (1959).

(H5) Hofreuter, D. H., Catcott, E. V., Keenan, R. G., and Xintaras, A. B. *Arch. Environ. Health* 3, 568 (1961).

(H6) Henderson, Y., and Haggard, H. W., "Noxious Gases." Reinhold, New York, 1943.

(J1) Jones, J. I., Schuck, E. A., Doyle, G. J., Endow, N., and Caldwell, R. G. "A Progress Report on the Chemistry of Community Air Pollution." Project P-3106, Stanford Research Inst., Menlo Park, California, 1962.

(K1) Kehoe, R. A. *In* "Report of the Surgeon General's Ad Hoc Committee on Tetraethyl Lead," pp. 56, 57. U.S. Govt. Printing Office, Washington, D.C., 1959.

(K2) Kehoe, R. A. Reported *in* "Technical Report of California Standards for Ambient Air Quality and Motor Vehicle Exhaust," p. 81. State of California Dept. Publ. Health, Berkeley, 1960.

(K3) Kettering Laboratory "Workshop on Beryllium." University of Cincinnati, Ohio, 1961.

(L1) Littman, F. E. Tech. Rept. No. IX, Project C-844. Stanford Research Inst., Menlo Park, California, 1955.

(L2) Leighton, P. A. "Photochemistry of Air Pollution." Academic Press, New York, 1961.

(L3) Linsky, B., and Wohlers, H. C. "Measuring Visibility Interference Due to Air Pollution on the West Coast." Presented at Am. Ind. Hyg. Assoc. Conference, Washington, D. C., 1962.

# Toxicity of Air Pollutants

315

(L4) Lawther, P. J. *Lancet* ii, 745 (1953).
(L5) Lawther, P. J. *Proc. Roy. Soc. Med.* 51, 262 (1958).
(M1) Mallette, F. S., ed. "Problems and Control of Air Pollution." Reinhold, New York, 1955.
(M2) Meetham, A. R. "Atmospheric Pollution," 2nd ed. Pergamon Press, New York, 1956.
(M3) Magill, P. L., Holden, F. R., and Ackley, C., eds. "Air Pollution Handbook." McGraw-Hill, New York, 1956.
(M4) Middleton, J. T., Kendrick, J. B., Jr., and Darley, E. F. *Proc. 3rd Natl. Air Pollution Symp., Los Angeles, California* (1955).
(M5) Matzen, R. N. *Am. J. Physiol.* 190, 84 (1957).
(M6) Manos, N. "Comparative Mortality Among Metropolitan Areas of the U.S." *Public Health Serv., Public Health Bull.* 562 (1957).
(M7) Motley, H. L., Smart, R. H., and Leftwich, C. I. *J. Am. Med. Assoc.* 171, 1469 (1959).
(N1) National Academy of Science. "The Fluorosis Problem in Livestock Production." *Natl. Acad. Sci. Publ.* 381, 85 pp. (1955); 824, 37 pp. (1960).
(P1) Phillips, P. H. *In* "Air Pollution Handbook" (P. L. Magill, F. R. Holden, and C. Ackley, eds.). McGraw-Hill, New York, 1956.
(R1) Renzetti, N. A., ed. *Air Pollution Found. (Los Angeles) Rept.* 9 (1955).
(R2) Robinson, E. R. *In* "Air Pollution" (A. C. Stern, ed.), Vol. 1. Academic Press, New York, 1962.
(R3) Renzetti, N. A., and Doyle, G. J. *Intern. J. Air Pollution* 2, 327 (1960).
(R4) Roholm, K. "Fluoride Intoxication." Lewis, London, 1937.
(S1) Stanford Research Institute "The Smog Problem in Los Angeles." Western Oil & Gas Assoc., Los Angeles, California, 1954.
(S2) State of California "Technical Report of California Standards for Ambient Air Quality and Motor Vehicle Exhaust." State of California Dept. Public Health, Berkeley, 1960.
(S3) Stephens, E. R., Hanst, P. L., Doerr, R. C., and Scott, W. E. *Ind. Eng. Chem.* 48, 1498 (1956).
(S4) Schuck, E. A., *Air Pollution Found., San Marino, California Rept.* 18 (1957).
(S5) Schuck, E. A., and Doyle, G. J. *Air Pollution Found., San Marino, California Rept.* 29 (1959).
(S6) Stephens, E. R., Darley, E. F., Taylor, O. C., and Scott, W. E. *Proc. Am. Petrol. Inst.* 40, III (1960).
(S7) Stokinger, H. E. *A.M.A. Arch. Ind. Health* 9, 366 (1954).
(S8) Stokinger, H. E. *A.M.A. Arch. Ind. Health* 15, 181 (1957).
(S9) Svirbely, J. L., Dobrogarski, O. J., and Stokinger, H. E. *J. Am. Ind. Hyg. Assoc.* 22, 21 (1961).
(S10) Stokinger, H. E. *A.M.A. Arch. Ind. Health* 15, 181 (1957).
(S11) Stokinger, H. E. Unpublished data reported *in* "Technical Report of California Standards for Ambient Air Quality and Motor Vehicle Exhaust." State of California Dept. Public Health, Berkeley, 1960.
(S12) Simm, V. M., and Prattle, R. E. *J. Am. Med. Assoc.* 165, 1908 (1957).
(S13) Sussman, V. H., Lieben, J., and Cleland, J. G. *Am. Ind. Hyg. Assoc. J.* 20, 504 (1959).
(S14) Stanford Research Institute "Final Report, Literature Review of Metropolitan Air Pollutant Concentrations." Menlo Park, California, 1956.
(S15) Sawicki, E., Elbert, W. C., Hauser, T. R., Fox, F. T., and Stanley, T. W. *Am. Ind. Hyg. Assoc. J.* 21, 443 (1960).

(S16) Stocks, P., and Campbell, J. M. *Brit. Med. J.* ii, 923 (1955).
(S17) Schoettlin, C., and Landau, E. "Air Pollution and Asthmatic Attacks in the Los Angeles Area." *Public Health Repts.* (*U.S.*) **76**, 545 (1961).
(T1) Thring, M. W., ed. "Air Pollution." Butterworths, London, 1957.
(V1) Van Ordstrand, H. S. *Ann. Internal Med.* **35**, 1203 (1951).
(W1) Wanta, R. C. *In* "Air Pollution" (A. C. Stern, ed.), Vol. 1. Academic Press, New York, 1962.
(W2) Wagner, W. D., Dobrogarski, O. J., and Stokinger, H. E. *Arch. Environ. Health* **2**, 534 (1961).
(Z1) Zimmerman, S. *Proc. 1st Natl. Air Pollution Symp., Stanford Research Inst., Pasadena, California*, p. 135 (1949).

# Analytical Methods for Air Pollutants

by MILTON FELDSTEIN

*Bay Area Air Pollution Control District, San Francisco, California*

## I. Introduction

Analysis of the ambient atmosphere may often require procedures capable of identifying and quantitating relatively small concentrations of specific pollutants. Generally, the sensitivity of the method must be greater than the sensitivity required for analysis of contaminants in workroom atmospheres. Table I indicates the concentration of various pollutants which may be found in polluted and nonpolluted air.

317

TABLE I

CONCENTRATION OF POLLUTANT

| Pollutant | Nonpolluted air (ppm) | Polluted air (ppm) |
|---|---|---|
| Carbon monoxide | 10–15 | 25–50 |
| NO | 0–0.5 | 0.5–3.5 |
| NO₂ | 0–0.1 | 0.1–1.0 |
| Oxidant | 0–0.15ᵃ | 0.15–1.0ᵃ |
| Total hydrocarbon | 0–2ᵇ | 2–50ᵇ |
| SO₂ | 0–0.2 | 0.2–5 |
| Fluoride (as HF) | 0–0.04 | 0.08 |
| H₂S | 0–0.05 | 0.9 |
| Beryllium | 0 | 0.1 ($\mu$g/m³) |
| Pb | 0–10 ($\mu$g/m³) | 30–40 ($\mu$g/m³) |

ᵃ Potassium iodide method.
ᵇ Calculated as $CH_4$, Flame Ionization Detector.

Three categories of pollutants have been considered in presenting the specific methods which are to be described:

( *a* ) Pollutants which may have a direct toxic effect if present in the atmosphere in sufficient concentration for a sufficient period of time. These include fluoride, carbon monoxide, sulfur dioxide, beryllium, and lead. The toxic effects which may be manifested include direct toxicity on man, toxic effects on vegetation, or indirect toxic effects on cattle foraging on vegetation which has absorbed or been dusted with the contaminant.

( *b* ) Pollutants which may not be present in the atmosphere in sufficient concentration to cause toxicity, but which create nuisance problems due to odor. These include hydrogen sulfide and mercaptans.

( *c* ) Pollutants which are involved in the photochemical process which occurs in the ambient atmosphere and which leads to the formation of reaction products which are eye-irritating, vegetation-damaging, and visibility-reducing. These pollutants include nitrogen dioxide, nitric oxide, and hydrocarbons. Of interest in this area is the measurement of ozone or "oxidant" which occurs as a by-product of the photochemical process.

## II. Analysis of Pollutants Which May Have a Direct Toxic Effect if Present in the Atmosphere in Sufficient Concentration for a Sufficient Period of Time

### A. Carbon Monoxide

#### 1. INFRARED METHOD (R1)

Samples may be collected in the field, in evacuated, stainless steel

34-liter tanks (F1). The contents of the tank are transferred to the evacuated 10-meter path length infrared cell, and the spectrum from 4 to 5 $\mu$ recorded. The concentration of carbon monoxide is calculated from the absorbance at 7.6 $\mu$ after calibration with known concentrations of the gas. The minimum detectable concentration under these conditions (10-meter path length cell and 3.85 liters of sample) is 5 ppm.

## 2. INDICATOR TUBE METHOD (J1)

Air samples are drawn through U. S. National Bureau of Standards (NBS) carbon monoxide indicator tubes with the aid of a small pump and flow meter. Sampling rate is adjusted to 100 ml/minute, and sampling is continued until the first perceptible change in color of the indicator from yellow to green is noted. Calibration may be accomplished by drawing a standard of 10 ppm carbon monoxide through an NBS tube at a rate of 100 ml/minute until the first perceptible color change from yellow to green occurs. Calculation of the CO concentration in the sample is then made as follows:

$$\text{CO concentration (ppm)} = 10 \times (T_2/T_1)$$

where $T_2$ is the time required for the sample, and $T_1$ is the time required for the standard to effect the color change.

## B. Fluoride

### 1. PARTICULATE AND GASEOUS FLUORIDES

Particulate and gaseous fluorides are effectively collected in a standard Greenburg–Smith impinger. Sampling at 1 cfm for 30–60 minutes will provide sufficient sample for analysis. Collection medium used is distilled water. After collection, the fluorides are isolated from interfering substances by a modification of the Willard and Winter distillation procedure (W1).

*Reagents*
1. Silver sulfate, C.P. crystals
2. Perchloric acid (72%)
3. 1:4 perchloric acid in water
4. Thorium nitrate, 0.005 $N$: Dissolve approximately 0.87 gm $Th(NO_3)_4 \cdot 12H_2O$ in distilled water and dilute to 1 liter.
5. Standard fluoride containing 5 $\mu$g F$^-$ per ml: Dry C.P. NaF, weigh out 0.2210 gm, and dilute to 1 liter; 1 ml = 0.1 mg F$^-$. Make proper dilutions.
6. Sodium hydroxide solution, 0.05 $N$
7. Hydrochloric acid, 0.05 $N$

8. Alizarin red S indicator, 0.05% in water
9. Buffer solution: Dissolve 2.0 gm of sodium hydroxide in 40 ml of distilled water. Dissolve 9.50 gm of monochloroacetic acid in 60 ml of distilled water. Slowly add the NaOH solution with stirring to the monochloroacetic acid solution. This solution is stable for 5 days (pH 3.0).

*Apparatus*

1. Steam generator: Add sufficient calcium hydroxide to the water to form a supersaturated solution.
2. Distillation apparatus:
   a. Distillation flasks, Claisen, modified
   b. Electric heater
   c. Condenser

*Procedure.* Transfer the sample to a clean Claisen distilling flask. Add 8 to 10 glass beads and sufficient silver sulfate to precipitate all the chloride present in the solution. Add 50 ml of concentrated perchloric acid. Add distilled water to bring volume to about 100 ml. Wash down the neck of the flask and connect to the condenser. Insert two-hole stopper containing the steam tube and thermometer into the neck of the flask. Close the rubber tube from the steam generator and heat the distilling flask to boiling. Allow steam to enter flask and collect the distillate in 500-ml bottles. Maintain the temperature in the flask at 132°C. Collect 400-ml distillate.

*Titration.* Standardization of 0.005 N thorium nitrate. Pipette samples of standard sodium fluoride solution directly into 500-ml flasks. Use concentrations of 10, 25, 50, and 100 μg of fluoride. Dilute to 200 ml with distilled water. Add 1.0 ml of 0.05% alizarin red indicator and restore the pink color by adding 0.05 N sodium hydroxide solution drop by drop. Discharge the pink color by addition of 0.05 N hydrochloric acid.

[*Note:* The pH is critical. Add 1.0 ml of monochloroacetic acid buffer solution and titrate with 0.005 N thorium nitrate solution until the appearance of a faint pink color. Titrate a reagent blank similarly. Titrate a 200-ml aliquot of sample distillate in a similar fashion.]

## 2. COLLECTION AND ANALYSIS OF FLUORIDE ON LIMED PAPER (A1)

Atmospheric concentrations of fluoride may be surveyed by the limed paper technique. Papers are prepared by soaking $1 \times 5$ inch strip of Whatman No. 4 paper in a saturated solution of low fluoride CaO. After drying, the papers are exposed in the field for periods of 1 month or more. A convenient shelter box may be constructed from 1-qt freezer cartons. The papers are stapled across the top of the box about 1 inch from the opening. The boxes are tacked inverted to convenient supports in the field about 3–6 ft from the ground.

Analysis of limed paper for fluoride:

*Reagents*
1. Amberlite IR-120, strongly acidic cation-exchange resin
2. 6 N HCl
3. 2 N HCl
4. Standard fluoride solution containing 5 $\mu$g F⁻ per ml: Dry C.P. NaF, weigh out 0.2210 gm and dissolve in 1 liter of distilled water (1 ml = 0.1 mg F⁻), and make proper dilution.
5. Th(NO$_3$)$_4$ solution, 0.005 N: Dissolve approximately 0.87 gm of Th(NO$_3$)$_4$·12H$_2$O and dilute to 1 liter.
6. Alizarin red S, 0.05% aqueous solution.
7. Monochloroacetic acid buffer solution: Dissolve 2.0 gm of sodium hydroxide in 40 ml of water and add to 9.45 gm of monochloroacetic acid dissolved in 60 ml of water. Monochloroacetic acid buffer solution is stable for 1 week (pH 3.0).

*Preparation of Column.* Soak the resin well in water, decanting any fines which rise to the top, and take enough resin to fill a column of 10 mm ID to a height of 13–15 cm. Transfer resin to column from its water bath being very careful not to entrain any air bubbles in the transfer; from this point, the column should not be allowed to dry. A few milliliters of solution should always cover the resin bed. Glass wool plugs are conveniently placed at the top and bottom of the resin bed.

*Recharging Column.* To wash the column pass through 200 ml of 6 N HCl at the rate of 0.5 ml/minute, then 200 ml of 2 N HCl at full flow through column, then 200 ml of distilled water at full flow. The column is now ready for samples.

*Procedure.* To the calcium oxide papers which have been cut in small sections in a 100-ml beaker, add 50–75 ml of distilled water plus 0.5 ml of 0.1 N HCl. Swirl well and let sit for approximately 10 minutes, swirl well again, and pass the solution through the column at full flow, rinse beaker with 20 ml distilled water, then pass an additional 15 ml of water through the column. Collect effluent directly in a 500-ml Erlenmeyer flask. Add 1 ml of alizarin red S to the effluent and make just alkaline with 0.1 N NaOH. Adjust to acid with 0.1 N HCl (yellow). Add 1 ml buffer solution and titrate with thorium nitrate to a salmon pink end point. A blank titration should be run along with samples. Compare end point color with blank.

Fifteen to twenty samples may be run before column need be washed, using the same procedure as in the preparation of the column.

*Standardization.* The thorium nitrate is standardized by passing known quantities of fluoride in 100 ml of solution through the column, and then titrating as above.

### 3. ANALYSIS OF VEGETATION FOR FLUORIDE

*Reagents*
   1. Calcium oxide (low fluoride content)
   2. Sodium hydroxide pellets

*Procedure.* A representative aliquot of the vegetation sample is obtained by first mincing in a food chopper or reducing to small pieces with a pair of scissors. Mix thoroughly and remove one sample for moisture and a second sample for fluoride determination.

*For Moisture:* The size of the sample taken should be large enough to be representative of the material. An aliquot of 25 gm is usually satisfactory. Place aliquot in a crucible dried to a constant weight and dry sample in a drying oven at 105°C.

*For Fluoride Determination:* Place 25-gm aliquot in a porcelain crucible. Add 1 gm of calcium oxide for each 10 gm of sample. Add sufficient distilled water to cover the sample and mix well by stirring. Add a few drops of phenolphthalein to test for alkalinity. Add more calcium oxide, if necessary, to maintain an alkaline condition during evaporation. Place sample on hot plate and evaporate to dryness. Slowly introduce the sample containing the dry material into a muffle furnace at a temperature of *not more* than 400°C. With the muffle slightly open, raise the temperature to 600°C. Close muffle when smoke ceases and continue heating until the ash is light gray in color. Stir the contents of the dish occasionally with a spatula if ignition is not complete after 1 hour.

After ignition is complete, transfer the ash to a nickel crucible. Add 5–10 gm of sodium hydroxide pellets. Place the crucible in the muffle furnace for 10–15 minutes at a temperature of 600°C. *Carefully* swirl the contents of the crucible to facilitate mixing. Cool and add minimum amount of water to dissolve the melt. Transfer the solution to a distillation flask. Wash the crucible first with distilled water and finally with 1:4 perchloric acid. Keep the volume below 125 ml. Follow procedure as outlined in method for distillation of fluoride.

### C. Beryllium (S1)

Samples are collected by means of a high volume filter unit such as the AEC high volume sampler. Samples are usually collected for 24 hours. Use Whatman 8 × 10 inch filter paper for collection. Paper filters are decomposed by wet oxidation. Beryllium is then coprecipitated with aluminum. The fluorometric morin method is applied for quantitative measurement.

*Reagents*

1. 1:9 $HClO_4$–$HNO_3$
2. 1:3 $HClO_4$–$HNO_3$
3. 2% (v/v) $HClO_4$ in water
4. Aluminum solution, 4 mg/ml (55.5 gm $Al(NO_3)_3 \cdot 9H_2O$/liter)
5. Mercaptoacetic acid, 60 or 70%
6. 25% ammonium chloride solution
7. Wash water: 10 ml concentrated hydrochloric acid neutralized with ammonium hydroxide to a pH of 8.5
8. 0.1% quinine solution in water
9. Standard quinine: 50 ppm in 0.1 N sulfuric acid
10. Triethanolamine-EDTA (ethylenediaminetetraacetic acid): Dissolve 5 gm EDTA (reagent grade) plus 3 ml of *colorless* triethanolamine (TEA) in water. Dilute to 100 ml.
11. Sodium hydroxide, 2 N
12. Alkaline stannite: Dissolve 2.4 gm sodium hydroxide in approximately 20 ml of distilled water. Add 1.5 gm of stannous chloride to 5 ml of water. Add stannite solution to sodium hydroxide with stirring and dilute to 50 ml.
13. Piperidine buffer: Dissolve 10 gm of hydrazine sulfate and 5 gm of EDTA in 30 ml of water, add 50 ml piperidine (*redistilled* if practical grade), and dilute to 500 ml.
14. Morin: Use analytical grade only, or purify technical grade. Weigh 7.8 mg, add to 100 ml of ethyl alcohol, store in a brown bottle.
15. 8.2 N sodium hydroxide: Dissolve 165 gm sodium hydroxide in water, cool, filter through glass wool, and dilute to 500 ml.

*Procedure. Oxidation:* Cut one-eighth high volume paper in small pieces into a 100-ml beaker. Place on hot plate and when hot add 30 ml 1:9 $HClO_4$–$HNO_3$ mixture. When 3 ml remain in beaker, add a few drops of 1:3 $HClO_4$–$HNO_3$ (perchloric acid–nitric acid) if oxidation is not complete. When 2–3 ml remain, remove beaker and cool.

*Separation:* To the cooled solution, add 1 ml aluminum solution (4 mg/ml), 1 ml 25% ammonium chloride solution, and 0.75 ml mercaptoacetic acid. Transfer from the beaker with 2% perchloric acid into a *fine* sintered glass funnel which contains approximately 0.2 gm celite and 3–4 ml ammonium hydroxide (concentrated). Stir the contents with a glass rod and adjust the pH to 8.0 if not so already. Rinse the stirring rod with 2% perchloric acid and vacuum-filter the sample. Wash the resulting precipitate until a clear filtrate is obtained, using the following solution: 2 ml of mercaptoacetic acid adjusted to a pH of 8 with concentrated ammonium hydroxide and diluted to 100 ml.

Then wash the precipitate with water to remove the mercaptoacetic acid. Discard all filtrates. Place a 25-ml graduated test tube, or a volumetric flask, below the funnel. With the vacuum off, add 2.5 ml of concentrated perchloric acid to the funnel and stir with a stream of 2% perchloric acid. Turn the vacuum on and collect the filtrate. Wash the funnel further with 2% perchloric acid, being careful not to *exceed* 12 ml in the receiving flask.

*Fluorescence Development:* To all samples and blanks, add 1 drop of 0.1% quinine and, using an ultraviolet lamp, add concentrated perchloric acid until fluorescence occurs. Defluoresce with $2 N$ sodium hydroxide, then add 2–3 drops in excess to dissolve the aluminum and beryllium hydroxides. Add in order 0.5 ml TEA and EDTA, shake, 0.5 ml alkaline stannite, shake, and finally 5.0 ml piperidine buffer. Add 1.0 ml morin solution. Adjust volume to 25.0 ml with water, mix, and read in fluorimeter at once. (The stannite must be made fresh just before using.)

*Calibration:* A series of standards containing 0.05, 0.1, 0.2, and 0.3 $\mu$g of beryllium should be added to one-eighth clean filter paper and carried through the complete procedure.

## D. Sulfur Dioxide (W2)

*Reagents*
1. Sodium tetrachloromercurate, 0.1 $M$: Dissolve mercuric chloride (0.1 mole, 27.2 gm) and 0.2 mole (11.7 gm) of sodium chloride and dilute to 1 liter.
2. Hydrochloric acid–bleached pararosaniline, 0.04%: Mix 4 ml of a 1% aqueous solution of pararosaniline hydrochloride and 6 ml of concentrated hydrochloric acid and dilute to 100 ml.
3. Formaldehyde, 0.2%

*Procedure.* Collect a 30- to 40-liter sample in 10 ml of sodium tetrachloromercurate in a fritted glass bubbler. To the sample add 1 ml of acidic pararosaniline and 1.0 ml of the formaldehyde solution. Treat a 10-ml portion of unexposed sodium tetrachloromercurate in the same manner. Allow to stand 20 minutes for full color development. Read in a spectrophotometer at 560 m$\mu$. Read the micrograms of sulfur dioxide from a standard curve prepared by using dilutions of standard sodium bisulfite in sodium tetrachloromercurate.

*Standardization.* Weigh 400 mg sodium *meta*-bisulfite (assay 55.5% as $SO_2$) and dissolve in 1 liter of water (0.26 mg $SO_2$/ml).

Standardize against $0.01 N \ I_2$. Dilute the standard $SO_2$ solution to obtain a solution containing 26.0 $\mu$g of $SO_2$ per ml. Add graduated amounts of the dilute standard up to 1 ml to a series of 10-ml flasks and dilute to the mark with the sodium tetrachloromercurate solution.

Add 1 ml pararosaniline dye and 1 ml formaldehyde solution and allow time for full color development. Plot the per cent transmittance on semilog paper vs the microgram of $SO_2$.

*Calculations.* (2.6 $\mu$g $SO_2$ per liter of air = 1 ppm $SO_2$). To calculate ppm of $SO_2$ in the sample:

$$\frac{\text{total micrograms of } SO_2 \text{ in sample}}{2.6 \times \text{volume of air sample (in liters)}} = \text{ppm } SO_2$$

*Note:* The procedure is based upon the use of exactly 10 ml of sampling medium in the bubbler.

## E. Lead (S2)

Samples are collected on high volume samplers of the AEC type. Collection is made on $8 \times 10$ inch Whatman filter paper over periods of 24 hours. The filter paper is cut into small pieces and ashed in a porcelain crucible at 600°C. The cooled ash is dissolved in 5 ml of hot 1:10 HCl, filtered, and diluted to 100 ml. (A blank filter paper should be carried through the entire procedure. Because of the relatively small quantities of lead collected in the normal atmosphere, it is necessary to use extreme caution to prevent contamination. If the reagent blank for lead is too high, it will be necessary to delead the reagents.)

*Reagents*
1. Phenol red indicator: Dissolve 1 gm of phenol red (phenol-sufonphthalein) in 20 cc of ethyl alcohol. Dilute this solution up to 250 ml with distilled water.
2. Ammonium hydroxide: $NH_4OH$, 28%
3. 40% ammonium citrate solution: To 400 gm of C.P. citric acid in a 2-liter beaker, add approximately 20 ml of distilled water and 5–10 drops of phenol red indicator. Neutralize the solution with ammonium hydroxide to a pH of 8.5 (the neutralization requires between 500 and 1000 ml of ammonium hydroxide). Add the hydroxide in 20- to 50-ml portions. Cool and extract with dithizone solution (I) until the chloroform layer remains green. Remove all dithizone by extracting the aqueous layer with 50-ml portions of chloroform until the chloroform layer is colorless. Dilute the aqueous ammonium citrate solution to 1 liter with distilled water.

4. 10% potassium cyanide solution: Dissolve 100 gm of C.P. potassium cyanide in approximately 75 ml of distilled water. Extract the aqueous solution with dithizone solution (I) until the chloroform layer remains green. Discard $CHCl_3$ layer. Wash aqueous layer with $CHCl_3$ until colorless. Dilute the potassium cyanide solution to 1 liter with distilled water.
5. *m*-Cresol purple indicator (used for the hydroxylamine hydrochloride purification): Dissolve 1 gm of *m*-cresol purple (*m*-cresol sulfonphthalein) in 20 ml of ethyl alcohol and make up to 200 ml with distilled water.
6. 4% sodium diethyldithiocarbamate (used for the hydroxylamine hydrochloride purification): Dissolve 4 gm of sodium diethyldithiocarbamate in 100 ml of distilled water.
7. 20% hydroxylamine hydrochloride solution: Dissolve 20 gm of hydroxylamine hydrochloride in about 65 ml of distilled water. Add 5 drops of *m*-cresol purple indicator and ammonium hydroxide until a yellow color appears. Add 1 ml of the sodium diethyldithiocarbamate solution. Extract the orange complex with 10-ml portions of chloroform until the chloroform extracts are colorless. Save the last chloroform extract and check for excess diethyldithiocarbamate by shaking with a small amount of copper salt solution. If the chloroform layer shows no color, all the excess diethyldithiocarbamate has been removed. When all the excess carbamate has been extracted, add concentrated hydrochloric acid to the aqueous solution of hydroxylamine hydrochloride until the indicator turns pink and dilute to 100 ml with water.
8. 0.5% hydroxylamine hydrochloride solution: Neutralize 2.5 ml of 20% hydroxylamine hydrochloride solution with ammonium hydroxide to a pH of 7.5, using 2 drops of phenol red indicator (indicator pink). Dilute the solution to 100 ml with distilled water.
9. Treated chloroform: In most cases, commercial C.P. or reagent grade chloroform ($CHCl_3$) may be used without treatment for dithizone determinations. It is preferable to use chloroform packaged in 5-lb glass bottles rather than the large drums. Test each new bottle of chloroform by diluting 10 ml of dithizone solution (II) with 10 ml of the new chloroform. Let the solution stand for 1 hour. If there is no change in color, the chloroform may be used without treatment. If the dithizone solution shows a color change, treat the chloroform as follows: Shake 1 liter of chloroform with 100 ml of 0.5% hydroxylamine hydrochloride

solution in a separatory funnel. Discard the aqueous phase and filter the chloroform through a thick cotton layer to remove excess water. Store the chloroform in a cool, dark place.

10. Ammonium-cyanide solution (lead buffer solution): Dilute 80 ml of concentrated ammonia and 40 ml of purified 10% potassium cyanide solution to 2 liters with distilled water.

11. 0.1% nitric acid: Add 1 ml of concentrated nitric acid (assay 69.6%) to 695 ml of distilled water. (If high blanks are obtained, check the redistilled water used and the nitric acid by extracting with dithizone. If the nitric acid is contaminated, distill the acid. The acid should be distilled in an all-glass apparatus using a Glascol heating mantle for constant temperature. Discard the first and last third of the distillate using only the middle third for dithizone determinations.)

12. Dithizone solutions: These solutions are stable for an indefinite period if stored in a dark, cool place. Check dithizone solutions (II) and (III) daily by comparing their spectral transmission against chloroform. The per cent transmission should be constant from day to day. If it drops by more than 3%, solution should be discarded.

    *a.* Stock dithizone solution: Place 125 mg of dithizone (diphenyl-thiocarbazone, $C_6H_5N:N\cdot CS\cdot NH\cdot NH\cdot C_6H_5$—Eastman Organic Chemicals) in a 250-ml volumetric flask and dilute to 250 ml with treated chloroform (1 ml = 0.5 mg of dithizone).

    *b.* Dithizone solution (I): Dilute 40 ml of stock dithizone solution to 1000 ml with treated chloroform. The solution contains 20 mg of dithizone per liter.

    *c.* Dithizone solution (II): Dilute 8 ml of stock solution to 1000 ml with treated chloroform. The solution contains 4 mg of dithizone per liter.

    *d.* Dithizone solution (III): Dilute 16 ml of stock solution to 1000 ml with treated chloroform. The solution contains 8 mg of dithizone per liter.

13. Stock lead standard: Place 1.5985 gm of recrystallized lead nitrate in a 1-liter volumetric flask and dissolve in a few milliliters of 0.1% nitric acid. Make up to volume with 0.1% nitric acid. This solution is quite stable. It should be discarded if any cloud or sediment forms. The solution contains 1 mg of lead per ml.

14. Intermediate lead standard: Dilute 100 ml of stock lead standard to 1 liter with 0.1% nitric acid. The solution contains a 100 $\mu$g of lead per ml.

15. High working lead standard: Dilute 50 ml of intermediate

working standard to 500 ml with 0.1% nitric acid. This solution contains 10 $\mu$g of lead per ml. This standard should be made up as needed.

16. Working lead standard: Dilute 50 ml of the high working lead standard to 500 ml with 0.1% nitric acid. The solution contains 1 $\mu$g of lead per ml. This standard should be made up as needed.

*Procedure*

1. To an aliquot of the sample and reagent blank in separatory funnels, add 10 ml of ammonium citrate solution, 2 drops of phenol red, 1 ml of 20% hydroxylamine hydrochloride solution, 5 ml of 10% potassium cyanide solution. Mix and adjust the pH of the solution to 9.0 (indicator red) by titrating with ammonium hydroxide.

2. Let the solution cool and add 5 ml of dithizone solution (I). Shake the funnel for 30 seconds. Allow the chloroform layer to separate and drain into a second 125-ml separatory funnel. Continue adding 5-ml portions of dithizone solution (I) and extracting until the green color of the dithizone solution is unchanged. Combine all the chloroform extracts in the second separatory funnel.

3. To the combined chloroform extracts add 50 ml of distilled water and shake for 1 minute. Drain the chloroform layer into a third separatory funnel.

4. To the chloroform extract add 50 ml of 0.1% nitric acid and shake for 1 minute.

5. Drain and discard the dithizone layer.

6. Add 2–3 ml of chloroform to the aqueous acid phase and shake for 1 minute. Discard the chloroform extracts. Repeat these chloroform extractions until the aqueous phase is free from dithizone (chloroform colorless). Discard these washings. Shake down the globules of chloroform and allow to separate for a few minutes. Draw off the chloroform layer as completely as possible.

7. To the aqueous phase, add 0.1 N hydrochloric acid to give a total volume of 50 ml.

8. To each solution add 10 ml of ammonia-cyanide solution, 1 ml of 40% ammonium citrate solution, and 1 ml of 20% hydroxylamine hydrochloride solution and mix. To each solution, add 10 ml of dithizone solution (III).

9. Shake the funnels for 1 minute. Let stand for 2 minutes to insure complete separation of the two phases. [If the color of the dithizone layer is red, add 10 more milliliters of dithizone (III) solution.] Filter through a cotton plug into cuvette.

10. Read in the spectrophotometer within 10 minutes at 510 m$\mu$ against $CHCl_3$.

*Standardization.* Treat a series of Pb standards as described above and prepare standard curve. Standards should contain 0–15 $\mu$g of lead.

*Calculation.* Read concentration of samples from curve. Subtract value of reagent and filter paper blank. If an additional 10 ml of dithizone was added in step 9, multiply results by 2. Finally, multiply by total volume of original digest/volume of aliquot taken for analysis.

# III. Analysis of Pollutants Which May Not Be Present in the Atmosphere in Sufficient Concentration to Cause Toxicity but Which May Create Nuisance Problems Due to Odor

## A. Hydrogen Sulfide (J2)

The method is based on the absorption of sulfides by a solution of $Cd(OH)_2$ and the subsequent formation of methylene blue by the addition of N,N-dimethyl-p-phenylenediamine.

*Reagents*
1. Absorption mixture: Dissolve 2.7 gm of anhydrous cadmium sulfate in approximately 100 ml of water. Dissolve 0.3 gm of sodium hydroxide in approximately 25 ml of water and add to the cadmium solution and dilute to 1 liter.
2. Stock amine solution: Add 50 ml of concentrated sulfuric acid to 30 ml of water and cool. Add 12 gm of N,N-dimethyl-p-phenylenediamine. Stir until solution is complete.
3. Test amine solution: Dilute 25 ml of the stock to 1 liter with 1:1 sulfuric acid.
4. Ferric chloride solution: Dissolve 100 gm of $FeCl_3 \cdot 8H_2O$ in enough water to make 100 ml of solution.

*Procedure.* Shake the absorption solution well and place 10 ml in a bubbler. Sample at 2.8 liters/minute for 15 minutes. After sampling is complete add an additional 10 ml of absorption solution to the bubbler. Mix. Add 0.6 ml of amine test solution and stir well to dissolve all the $Cd(OH)_2$. Then add 1 drop of $FeCl_3$ solution and stir well. Bring to a total volume of 25 ml with distilled water and allow to stand for 30 minutes. A blank containing all the reagents should be run along with the samples. Read at 670 m$\mu$ against blank.

*Preparation of Standard Curve.* Dissolve 0.71 gm of $Na_2S \cdot 9H_2O$ in 1 liter of water. Standardize with iodine and thiosulfate. Make proper dilution to obtain a solution containing 1 $\mu$g $H_2S$/ml.

Add 0, 1, 2, 3, and 4 $\mu$g of $H_2S$ respectively to 20-ml portions of absorption solution in 25-ml graduated test tubes. Add 0.6 ml amine solution; stir well. Add 1 drop of $FeCl_3$ solution and stir well. Dilute to 25 ml with distilled water and allow to stand for 30 minutes for color development. Set instrument at 670 m$\mu$ and adjust to 100% transmission with the 0 $\mu$g H$_2$S sample. Take respective readings and make a plot of transmission versus concentration to obtain the standard curve:

$$\frac{\mu\text{g H}_2\text{S from curve} \times 10^3}{\text{total air volume (in liters)} \times 1.4} = \text{ppb (parts per billion) H}_2\text{S}$$

## B. Mercaptans (M1) (Modified)

*Reagents*

1. Absorption solution: 5% mercuric acetate in water
2. Amine solution: Dissolve 0.50 gm of *N,N*-dimethyl-*p*-phenylene-diamine in 100 ml of concentrated hydrochloric acid. This solution should be clear; if tinted check its absorbance at 500 m$\mu$; a value of 0.04 or less is acceptable. The technical grade reagent is of insufficient purity. Eastman No. 492 was found to be satisfactory. If protected from light the solution is stable for weeks.
3. Reissner solution: Dissolve 6.8 gm of ferric chloride hexahydrate in distilled water, dilute to 50 ml, and mix with 50 ml of a nitric acid solution containing 7.2 ml of concentrated nitric acid. This solution is stable indefinitely.

*Procedure.* To each of two impingers in series add 6.0 ml of the absorption solution. Draw air through at a rate of 2.8 liters/minute for 45–60 minutes depending on the concentration of mercaptans.

To each impinger add 1.5 ml of amine solution and 2 drops of Reissner solution. Shake well and let stand for 30 minutes. A blank containing reagents alone is also run. Read in a spectrophotometer at 500 m$\mu$ (which is set at 100% transmission with blank). Convert reading to micrograms methyl mercaptan from a standard curve.

*Standardization.* Crystalline lead methyl mercaptide is used as the standard for methyl mercaptan. Transfer 0.100 gm to a 500-ml volumetric flask, add about 300 ml of distilled water, followed by 0.5 ml of 3 $N$ HCl, and dilute to mark with water. This solution will be equivalent to 60 $\mu$g methyl mercaptan/ml.

To a series of graduated tubes add 5 ml of mercuric acetate, then 10-, 20-, 30-, and 50-$\mu$g aliquots of standard mercaptan. Bring each tube to 6.00 ml with mercuric acetate and allow the color to develop. A plot of transmission vs micrograms of methyl mercaptan on semilog paper yields the standard curve used in analysis.[1]

---

[1] The lead mercaptide salt is made according to the procedure of Sliwinski and Doty [*J. Agr. Food Chem.* **6**, 41 (1958).]

## IV. Analysis of Pollutants Involved in the Photochemical Process

Pollutants involved in the photochemical process may occur in the ambient atmosphere, leading to the formation of reaction products which are eye-irritating, vegetation-damaging, and visibility-reducing. Ozone or "total oxidant" is a by-product of the reaction.

### A. Nitrogen Dioxide (S3)

*Reagent*

Absorbing reagent: Dissolve 2.5 gm of sulfanilic acid in about 500 ml $H_2O$. Add 70 ml glacial acetic acid and 10 mg N-(1-naphthyl)-ethylenediamine dihydrochloride. Dissolve and dilute to 1 liter. Reagent is stable for several months if left refrigerated in the dark.

*Procedure.* Place 10 ml of absorbing reagent in a bubbler equipped with a fine porosity fritted tube. Draw air sample through at a rate of 0.4 liters/minute for 20 minutes. Read the color against a blank at 550 m$\mu$.

*Preparation of Standard Curve.* Weigh, dissolve, and bring to 1 liter 0.203 gm of sodium nitrite, C.P. Dilute 10 ml of this solution to 1 liter. One milliliter of this diluted standard contains the equivalent of 0.4 $\mu$l or 1.36 $\mu$g of nitrogen dioxide.

Set up a series of six 25-ml graduated test tubes, add respectively 0, 1, 2, 3, 4, and 5 ml of the diluted standard, bring each to volume with absorbing reagent, stopper, shake well, and let stand for 15 minutes for color development. Take respective readings at 550 m$\mu$ against a blank.

Using semilog paper plot the transmission versus micrograms nitrogen dioxide.

*Calculation*

$$\text{ppm } NO_2 = \frac{\text{micrograms from chart}}{1.36 \times \text{volume of air in liters}}$$

### B. Nitric Oxide

Nitric oxide is determined by difference between total nitrogen oxides and nitrogen dioxide. Total nitrogen oxides are determined by bubbling the air sample first through a 5% solution of $KMnO_4$ in 5% $H_2SO_4$ and then into the absorbing reagent described for nitrogen dioxide determination. In practice it is convenient to set up a train as follows: fritted bubbler containing absorbing reagent; fritted bubbler containing $KMnO_4$ solution; fritted bubbler containing absorbing reagent. The air sample is drawn through the train at 0.4 liters/minute for 20 minutes. The first bubbler measures the $NO_2$ and the third bubbler measures NO (after being oxidized to $NO_2$ by the $KMnO_4$). Calibration and standardization are as described under nitrogen dioxide.

## C. Ozone or "Oxidants"

Ozone is formed during the photochemical reaction which occurs in the atmosphere between nitrogen oxides and olefinic hydrocarbons. In addition, subsequent reactions between ozone and olefinic hydrocarbons result in the production of organic peroxy compounds which are also oxidizing in nature. Most of the chemical methods for the determination of ozone measure to a greater or lesser degree the oxidizing capacity of the atmosphere. The term "total oxidant" is often substituted for the term ozone in such chemical determinations.

Two methods will be described. The first or "neutral buffered potassium iodide method for total oxidant" is less responsive to organic peroxides and $NO_2$ than is the second or "phenolphthalin" method. Hence, when analyzing a mixture of polluted atmosphere, the KI method will give values which are generally lower than values obtained with the phenolphthalin method. There has not as yet been established a correlation factor between the two methods, although a first approximation indicates that the phenolphthalin method gives results which are twice those obtained by the KI method. It should be pointed out that in the presence of relatively large amounts of $SO_2$ (0.1–0.3 ppm) the net ozone or oxidant level in the atmosphere may be inordinately low (a few ppb).

1. NEUTRAL BUFFERED POTASSIUM IODIDE METHOD FOR
   TOTAL OXIDANT IN AIR (C1)

*Principle.* The method is based upon the oxidation of potassium iodide with the attendant release of free iodine in neutral buffered potassium iodide solution. The resulting characteristic color of triiodide ion is measured in a spectrophotometer at 352 m$\mu$. The intensity of the yellow color is directly proportional to the concentration of oxidant in the atmosphere sampled.

A calibration curve of absorbancy vs concentration of ozone is plotted using a standard solution of iodine.

*Preparation of Reagents*

    1. 2% neutral buffered KI: Dissolve the following in water sufficient to make 1 liter of solution:

        20 gm KI
        36 gm $Na_2HPO_4 \cdot 12H_2O$
        14 gm $KH_2PO_4$

    2. 0.1 N iodine solution: Dissolve 12.7 gm iodine in 1 liter of 2%

potassium iodide. Standardize versus 0.1000 $N$ sodium thiosulfate. The above standardized solution of 0.1 $N$ $I_2$ is diluted 1:10 to produce a solution containing 0.01 eq/liter. This solution is in turn diluted 1:100 to yield a solution containing 0.0001 eq/liter or 100 $\mu N$ $I_2$. This latter solution becomes the working solution from which the calibration curve is constructed.

*Relation of I to $O_3$*

I is equivalent to $\frac{1}{2}$ $O_3$ at 25°C: (24.5 liters/2) = 12.25 liters.

1 $\mu$eq of $O_3$ at 25°C = 0.01225 ml or 1.225 × $10^{-2}$ ml.

1 ml of 1 $\mu N$ $I_2$ contains (1/1000) $\mu$eq $I_2$ = 1 × $10^{-3}$ $\mu$eq $I_2$.

1 ml of 1 $\mu N$ $I_2$ is equivalent to 1 × $10^{-3}$ (1.225 × $10^{-2}$) = 1.225 × $10^{-5}$ ml of $O_3$.

Therefore: 1 ml of 1 $\mu N$ $I_2$ represents 1.225 × $10^{-5}$ ml of $O_3$ per liter of air.

Since 10 liters of air will be sampled, 1.225 × $10^{-4}$ ml of $O_3$ would be collected if the atmosphere were originally at 1.225 pphm (parts per hundred million) of $O_3$. Therefore, a solution of 1 $\mu N$ $I_2$ represents an ozone concentration of 1.225 pphm (parts per hundred million).

The solutions for determination of the calibration curve are freshly prepared immediately before use as the action of light produces free $I_2$.

*Calibration.* Returning to the 100 $\mu N$ $I_2$ solution, serial dilutions are prepared with 2% buffered KI as follows:

Dilute 10 ml 100 $\mu N$ $I_2$ to 100 ml yielding the equivalent of 12.25 pphm.

Dilute 20 ml 100 $\mu N$ $I_2$ to 100 ml yielding the equivalent of 24.50 pphm.

One hundred milliliters of 100 $\mu N$ $I_2$ yields the equivalent of 1.225 ppm.

Measure the absorbance in a spectrophotometer at 352 m$\mu$.

Plot absorbance against ppm of $O_3$.

*Sampling Procedure.* Place 10 ml of neutral buffered KI in a midget impinger. Draw air through the bubbler at a rate of 1 liter/minute for 10 minutes. Read absorbance at once at 352 m$\mu$ with the absorption solution used as a blank. The absorbance is converted to ppm ozone or oxidant by reference to the calibration curve previously prepared.

2. PHENOLPHTHALIN METHOD (C1)

*Principle.* The method is based upon the oxidation of phenolphthalin by oxidants present in the air to phenolphthalein.

*Reagents*

1. Concentrated phenolphthalin: Reflux 1 gm of phenolphthalein, 10 gm of NaOH, 5 gm of zinc dust, and 20 ml of distilled water

on a steam bath for 2 hours until colorless, then filter through a sintered glass filter and dilute with 50 ml of distilled water. Keep the concentrated solution over granulated zinc in a closed bottle in a refrigerator.

2. Stock phenolphthalin: Dilute 10 ml of concentrated phenolphthalin solution with 30 ml distilled water, and keep refrigerated.

3. Stock $CuSO_4$ (0.01 $M$): Weigh out 0.16 gm $CuSO_4$ and dilute to 100 ml.

4. Test phenolphthalin: Dilute 1 ml of the stock solution with about 50 ml of water. Add 1 ml of 0.01 $M$ copper sulfate and dilu$^t$e the final volume to 100 ml; mix well. The test phenolphthalin solution should be kept refrigerated and prepared fresh each week. When used in the field keep immersed in ice until placed in bubbler.

*Procedure.* Place 10 ml of the test reagent (No. 4) in an all glass impinger and draw 10 liters of air at a rate of 1 liter/minute. After obtaining sample let stand at room temperature for 15 minutes. Transfer sample to cuvette and read transmittance at 530 m$\mu$ against the test reagent used as a blank.

(*a*) *Calibration.* Since the end product measured in the reaction is phenolphthalein, this substance may be used to calibrate the spectrophotometer.

*Reagents*

1. Sodium hydroxide solution: Dissolve 1.25 gm of sodium hydroxide in 1 liter of distilled water.

2. Phenolphthalein solution stock: Dissolve 0.1000 gm of phenolphthalein in 200 ml of isopropyl alcohol and bring to volume in a 1-liter volumetric flask with distilled water.

3. Phenolphthalein working solution: 10 $\mu$g/ml, made by diluting 25 ml of the stock to 250 ml with distilled water. Keep refrigerated.

*Procedure.* To a series of graduated 25-ml tubes add, respectively, 1, 2, 3, 4, 5, and 6 ml of the phenolphthalein working solution. Bring each to a volume of 15 ml with the sodium hydroxide solution. Transmittance readings should be taken within 5 minutes at 530 m$\mu$ using distilled water as a blank. The 1- through 6-ml standards are equivalent to 0.1 through 0.6 ppm(v/v)$H_2O_2$, when 10 ml of phenolphthalein solution are used at the conventional 1 liter/minute rate for 10 minutes as described in the sampling procedure. A plot is made using semilog paper of transmittance vs concentration.

(*b*) *Alternate Calibration.* This procedure uses $H_2O_2$ to oxidize the phenolphthalein.

*Reagents*

1. Dilute $H_2O_2$: Dilute 3–4 ml 30% $H_2O_2$ to 1000 ml (approxi-

mately 0.1% $H_2O_2$). Standardize with KI and $0.1000 N$ $Na_2S_2O_4$.
2. Working $H_2O_2$: Dilute the standardized $H_2O_2$ so that 1 ml will contain 1 $\mu$g of $H_2O_2$.

*Calibration.* Place suitable aliquots of the 1 $\mu$g/ml $H_2O_2$ in a series of test tubes, add 0.1 ml of 0.01 $M$ $CuSO_4$, followed by 2–3 ml $H_2O$ and 0.1 ml of the stock phenolphthalein solution. Bring the volume to 10 ml with distilled water. The curve should contain at least five points in the range of 0–1 $\mu$g $H_2O_2$.

Fifteen minutes should be allowed for color development before reading the per cent transmittance at 530 m$\mu$ using a blank of distilled water. Plot and per cent transmission vs micrograms $H_2O_2$ to obtain standard curve.

*Calculation*

$$\text{total oxidant in ppm}(v/v)H_2O_2 = \text{micrograms } H_2O_2/14$$

# V. Continuous Automatic Measurement of Air Contaminants (S4)

Brief mention should be made of the development of continuous automatic recording instruments for the measurement of certain air contaminants. Pioneer work in this field was done by such organizations as the Los Angeles Air Pollution Control District, Stanford Research Institute, and others. Because of the variation in concentration of air pollutants with distance from sources, meteorological factors, and reaction in the atmosphere, a more comprehensive picture of the exposure concentrations is afforded by continuous monitoring. Mention here will be made only of those instruments which are sensitive enough to measure the contaminants in concentrations in which they occur in the atmosphere, and which are commercially available.

## A. Carbon Monoxide (W3)

The main type of instrument for the continuous analysis of carbon monoxide is based on nondispersive infrared spectrometry. The air sample is introduced into the path of an infrared beam in a sample cell. Carbon monoxide present in the air sample attenuates the beam in proportion to its concentration. Commercial instruments utilizing this principle are available. This method is most satisfactory for continuous monitoring because it measures a physical property of the substance and is nondestructive.

## B. Hydrocarbons

Nondispersive infrared instruments for the measurement of hydrocarbons are also available (L1). One of the difficulties involved in the measurement of hydrocarbons concerns the type of hydrocarbon it is desired to measure. The nondispersive infrared instrument is usually sensitized with hexane, so that it responds to saturated hydrocarbons more strongly than to unsaturated or oxygenated hydrocarbons. Hexane absorbs strongly at $3.4\,\mu$ whereas olefins, aromatics, and oxygenated compounds do not absorb as strongly on a mole for mole basis.

A compromise solution using mixtures of saturated, unsaturated, and aromatic compounds as the sensitizing gas has been used, but again reveals only a partial indication of the nature of the hydrocarbons being analyzed.

Recent introduction of Flame Ionization Detectors (B1) has extended the sensitivity of hydrocarbon detection, but this system is not without its drawbacks. Since all compounds containing a C—H group respond, and since ethane gives twice the response and propane three times the response of methane, the net measurement gives no indication of the nature of the hydrocarbons present in the sample.

If one is concerned with the measurement of olefinic compounds, which are the most reactive in the photochemical process, total hydrocarbons by flame ionization offer no clue as to the relative concentration of olefinic compounds present.

An instrument which measures olefinic hydrocarbons by reaction with bromine has recently been introduced (M2). However, insufficient experience with this instrument has been accumulated to determine whether or not it measures only olefins and whether or not certain olefins are more reactive than others.

The ideal presentation of hydrocarbon monitoring data might utilize gas chromatographic separation and flame ionization detection of the separated components. Such systems are presently available for batch-type analysis, but have not as yet been incorporated into a continuous monitoring system.

## C. Sulfur Dioxide

Two general types of automatic recording instruments for $SO_2$ are available. One measures the conductivity generated by the absorption and oxidation of $SO_2$ in a weakly acidic $H_2O_2$ solution (T1). A variation of this type measures the conductivity of $SO_2$ dissolved in ion-free water. It should be pointed out that these instruments measure the total conductivity of the absorbing solution and that any ion-forming substance will add to the apparent $SO_2$ concentration.

A second type of $SO_2$ analyzer is based on automatic bromometric titration (S5). Oxidizable compounds containing sulfur are titrated with a solution in which bromine is generated electrolytically. The rate of bromine generation is maintained equal to the rate of bromine utilization so that the generating current is a function of bromine used up in the reaction. In addition to $SO_2$, other oxidizable sulfur compounds will respond including $H_2S$ and mercaptans. High concentrations of olefins also react with bromine. A filter has recently been developed containing $HgCl_2$ adsorbed on filter paper which removes $H_2S$ from the air stream without affecting the $SO_2$ concentration (F2). This makes the instrument a little more specific for $SO_2$.

## D. Nitrogen Oxides (T2)

Nitrogen dioxide is measured colorimetrically by reaction with Saltzman reagent. Air is mixed in a contactor column with reagent and the resulting color is measured in a photometer incorporated into the instrument. The difference in signal between the absorption caused by colored and blank reagent, is recorded. For total nitrogen oxides the incoming air stream is split, and one portion is used to measure $NO_2$. The other portion is exposed to ozone which converts NO to $NO_2$ and total oxides are then measured as described for $NO_2$. Nitric oxide is determined as the difference between the two signals.

## E. Ozone or Oxidants (L2)

Total oxidant is measured colorimetrically by liberation of iodine from a neutral buffered KI solution. Air containing ozone or oxidizing compounds is contacted by the reagent in a contacting column and the transmittance of the yellow triiodide solution is measured photoelectrically. The signal is continuously recorded.

A recent development utilizes the coulometric measurement of current generated in the oxidation of iodide to iodine by ozone (M1). This instrument is said to be more specific for ozone and has the advantage of being truly portable.

## REFERENCES

(A1)  Adams, D. F. *J. Air Pollution Control Assoc.* **7**, 88 (1957).
(B1)  Beckman Instrument Company, Fullerton, California, 1961.
(C1)  Recommended Methods in Air Pollution Measurements, Air and Industrial Hygiene Laboratory. California State Dept. of Public Health, Berkeley, California, 1961.
(F1)  Feldstein, M., Coons, J., Johnson, H., and Yocom, J. E. *Am. Ind. Hyg. Assoc. J.* **20**, 374 (1959).
(F2)  Feldstein, M., and Levaggi, D. A. L. Paper Presented at American Chemical Society 140th Annual Meeting, Chicago, Illinois, September, 1961.
(J1)  Jacobs, M. B. "The Chemical Analysis of Air Pollutants." Wiley (Interscience), New York, 1960.
(J2)  Jacobs, M. B., Braverman, M. M., and Hochheiser, S. *Anal. Chem.* **29**, 1349 (1957).

(L1)  Littman, F. E., and Denton, J. Q. *Anal. Chem.* **28**, 945 (1956).
(L2)  Littman, F. E., and Benoliel, R. W. *Anal. Chem.* **25**, 1480 (1953).
(M1)  Moore, H., Helwig, H. L., and Grave, R. J. *Am. Ind. Hyg. Assoc. J.* **21**, 466 (1960).
(M2)  Mast Development Co., Davenport, Iowa, 1962.
(R1)  Renzetti, N. A. *Air Pollution Found.* (*Los Angeles*) *Rept.* **16** (1956).
(S1)  Sill, C. W., and Willis, C. P. *Anal. Chem.* **31**, 598 (1959).
(S2)  Sandell, E. B. "Colorimetric Determination of Traces of Metals," Chapter 23. Wiley (Interscience), New York, 1959.
(S3)  Saltzman, B. E. *Anal. Chem.* **26**, 1949 (1954).
(S4)  Stern, A. C., ed. "Air Pollution," Vol. I, Chapter 17. Academic Press, New York, 1962.
(S5)  Shaffer, P. A., Jr., Briglio, A., and Brockman, J. A. *Anal. Chem.* **20**, 1008 (1948).
(T1)  Thomas, M. D., and Cross, R. J. *Ind. Eng. Chem.* **20**, 645 (1928).
(T2)  Thomas, M. D., MacLeod, J. A., Robbins, J. A., Gettlemen, R. C., Eldridge, R. W., and Rogers, L. H. *Anal. Chem.* **28**, 1810 (1956).
(W1)  Willard, H. H., and Winter, O. B. *Ind. Eng. Chem. Anal. Ed.* **5**, 7 (1933).
(W2)  West, P. W., and Gaeke, G. C. *Anal. Chem.* **28**, 1816 (1956).
(W3)  Waters, J. L., and Hartz, N. W. Conference of Instrument Society of America, Houston, Texas, 1951.

# Poisonous Mushrooms

by Varro E. Tyler, Jr.

*College of Pharmacy, University of Washington, Seattle, Washington*

## I. Introduction

The study of poisonous mushrooms is not yet an exact science, nor will it be for some time. Comprised of nearly equal parts of three sciences, it suffers the limitations imposed by the empirical nature of toxicology, the subjective nature of systematic mycology, and the scanty application of chemical analysis to these plant tissues. Consequently, much of the pertinent literature is characterized by misstatements, speculations, and omissions. This is particularly true of the English language coverage of the subject, which, due to lack of interest in the field, has consisted for nearly 40 years of little more than clinical observations of poisoning victims and plagiarized generalities. With certain notable exceptions, practically every aspect of the existing literature on poisonous mushrooms must be re-evaluated critically in order to determine its validity.

For many years it has been the custom to introduce contributions on this subject with a listing of famous personages who lost their lives by the accidental ingestion of poisonous mushrooms. V. P. and R. G. Wasson (W4) recently examined these alleged cases and concluded that mycologists are prone to exaggerate the importance of mushroom poisoning in history. Attribution of the death of Euripides' wife and children to this cause is apparently based on a misreading of Athenaeus. Historical records do not support the contention that Pope Clement VII and Tsar Alexis of Russia, or his widow, were victims. Emperor Claudius probably died from poisoned, not poisonous, mushrooms, but the Wassons present a convincing argument that the poison employed was actually *Amanita phalloides*. The German Emperor Charles VI may actually have succumbed to accidental mushroom poisoning, since he ate mushrooms at a meal 10 days prior to his death, and the clinical details are compatible with *Amanita phalloides* poisoning.

In spite of the lack of definite proof, these alleged cases do indicate that mushroom poisoning has been a continuing problem down through the ages. It is a more acute problem in certain European countries, such as France, where wild mushrooms are avidly sought for culinary purposes, but its very infrequence in the United States and other mycophobic nations actually increases its danger through lack of adequate knowledge.

## A. Occurrence of Mushroom Poisoning

The first report of fatal mycetismus in the United States (J2) is recorded on a tombstone in the cemetery of Trinity Episcopal Church, Fishkill, Dutchess County, New York, which indicates that in October, 1838, William Gould, his wife, and son were "Poisoned by eating Fungi (toadstools)." Since that time there have been numerous reports of fatal and nonfatal poisonings in the pertinent American literature (A1, C1, C2, C5, C6, C9, C10, C14, D1, D2, D3, D6, F1, G4, H3, H8, J1, K2, M1, M5, P5, R3, T2, V1). A number of more or less comprehensive reviews of mushroom poisoning have also appeared (B9, C16, F3, F4, F7, F9, F12). In 1918, Fischer (F2) estimated that less than 10% of the cases in this country find their way into the medical literature, and the figure is probably only slightly different at the present time.

Cann and Verhulst (C2) indicate that accidental ingestion of unidentified or misidentified mushrooms accounts for less than 2% of cases reported from local control centers to the National Clearinghouse for Poison Control Centers in Washington, D. C. During the period 1958–1959, 29,980 accidental ingestions of poisonous substances were reported to this agency. Of these, 256 (0.9%) were due to mushrooms. Children under 5 years of age accounted for 25,308 of the total cases and 185 (72%) of the mushroom ingestions. The National Office of Vital Statistics recorded eight deaths from mushroom poisoning in the United States during 1957, four deaths in 1958, and two in 1959 (V2). Even this relatively low frequency is sufficient to alert physicians to the dangers of mycetismus.

Fatal poisoning by mushrooms is also comparatively infrequent in Great Britain. Thirty-eight fatalities in England and Wales were officially recorded between 1920 and 1945 (B2). The London daily press recorded twenty-one cases of poisoning, including fourteen fatalities, in the 15-year period ending in 1945 (D7).

Of all the continental European countries, the most complete records of mushroom poisoning are available from Switzerland where, since 1919, data concerning every recognizable case have been collected and analyzed statistically. During the 40-year period ending in 1958, 1980 cases were recorded, of which 96 (4.85%) were fatal (A3, A4). The occurrence of this number of cases in a small country, in spite of an official organization, *Vereinigung der amtlichen Pilzkontrollorgane der Schweiz* (VAPKO), which disseminates information on toxic and edible mushrooms and maintains qualified personnel who advise amateurs on the edibility of their collections, is indicative of the magnitude of the poisonous mushroom problem in other mycophilic countries such as France, Italy, and Germany.

## B. Problems in Identifying Poisonous Mushrooms and Mushroom Poisons

All rules of thumb for determining the edibility of mushrooms—the inability to tarnish a silver spoon during cooking, the peelability of the surface layer of the pileus, and/or the failure to turn color when broken —are inaccurate. Outside of eating them, which is a certain test but may be a dangerous one, the only sure method of detection of poisonous mushrooms is by their botanical characteristics.

This is not a simple matter. Although Elias Fries (1794–1878), the founder of mushroom taxonomy, shunned the use of a microscope and developed a classification scheme based solely on macroscopic characteristics, more recent studies have relied heavily upon microscopic features. Hennig (M4) estimates that of the approximately 3000 species of mushrooms found in central Europe only 800 can be differentiated without a microscope. Exact species identification is, therefore, difficult, requiring a careful examination of such gross characteristics as the general color and form of the carpophore with special attention to the surface of the pileus, the presence of gills and their nature, and the presence of velar structures. In addition, microscopic examination of the spores to determine their color, size, and shape, as well as a detailed study of the anatomy of the gills (or other type of hymenophore), the nature of the basidia, and the presence and type of cystidia, are characteristics which must be accurately determined. Once these features have been established, the findings must be compared with descriptions in the mycological literature; this is no easy task, since reasonably complete collections are not numerous, and many key works have long been out of print.

For example, the standard color reference frequently referred to in American mycological writings is Ridgway's *Color Standards and Color Nomenclature,* published in 1912 (R2). Without this volume, now classified as a rare book, one can only guess at the exact meaning of color terminology derived from it. One of the most comprehensive works containing accurate descriptions and illustrations of the poisonous mushrooms, together with an extensive bibliography, is *Les Champignons Toxiques* by Dujarric de la Rivière and Heim (D8). Published in 1938, it is practically unobtainable and is avidly sought by mycological bibliophiles. Other general treatments are outdated (F7, P4, S1).

The use of chemical tests to identify mushroom poisons holds some promise but is at present in its infancy. With few exceptions, literature devoted to the chemical detection of specific poisonous principles in mushrooms is practically nonexistent, a fact not surprising in view of the general lack of chemical attention devoted to this area. The most recent comprehensive survey of the chemical constituents of the higher fungi is Zellner's *Chemie der höheren Pilze,* published in Leipzig in 1907 (Z2) Reviews since that time have been restricted to a limited number of types of compounds, but some are pertinent (L3).

Even if botanical identification of poisonous mushrooms requires expert knowledge not readily accessible to every physician, and if chemical tests are lacking for many poisonous species, fortunately the principal mushroom poisons may be differentiated on the basis of symptomatology. The length of the latent period following ingestion but preceding the onset of symptoms and the course of the ensuing illness furnish valuable clues which permit the physician to distinguish in most cases the type of poison involved and the proper treatment.

Section II of this chapter is devoted to a discussion of the chemistry and properties of the various mushroom toxins. Wherever chemical methods for their detection are known, the detailed procedures are included. Section III presents a summary of the symptoms, diagnosis, and treatment of mushroom poisoning. Since comprehensive listings of the principal poisonous mushrooms of the United States are not readily available, Section IV comprises an enumeration of their scientific names, outstanding botanical features, references to good illustrations of them, and the types of poison which they contain.

## II. Chemistry and Methods of Detection of Mushroom Poisons

### A. Systems of Classification

A number of systems have been proposed by different authors for the classification of mushroom poisons. Ford (F8) recognized five different types of mycetismus which he labeled: (1) *gastro-intestinalis;* (2) *choleriformis;* (3) *nervosus;* (4) *sanguinareus;* and (5) *cerebralis.* A more recent classification by Alder (A4) recognizes three principal types of poisonous mushrooms: (1) fungi producing irritation of the digestive organs; (2) those causing neurological symptoms; and (3) those effecting cellular degeneration of the vital organs.

In the light of present knowledge, it seems useful to accept the three basic divisions of Alder with minor modifications and one additional category. Four basic varieties of mushroom toxins are thus recognized:

1. Protoplasmic poisons
   *a.* amanita toxins
   *b.* helvella poisons
2. Compounds exerting neurological effects
   *a.* muscarine
   *b.* "pilzatropine"
   *c.* psilocybin
3. Gastrointestinal irritants
4. Disulfiram-like constituents

All of the known poisonous mushrooms contain principles with at least one of these activities, but the clinical picture is sometimes complicated in the case of those which contain two such constituents which may exert antagonistic actions. The basic classification does not include poisonings resulting from hypersensitivity to mushroom protein or from eating mushrooms which have been partially decomposed by the action of microorganisms.

### B. Protoplasmic Poisons

#### 1. Amanita Toxins

*a. Structure and Activity.* The most common type is an extremely poisonous mixture of toxins which occurs in *Amanita phalloides, A. verna,*

*A. virosa,* and related species of the so-called deadly amanitas; also possibly (based on symptoms) in *Galerina venenata* and perhaps in *Lepiota cretacea* (insubstantial chromatographic evidence). Five related cyclopeptides designated collectively as *amanita toxins* have been isolated from *A. phalloides,* and the structures of four of them have been established (W6).

Phalloidin and phalloin (Fig. 1) differ chemically only in the substitu-

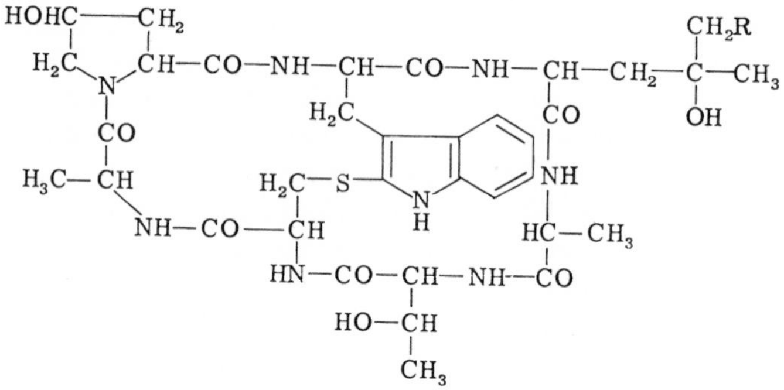

HOHC——CH₂
H₂C    CH—CO—NH—CH—CO—NH—CH—CH₂—C—CH₃ (with CH₂R, OH)
   N                      H₂C.              CO    OH
   CO                                        NH
H₃C—CH        H₂C—S             HC—CH₃
   NH—CO——CH      H    HN—CO—CH—NH—CO
                      HO—CH
                        CH₃

Phalloidin  (R = OH)

Phalloin    (R = H)

Fig. 1. Structure of amanita toxins.

tion of a hydrogen atom in the latter for a hydroxy group in the former. On intraperitoneal injection in the white mouse the LD$_{50}$ of phalloidin was found to be 1.9 mg/kg, of phalloin 1.4 mg/kg.

The relationship of α- to β-amanitin (Fig. 2) is that of an acid amide to its respective carboxylic acid. The structure of γ-amanitin has not yet

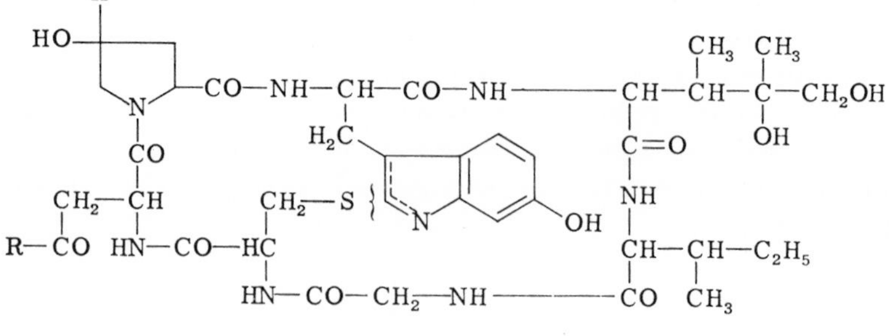

HO—[ring with H]
   N—CO—NH—CH—CO—NH——CH—CH—C—CH₂OH (with CH₃ CH₃, OH)
   CO            H₂C.                C=O
CH₂—CH      CH₂—S               NH
R—CO HN—CO—HC        OH        CH—CH—C₂H₅
         HN—CO—CH₂—NH——————CO  CH₃

α-Amanitin  (R = NH₂)

β-Amanitin  (R = OH)

Fig. 2. Structure of amanita toxins.

been determined. These compounds have an $LD_{50}$ in the white mouse of 0.1, 0.4, and 0.8 mg/kg, respectively.

Spectrophotometric assay following paper chromatographic separation and elution of the toxins revealed the following quantities of toxins in 100 gm of fresh A. *phalloides:* phalloidin, 10 mg; $\alpha$-amanitin, 8 mg; $\beta$-amanitin, 5 mg; $\gamma$-amanitin, 0.5 mg; phalloin, traces (W8). It is apparent that in this mixture $\alpha$-amanitin is largely responsible for the toxic effect. It is not only approximately twenty times more toxic than phalloidin, but a fatal dose requires about twenty times longer to kill an experimental animal. Conceivably, a mushroom weighing 50 gm contains sufficient toxin to kill a human being.

Studies with purified toxins have revealed that hepatic glycogen mobilization associated with blood glucose elevation is the first demonstrable change in both amanitin and phalloidin poisoning. Acting rapidly, phalloidin begins to inhibit important enzymes of carbohydrate, fat, and protein metabolism within 1 hour after administration. Fatty degeneration of the liver and other vital organs is undoubtedly a secondary, nonspecific process, but the severe liver hemorrhages which are regularly observed in rats and mice poisoned with phalloidin are probably direct results of the toxin. Phalloidin also inhibits the formation of energy-rich phosphate *in vitro*, but attempts to understand the role of this function are, as yet, speculative.

The chemical mechanism of toxin action is also obscure but must be highly specific since rupture of the S bridge in the cyclopeptides causes loss of activity. Unfortunately, no enzyme capable of degrading amanitin or phalloidin has been discovered. All available data indicate that the amanita toxins do not act directly upon enzymatic proteins; rather, their lethal activity depends on the ability to disturb the integrity of cellular membranes, possibly by becoming affixed at certain sites where they disrupt vital life processes.

*b. Detection.* Amanita toxins in mushroom tissue may be detected by paper chromatography as described by Block *et al.* (B3). Place the minced mushroom (0.1 gm fresh weight) in a beaker and cover with several volumes of methanol. Heat to boiling and keep the mixture hot for at least 2 minutes. During this time stir and press the tissue fragments with a glass rod. Filter and express the remaining solvent from the tissue. Evaporate the extract to dryness on a steam bath.

Dissolve the residue in a minimal quantity (few drops) of methanol. Using a micropipette, apply the total volume, in small portions, to a spot 1 inch from the bottom of a 1-inch × 10-inch strip of Whatman No. 1 or S. & S. 2043b filter paper. Suspend the strip in a suitable chromatographic chamber so that the lower end is immersed to a depth of 0.5

inch in a solvent system composed of methyl ethyl ketone:acetone: water:n-butanol (20:6:5:1). Form ascendingly for 40 minutes.

Remove the strip and permit it to air-dry. Spray lightly with a solution of 1% cinnamaldehyde in methanol. Again allow to dry and suspend the strip in a stoppered tube above concentrated hydrochloric acid for 5–10 minutes. The strip may then be removed and examined. One or more violet- or blue-colored spots are indicative of the presence of amanita toxins. Orange, yellow, brown, or pink spots are not significant.

If time permits, three modifications will facilitate separation of the individual toxins. Extend the original extraction time of the mushroom tissue to 1 hour or longer. Evaporate the methanol extract and redissolve the residue three times to coagulate the polypeptides. Employ a 14-inch paper strip and form the chromatogram for 2 hours.

The amanita toxins most likely to be detected by this simple chromatographic separation of relatively unconcentrated extracts are α- and β-amanitin which form violet spots with average $R_f$ values of 0.43 and 0.17 respectively. γ-Amanitin is present in *A. phalloides* only in traces, and the cinnamaldehyde–hydrochloric acid color reaction is ten times less sensitive for phalloidin and phalloin than for the amanitins. Since α-amanitin is recognized as the principal toxic compound in *A. phalloides*, the procedure is a generally satisfactory one for the characterization of amanita toxin–containing mushrooms.

## 2. Helvella Poisons

*a. Properties.* A second type of protoplasmic poison, less dangerous than the amanita toxins but still capable of producing fatal results, occurs in certain false morels (*Helvella esculenta, H. gigas,* and *H. underwoodii*). Helvellic acid, a hemolytic poison, was isolated from *H. esculenta* by Boehm and Külz in 1885 (B6), but it is now recognized that the fungus exerts only slight hemolytic activity in man (S17), the importance of this action being overemphasized due to the results of early studies on unsuitable test animals (dogs). Furthermore, helvellic acid is heat-labile and cannot be the cause of poisoning in those cases involving cooked mushrooms (D4).

Even though the exact identity and the chemical nature of the toxic principle(s) of *Helvella* species remain unknown, the activity is essentially hepatotoxic, with additional effects on the hematopoietic system and the central nervous system (F13). It may therefore be classified as a protoplasmic poison, although its ready solubility in boiling water, its instability in the dried mushroom, and its generally less drastic physiological effects distinguish it from the amanita toxins.

Some authorities believe that the poisonous nature of false morels is not due to an inherent toxic principle but results from decomposition of the protein in older specimens. This would explain the apparently irregular occurrence of the toxin in different specimens, but it does not explain the apparent resistance of certain individuals to the poison. For a detailed discussion of these matters, see Pilát and Ušák (P2).

b. *Detection.* The Reif test (F13) may be employed to distinguish tissues of toxic *Helvella* species from edible *Morchella* species (morels). Finely chopped fresh tissue (10 gm) or pulverized dried material (1 gm) is placed in a 500-ml flask together with 40 ml of water, 10 ml of 10% sodium hydroxide solution, 5 gm of sodium chloride, and a few glass beads. After thorough mixing, a condenser is attached and the flask heated until 30 ml of distillate are collected. Heat must be applied cautiously to prevent excessive foaming.

To 15 ml of the distillate are added 15 drops of a reagent prepared by dissolving 0.5 gm of selenious acid in 100 ml of concentrated sulfuric acid. The mixture is warmed on a steam bath for 15 minutes. A positive test (*Helvella* species) is indicated by the formation, beginning after about 5 minutes, of a precipitate of amorphous red selenium. Tissues of *Morchella* species do not produce this color reaction.

## C. Substances Exerting Neurological Effects

These may be classified into three basic subtypes: (1) muscarine; (2) "pilzatropine"; and (3) psilocybin. The first two compounds exert physiological effects which are opposite, even antagonistic; the activities of the latter two are similar in certain respects, different in others.

### 1. MUSCARINE

a. *Structure and Activity.* Muscarine is a chemical compound which derives its name from the plant from which it was first obtained, *Amanita muscaria* (S2). It occurs in that species and in the closely related *A. pantherina* in extremely small amounts and is not the principal toxic agent in these mushrooms. It is reported to be present in certain species of *Boletus, Clitocybe, Lepiota, Hebeloma, Russula,* etc. (A2), but verification is required (E5). Certain species of *Inocybe* remain the richest source of muscarine; concentrations ranging up to 0.73% of dry weight have been detected chromatographically in some of them (B8).

In spite of the isolation of muscarine in impure form nearly 150 years ago, determination of its structure proved to be a particularly difficult problem but of sufficient interest to attract the attention of a number of chemists. As Wilkinson (W10) has pointed out in his excellent review of the subject, several groups of workers realized almost simultaneously the importance of isolating a sufficient quantity of pure muscarine to permit comprehensive chemical and physical analyses. Credit for describing the first pure crystalline muscarine chloride belongs to Eugster and Wasser (E7) who later provided chemical and pharmacological details (E2, W1). X-ray crystallographic studies conducted by Jellineck in Kögl's laboratory (K4) revealed that muscarine chloride is the quaternary ammonium salt of 5-aminomethyltetrahydro-3-hydroxy-2-methylfuran (Fig. 3), a structure subsequently verified by synthesis (E4, K3).

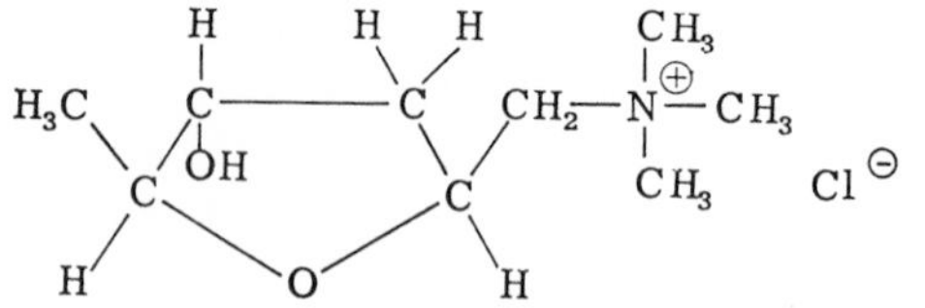

FIG. 3. Structure of muscarine chloride.

The entantiomorphs of (±)-muscarine differ greatly in potency, which is almost exclusively associated with the naturally occurring (+) isomer. It has a highly specific, peripheral parasympathetic action due to its effect on postganglionic, parasympathetic effector sites. Inhibition of cholinesterase activity enhances muscarine activity markedly, indicating that compound might be converted in the body into an active acetyl ester. A number of isomers and derivatives of muscarine have been prepared and examined for their physiological activity. For the pertinent literature see Wilkinson (W10).

   *b. Detection.* Identification of muscarine in mushroom tissues is complicated by the presence of choline which almost always accompanies it. Brown (B8) developed a simple quantitative procedure for the estimation of muscarine in *Inocybe* species. After the muscarine was separated from choline and other quaternary compounds by paper chromatography, it was rendered visible by Thies and Reuther's reagent. A modification of Brown's procedure may be employed for the qualitative determination of muscarine in fresh or dried mushrooms.

   Place the mushrooms (50 gm fresh weight or 5 gm dry weight) in a Waring Blendor, add 100 ml of a mixture of absolute ethanol:10% ammonium hydroxide solution (19:1), and homogenize. Filter the resulting brei on a suction filter, return the marc to the Blendor, and repeat the extraction and filtration process two additional times. Combine the extracts and evaporate under reduced pressure at 50°C to a thick syrupy residue (approximately 2 ml).

   Dissolve the residue in successive small volumes of distilled water and combine (total 25 ml). Dissolve 3 gm of sodium hydroxide in this solution, then add 5 ml of a 13% solution of ammonium reineckate in methanol. Cool, centrifuge, and decant the supernatant liquid. Wash the precipitate with cold *n*-propanol (three 2-ml volumes) and dissolve the washed precipitate in a total of 7 ml of acetone.

Convert the quaternary reineckates thus obtained to the respective chlorides by adding 1.4 ml of distilled water, 5 ml of a saturated solution of silver sulfate, and 0.5 ml of a 20% aqueous solution of barium chloride. Cool, centrifuge, decant the supernatant liquid, and evaporate it to dryness under reduced pressure at 50°C. Dissolve the residue in the smallest possible quantity of absolute ethanol (<10 ml). This constitutes a purified extract of quaternary chlorides which is ready for chromatographic examination.

Buffer 20-cm² sheets of Whatman No. 1 filter paper at pH 4.5 by dipping in a solution prepared by mixing 10.92 parts of 0.1 $M$ citric acid solution with 9.09 parts of 0.2 $M$ disodium hydrogen phosphate solution. Allow the sheets to air-dry. Prepare a sheet for circular chromatography by placing it over the bottom section of a 150-mm Petri dish, then pressing down the lid in the usual manner. Remove the sheet which now conforms to the outline of the dish, and cut a 10-mm wide tongue from the edge to the center of the circular area. Cut this tongue to a length of approximately 5 cm. Place a pencil dot in the center of the tongue at the place where it is attached to the paper sheet.

With a micropipette spot approximately 50 $\mu$l (in 10-$\mu$l portions) of the purified extract on the pencil spot. Pour 50 ml of a solvent system composed of *n*-butanol:methanol:water (10:3:2) in the lower section of the dish, put the sheet in place, and relace the cover tightly. Form the chromatogram for approximately 2 hours.

Remove the sheet, dry in air, and spray with Thies and Reuther's reagent. This is prepared by heating 2.6 gm of bismuth subcarbonate and 7.0 gm of sodium iodide (dried over concentrated sulfuric acid for 24 hours) with 25 ml of glacial acetic acid for a few minutes. Let stand overnight; filter the clear filtrate from the crystals of sodium acetate. The filtrate constitutes a stable stock solution which may be preserved indefinitely in a tightly closed bottle. To prepare the spray reagent, mix 10 ml of the stock solution with 50 ml of glacial acetic acid and 120 ml of ethyl acetate. Add 10 ml of distilled water to the solution dropwise and with constant shaking.

As the reagent dries, muscarine and choline appear as dark orange-red semicircular zones on a light background with average $R_f$ values of 0.28 and 0.09 respectively. Acetylcholine, present in some mushrooms, is ordinarily hydrolyzed by the alkaline extraction procedure and does not interfere. If present on the chromatogram, it also produces an orange-red zone (average $R_f$, 0.23).

When conducted as described (50 gm fresh tissue, 10 ml of purified extract, 50 μl applied to the chromatogram), this test should detect >0.005% of muscarine in mushroom tissue. Its sensitivity may be increased by using a larger quantity of mushrooms, by further concentration of the purified extract, or by spotting a larger quantity of extract on the chromatogram.

### 2. "Pilzatropine"

It has long been recognized that ingestion of *Amanita muscaria* or *A. pantherina* produces symptoms which are not typical of muscarine but resemble the central nervous system stimulation induced by atropine. Explorers and travelers who toured Siberia in the early part of the eighteenth century reported the use of the fly agaric (*A. muscaria*) as a narcotic or intoxicant by the Koryak and neighboring tribes of Kamchatka. Vivid descriptions of orgies resulting from the use of this plant are recorded. See Ramsbottom (R1) for the pertinent literature.

The principle(s) responsible for this action, long designated "pilzatropine," remains unidentified. Tyler (T3) has reviewed the attempts to isolate this ambiguous compound through the year 1957. Since that time, an additional preliminary report has appeared (E5) which indicates that traces of indole derivatives, possibly 4-hydroxyindole compounds (psilocybin ?), exist in *A. muscaria,* but additional evidence for the identity of "pilzatropine" is required.

To complicate the situation further, these species also contain muscarine, but since it is present only in minute quantities the principal effects of poisoning are those of central nervous system stimulation. Since the chemical identity of "pilzatropine" is unknown, there are no chemical tests to determine its occurrence in mushrooms.

### 3. Psilocybin

*a. Structure and Activity.* Certain species of *Psilocybe, Panaeolus, Conocybe, Psathyrella,* and possibly *Russula* are capable of inducing psychotropic manifestations in the human being following ingestion (S6, S7, W3). Chemical investigations have revealed the presence of two 4-substituted tryptamine derivatives, psilocybin and psilocin (Fig. 4), in selected species of the first two genera (H2, H6). Based on their similar employment in native magico-religious ceremonies, it is possible that certain species of the three latter genera contain the same active principles.

Both psilocybin and psilocin have identical physiological actions, but the former is the more stable and generally occurs in larger proportions in mushrooms. *In vitro* studies utilizing rat and mouse tissue homog-

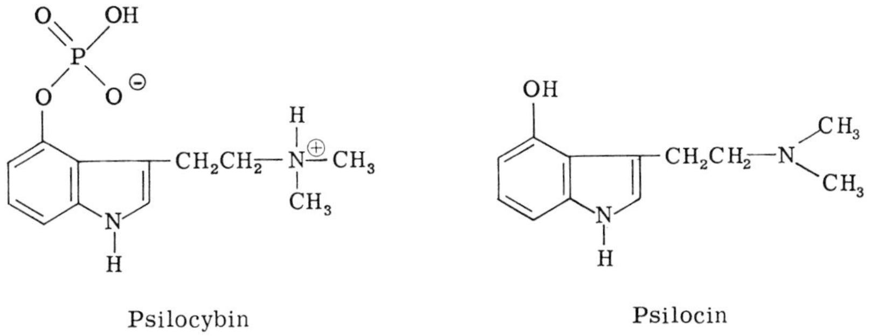

Psilocybin                          Psilocin

FIG. 4. Structure of 4-substituted tryptamine derivatives.

enates indicate that possibly in the intact animal psilocybin is rapidly dephosphorylated and is pharmacologically active as psilocin, while the duration of its effect might be controlled by the oxidation of the latter compound to an *o*-quinone type of structure (H7). The pharmacology of psilocybin has been reviewed by Cerletti (C4, H2).

*b. Detection.* Psilocybin and psilocin in mushrooms are readily detected by circular paper chromatography. An unbuffered, 20-cm² sheet of Whatman No. 1 filter paper is fitted over a 150-mm Petri dish, and a paper tongue is cut to the center of the disc as described previously under muscarine detection (Section II,C,1,*b*). Mushroom tissue (1 gm fresh weight, 0.1 gm dry weight) is extracted with 5 ml of cold methanol, either by grinding in a small mortar and pestle or by shaking the finely powdered tissue in a stoppered test tube. After centrifuging, the supernatant solution (50 μl in 10-μl aliquots) is applied to the chromatogram with a micropipette.

Resolution is carried out with water-saturated *n*-butanol for approximately 2 hours. The sheet is removed, air-dried, sprayed with a reagent consisting of 2% *p*-dimethylaminobenzaldehyde in 1 N hydrochloric acid, and dried in a stream of warm air. Psilocybin appears as a reddish violet semicircular zone (average $R_f$, 0.25), psilocin as a blue-violet zone (average $R_f$, 0.53). Since both these compounds are commercially available, mixed chromatograms, prepared by spotting reference compounds and the extract in admixture, may be employed to verify their identity.

## D. Gastrointestinal Irritants

Mushrooms containing compounds which have an irritating action upon the gastrointestinal tract include certain species of *Agaricus*, *Boletus*, *Cantharellus*, *Clavaria*, *Clitocybe*, *Lactarius*, *Lepiota*, *Paxillus*, *Rhodophyllus*, *Russula*, and *Tricholoma*. The chemical nature of the active principles of these species is not known, but they are generally presumed to be resin-like substances. No chemical tests for their detection are recorded in the literature.

### E. Disulfiram-like Constituents

Ingestion of *Coprinus atramentarius* and the subsequent ingestion of alcohol give rise, at least in certain persons, to physiological symptoms resembling those of the alcohol-disulfiram syndrome. The remarkable similarity between the two types of poisoning caused considerable speculation regarding the possible occurrence of disulfiram in the mushroom. In 1956, Simandl and Franc reported the isolation of disulfiram from *C. atramentarius* (S3). The reported finding of this unusual chemical compound in plant tissues prompted two independent reinvestigations of the mushroom, neither of which was able to verify the occurrence of disulfiram in it (L4, W9). Consequently, the identity of the active principles and chemical tests to establish their presence in mushrooms are unknown. Other species of *Coprinus,* such as *C. comatus,* apparently do not cause this type of poisoning (K7).

## III. Symptoms and Treatment of Mushroom Poisoning

Although there is no simple rule which permits a collector to distinguish readily and with exactitude between poisonous and edible mushrooms, there is a simple rule which may be used by the physician as a guide in the treatment of cases of mushroom poisoning. Basically, those cases in which symptoms appear from 6 to 12 or even 24 hours after ingestion of the mushrooms are caused by protoplasmic poisons; they are always severe and frequently fatal. Cases in which the symptoms appear approximately ½–2 hours after ingestion are caused by compounds exerting neurological effects, by gastrointestinal irritants, or by disulfiram-like constituents. Such poisonings are frequently mild, infrequently severe, and only in exceptional cases (children, invalids) are they dangerous to life.

### A. Species Containing Protoplasmic Poisons

#### 1. AMANITA TOXINS

Clinically, the outstanding characteristic of deadly amanita poisoning is the long (up to 24 hours), asymptomatic latent period. The symptoms (A4, L5) begin suddenly and are characterized by violent vomiting and continuous diarrhea leading to a loss of strength, desiccation, and muscle cramps. Circulatory disturbances include a feeble, rapid pulse; the patient is apathetic, and his general appearance is bad. During this period the senses are generally little affected. Children and adolescents often succumb during this stage of the poisoning, or at least become comatose. Collapse is caused primarily by loss of body fluids, which often amounts to 2–3 liters/day. Blood pressure falls due to decreases in its sugar and sodium chloride content. The residual nitrogen content of the blood increases, accompanied by a potassium deficiency and leucocytosis.

The poisoning shows a clear biphasic development. With proper treatment the patient usually survives this first stage, shows a slight improvement, then relapses. The liver is distended, and nearly one-third of the victims become jaundiced as a result of severe metabolic disturbance leading to fat deposition in the liver, kidneys, and heart. Other symptoms include cramps, drowsiness, dilation of the pupils, albuminuria, hemoglobinuria, oliguria, and anuria. Loss of consciousness, coma, and death may occur, usually as a result of acute hepatic necrosis.

Most fatalities occur within 3 to 5 days; in young people death is frequent after 2 days. Alder (A4) has reviewed the statistics on deadly amanita poisonings occurring during the last 40 years and concluded that the mortality rate varies from 34 to 63%.

There is no proven, specific antidote for this type of protoplasmic poison. Because of the insidious nature of the toxins, treatments designed to remove the fungus from the gastrointestinal tract (emetics, cathartics, gastric and colonic lavage) are often applied too late to prevent much absorption. Nevertheless, these measures should be instituted if the poisoning is diagnosed before vomiting and diarrhea commence. Further treatment is largely symptomatic and supportive. Clinical estimations of the sugar, potassium, sodium, chloride, alkali reserve, and urea content of the blood are essential in all severe cases and may be used as a guide to therapy.

Intravenous administration of dextrose (5%) and sodium chloride injection, up to 3 liters daily, should be begun. Treat collapse with stimulants; shock and a profound decrease in blood pressure with whole blood, plasma, or plasma extender; restlessness and pain with chlorpromazine, paraldehyde, or meperidine. Large doses of vitamins C, K, and the B complex should be injected. Oral administration of broad spectrum antibiotics (tetracycline) as soon as feasible may minimize hepatic necrosis. Corticosteroids should be administered, intravenously at first, later orally, and are believed by Alder (A4) to be of considerable value during the critical phase. Anuria, oliguria, and hepatic necrosis are treated by customary procedures. Hemodialysis with an Allwal artifical kidney has proved beneficial (E1).

Administration of an antidote composed of chopped, raw rabbit stomach and brains as recommended by Limousin and Petit (L2) has nothing to recommend it to persons already suffering from severe nausea. The effectiveness of the *sérum antiphallinique* prepared in France and alleged to be effective in the treatment of deadly amanita poisoning remains to be proven (L5, W8). Since it is not ordinarily available in the United States, it need not be given further consideration.

## 2. HELVELLA POISONS

There is a distinct latent period, rarely less than 6–10 hours, between ingestion of the mushrooms and the onset of symptoms which are very similar to, but generally less severe than, those produced by the amanita toxins.

The mortality rate in false morel poisoning ranges between 2 and 4% (A4). Although cases are comparatively common in Europe and often involve relatively large numbers of people (D4, S17), only a few fatal poisonings have been reported in the United States and Canada (D2, H3).

Treatment of helvella poisoning is similar to that recommended for deadly amanita poisoning.

## B. Species Exerting Neurological Effects

## 1. MUSCARINE

Symptoms appear quite rapidly, usually within 15 to 30 minutes, following the ingestion of mushrooms containing muscarine. Increased salivation, perspiration, and lachrymation are followed by nausea, abdominal pain, vomiting, and diarrhea. The pulse is slowed and irregular, the pupil is constricted, breathing becomes asthmatic. In uncomplicated muscarine poisoning, the victim's mental processes are ordinarily clear; he does not experience delirium or hallucinations. Death infrequently results in severe cases from cardiac or respiratory failure.

Treatment of muscarine poisoning involves gastric lavage, unless this has been rendered unnecessary by the emesis and diarrhea, and the hypodermic injection of atropine, a specific antidote. The dose of atropine sulfate is 0.5–1.0 mg, repeated in ½ hour if necessary. After vomiting has ceased, dilute saline solutions and glucose should be administerd orally in large amounts.

## 2. "PILZATROPINE"

Symptoms appear ½–2 hours after ingestion. Vomiting may not always occur. The victim passes into a state of excitement resembling advanced alcoholic intoxication and characterized by restlessness, confusion, delirium, disturbances of vision, and muscle spasms. Following this excited state, he becomes depressed, loses consciousness, and awakens with little or no memory of it.

Depending upon the muscarine content of the mushrooms and the quantity ingested, these "pilzatropine" symptoms may be accompanied to some extent by those of muscarine poisoning. Death seldom results and recovery is rapid, ordinarily within 24 hours.

Treatment consists of removal of the poisonous material by gastric lavage or emetics followed by cathartics. Atropine is best avoided in all cases characterized by excitement, but if muscarinic symptoms predominate it may be used with caution. Phenobarbital or chlorpromazine may be required during the excitement phase. As the patient becomes depressed, administer liquids, including caffeine beverages. Nikethamide may be employed during this stage as a stimulant. Further treatment is largely symptomatic (A4, J3).

### 3. Psilocybin

Following the ingestion of psilocybin-containing mushrooms, psychotomimetic symptoms resembling those induced by lysergic acid diethylamide (LSD) commence in about 30–60 minutes and continue for several hours. The patient displays anxiety and difficulty in concentration and understanding. Changes in sensory perception, including sensitivity to touch and distortion of tactile sensations, as well as changes in size, shape, color, and depth of vision with kaleidoscopic variations, are noted. The mood is altered: usually it is elevated, but depression may occur. Both elementary hallucinations, such as the appearance of colored lights and patterns on closing the eyes, and true hallucinations may be experienced.

Persons suffering from this type of mushroom poisoning ordinarily recover spontaneously and completely in 5–10 hours. Gastric lavage or emetics may hasten recovery; other treatment is symptomatic.

### C. Species Containing Gastrointestinal Irritants

Ingestion of mushrooms of this type generally produces symptoms in ½–2 hours. These include nausea, vomiting, and diarrhea and range from very mild to extremely severe disturbances. The latter are often accompanied by abdominal cramps and intense pain. In most cases, the symptoms terminate spontaneously within a few hours, and the patient's condition returns to normal in a day or two.

*Lactarius torminosus, Rhodophyllus sinuatus,* and *Tricholoma pardinum* (together with related species) may produce extremely violent poisoning under certain conditions and have caused fatalities, particularly among children. *R. sinuatus* has some hepatotoxic activity, and this property may extend to other mushrooms producing violent gastro-enteritis.

Treatment involves removal of the toxic material from the digestive tract, if this has not been rendered unnecessary by vomiting and diarrhea, followed by symptomatic treatment. Usually a period of bed rest and light diet are indicated (A4).

## D. Species Containing Disulfiram-like Constituents

Symptoms occur within ½–2 hours following the consumption of *C. atramentarius* and alcohol. These include flushing, palpitations, dyspnea, hyperventilation, and tachycardia, but vomiting and diarrhea are usually absent. The symptoms ordinarily last only a short time but vary in severity in accordance with the amounts of mushroom and alcohol consumed and the relative time interval.

In some cases, alcohol may be drunk with impunity immediately after eating the mushroom, but a reaction will occur if alcohol is consumed again 24 hours later. In other instances, the poisoning may occur at once following the meal and will reoccur, even after 48 hours, if more alcohol is consumed at that time. These, and other irregularities, are common in this type of poisoning. They may be the result of idiosyncrasies of the consumers, misidentifications, or strain variations of the mushroom (P2).

This type of poisoning is easily prevented by abstention from alcoholic beverages for a period of several days following the consumption of *C. atramentarius*. Recovery is ordinarily spontaneous and complete but in severe cases may be facilitated by gastric lavage or emesis followed by symptomatic treatment.

## IV. Names, Descriptions, and Relative Toxicities of Poisonous Mushrooms

## A. Explanation of Nomenclature

The proper nomenclature of the higher fungi is an extremely complex subject. Essentially, the complete proper name of any plant consists of its correct generic name and species epithet followed by the author citation (name of the botanist or botanists proposing the name). The generic name is always capitalized, but the species epithet may be written with a lower case initial letter; both names are italicized. An example of such a proper name is *Amanita silvicola* Kauff., in which Kauff. is the abbreviation for C. H. Kauffman, the distinguished American mycologist who named this mushroom.

According to the International Rules of Botanical Nomenclature, the validity of a name of a mushroom is determined on the basis of priority, starting with the publication of *Systema Mycologicum* by Elias Fries in 1821. If an author incorrectly places a species in a certain genus, another investigator may later discover this fact and desire to correct the error. Because of the priority system, he cannot assign an entirely new name to the species. Instead, he must employ the original species epithet, which is recognized as the valid one, and transfer it to the proper genus, thus making a new combination. In this case the name of the first author is placed in parentheses following the generic name and species epithet, and the name of the author of the new combination follows, outside of the parenthesis. Thus, the name *Amanita verna* (Fr.) Quél. indicates that this species was first assigned to a different genus (*Agaricus*) by Fries but that it was later characterized as a species of *Amanita* by Quélet. *Agaricus vernus* Fr. thus becomes a synonym for the recognized or accepted name of this mushroom. A list of standard abbreviations employed for the authors' names is found in Hennig (M4).

There are many details of plant nomenclature which cannot be dealt with in a brief introduction. In some cases authorities are not in agreement regarding the correct nomenclature of certain higher fungi. In the following, Singer (S5) has been employed as the authority, unless otherwise noted, for all species covered by him.

## B. Genera and Species

### 1. *Agaricus* SPECIES

The diagnostic characteristics of this genus include spores which are some shade of purple-brown to blackish brown. The gills are free from the stipe, and the latter separates easily and cleanly from the pileus. An annulus is present but not a volva. Some of the most desirable edible fungi belong to this genus. Although no deadly poisonous species are recorded, a number have been observed to produce toxic symptoms following ingestion by some individuals. The idiosyncratic nature of this response requires emphasis (Table I).

### 2. *Amanita* SPECIES

Members of this genus are characterized by their white spores, the presence of both an annulus and a volva, and typically free gills. Included are deadly species containing the amanita toxins, other toxic species which contain muscarine and/or an atropine-like principle, and still other species which are entirely harmless and are valued as esculents. Many conflicting statements are to be found in the literature regarding the identity and toxicity of *Amanita* species (Table II).

*Varro E. Tyler, Jr.*

TABLE I

CHARACTERIZATION OF *Agaricus* SPECIES

| Species | Outstanding botanical characteristics | Relative toxicity | Comments | References |
|---|---|---|---|---|
| *A. albolutescens* Zeller | Large, broad white pileus staining amber yellow. Flesh white. Gills free, close, unequal. Stipe with superior annulus. Odor of anise or amygdalin. Spores ovoid to ellipsoid, 5–6 (7) × 3.5–4.6 μ. Similar to *A. arvensis* but color is different. | ? | Poisonous, at least to some. | S10, Z1 |
| *A. arvensis* Schaeff. ex. Fr. var. *palustris* A. H. Smith. | White fibrillose pileus with dull pinkish gills becoming chocolate brown with age. White tissue tends to become yellow where bruised. Prominent double annulus, flattened stipe base. Spores usually ovoid, 7–8.5 (9) × 4.5–5 μ. | + | Poisonous to some, not to others. Ingestion of authenticated specimens produced two-day incapacitation (gastrointestinal disturbance) in one individual but no unusual symptoms in another. Differences in spores only distinguish this mushroom from *A. sylvicola* (Vitt.) Fr. which is considered edible. May account for contradictory statements. Illustration (S12). | S9, S10, S12 |
| *A. hondensis* Murr. | White smooth pileus becomes vinaceous brown with maturity. White flesh stains yellow to vinaceous when bruised. Annulus is white, striate above. Stipe thick at apex with rather abrupt bulb. Spores ellipsoid, 4.5–5.5 × 3–3.5 μ. | ? | Dangerous, probably similar to *A. arvensis* var. *palustris*. Illustration (S10). | S10 |
| *A. placomyces* Peck | Flat pileus with brownish to grayish fibrils or fibrillose scales over surface, the disc darker than marginal areas. Young gills fleshy pink color. Tissue of cap becomes pink with age. Double annulus. May have phenolic odor when crushed. Spores ellipsoid, 4.5–5.5 × 3.5–4.2 μ. | ? | Edible by some, probably not by others. Certain variants of the species (phenolic odor) may be responsible, or individual human beings may vary in sensitivity. Needs investigation. Illustration (S10, S12). | S10, S12 |

### 3. *Boletus* SPECIES

These fleshy pore fungi have typically central stipes, but, unlike the gill fungi, the hymenophore consists of a layer of tubes which is easily separable from the pileus. The individual tubes forming this layer are usually readily separable from each other. Species which possess red tube mouths or which turn blue when bruised are best avoided by the mycophagist, but only a few have been proved poisonous (Table III).

### 4. *Cantharellus* SPECIES

Members of this genus have a tubular or vase-shaped fleshy pileus, not always distinct from a central stipe. The hymenium on the under side of the pileus and on the upper portion of the stipe occurs in the form of foldlike, thick ridges, forked, sometimes with pronounced cross veins. Spores are white to ochraceous, nonamyloid, smooth or rough. Most species are edible, much sought after for culinary use. At least one species is mildly poisonous to some persons (Table IV).

### 5. *Clavaria* SPECIES

These are fungi with fleshy or gelatinous fruiting bodies, simple to repeatedly branched, often comprised of masses of brightly colored, upright branches. The hymenium is glabrous, rather uniformly distributed over the branches. A stipe is more or less distinct, often lacking basidia. Spores are variable. The peculiar growth habit is responsible for the name "coral mushrooms" commonly applied to species of this genus. With a few exceptions, most large corals are edible (Table V).

### 6. *Clitocybe* SPECIES

These species are characterized by typically white spore deposits, fleshy central stipes, and broadly adnate to decurrent gills. A universal or partial veil is absent. Certain species appear to contain muscarine or other toxic principles, but scientific investigation is required. The species tend to intergrade with those of other genera, and the problems of identification and proper nomenclature are complex. There is no taxonomic work available which adequately treats the North American species (S5, S10) (Table VI).

### 7. *Coprinus* SPECIES

These mushrooms are characterized by a dark-colored spore deposit, typically black, and by the free or slightly attached gills which deliquesce into a dark-colored fluid as the spores are discharged; hence, the name

TABLE II

CHARACTERIZATION OF *Amanita* SPECIES

| Species | Outstanding botanical characteristics | Relative toxicity | Comments | References |
|---|---|---|---|---|
| *A. agglutinata* (Berk. & Curt.) Sing. [*Amanitopsis volvata* (Peck) Sacc.] | Whitish to brownish pileus covered with fibrillose or floccose scales. No annulus. Very large, membranous brown volva. | ? | Injections of extract slowly fatal to guinea pigs and rabbits. No evidence of toxicity in human beings. Edible? Illustration (T1). | F6, K1, M2, T1 |
| *A. bisporigera* Atk. | Like *A. verna* except more slender and two-spored basidia. | +++ | Presence of protoplasmic poison suspected on basis of relationship to *A. verna*. Illustration (A5) Fig. 61 as *A. verna*, (S10) as *A. verna*. | A5, K1, S10 |
| *A. brunnescens* Atk. | Dark to brownish gray pileus (lighter with age) with few whitish warts on surface. Longitudinally split volva forms very shallow cup. | +++ | This American species was for years referred to as *A. phalloides*. Assumed to be deadly poisonous but injection not toxic to mice, and amanita toxins not detected chromatographically. Needs reinvestigation. Illustration (S12). | B4, S12 |
| *A. chlorinosma* (Peck) Sacc. | White to cream pileus with dense white floccose warts. Annulus fragile, may disappear. Volva densely floccose. Strong odor of chlorine. | ? | Conflicting opinions. Injection toxic to guinea pigs, but edible? by some human beings. Relatively rare occurrence. Illustration (H4). | F5, G1, H4, M2 |
| *A. citrina* Schaeff. ex S. F. Gray [*A. mappa* (Batsch ex Fr.) Quél.] | Pileus, usually yellow with tinge of green, possesses very even margin. White or pale brownish warts on surface. Volva adherent to bulb, but with free margin above. Odor of sprouting potatoes. | + | Considered mildly toxic but is devoid of deadly amanita toxins. Does contain bufotenine. Old reports of deadly character stem from confusion with *A. phalloides* (in Europe) and *A. brunnescens* (in United States). Illustration (M4). | K1, M4, T4, W7, W8 |
| *A. cothurnata* Atk. | Entirely white except for yellow tinge over disc of pileus. Warts may be few or | + | Caused severe gastrointestinal upset in human beings but muscarinic symptoms | B4, C2, D3, S10, S12 |

| Species | Description | Toxicity | Comments | References |
|---|---|---|---|---|
| | absent. Volva fits closely over bulb terminating in distinct inrolled collar. | | were absent. Injections of extract without effect in guinea pigs or mice. Illustration (S10, S12). | |
| A. excelsa (Fr.) Quél. | Pileus brownish gray with whitish gray, easily separating warts. Lower stem covered with concentric scales. Bulb when young somewhat marginate. | ? | Considered poisonous. Considerable confusion with A. spissa (see below). Needs investigation. | M2 |
| A. flavivolva Murr. | Pileus pale yellow with grayish disc, few flat volval patches. Large skirtlike annulus, white with flavous edge. Volva adnate to small ovoid bulb, flavous, soon fragmenting. Similar to A. gemmata, but yellow volva. | ++ | Injections of extract produced no effect in guinea pigs but produced symptoms typical of muscarine poisoning in mice. No amanita toxins detected chromatographically. | B4, C15, M9 |
| A. flavoconia Atk. | Pileus orange-yellow to yellow with pale to bright yellow warts. Floccose yellowish patches of universal veil tissue on base of stipe. Amyloid spores. | ? | Injections of extract nontoxic in mice. Amanita toxins not detected chromatographically. The A. frostiana examined by Ford may have been this species. If so, A. flavoconia is nontoxic. Illustration (H4, S10). | B4, F6, H4, S10 |
| A. flavorubescens Atk. | Similar to A. flavoconia but tissue stains reddish when bruised. | ? | Suspect, requires investigation. Illustration (K1). | K1, S10 |
| A. frostiana (Peck) Sacc. | Similar to A. muscaria but spores are globose, not broadly ellipsoid. | ? | Toxicity requires verification. See comment under A. flavoconia. Danger of confusion with A. muscaria is considerable. Illustration (A5). | A5, S10 |
| A. gemmata (Fr.) Gill. [A. junquillea Quél.] | Pale yellow pileus with white to pale brownish warts. Free-margined collar around apex of bulb. Often appears to intergrade with A. pantherina. | ? | May possess limited edibility, but danger of confusion with A. pantherina prohibits use as esculent. If poison is present, probably muscarine. Amanita toxins not detected chromatographically. Illustration (M4, S10). | C3, M4, S10 |

TABLE II (*Continued*)

| Species | Outstanding botanical characteristics | Relative toxicity | Comments | References |
|---|---|---|---|---|
| A. *morrisii* Peck | Pileus dark grayish brown or blackish brown. Annulus double, radially striate above, whitish buff beneath. Slight volva, fragmentary and disappearing or partly adhering near base of stipe. | ? | Injections of extract fatal to guinea pigs and rabbits, death resulting from chronic intoxication. Effect on human beings unknown. Illustration (M2). | F6, M2 |
| A. *muscaria* (L. ex Fr.) Pers. ex Gray | Blood-red to orange to yellow pileus (depending on variety) with whitish warts. Intergrown volval remnants on bulb. Spores broadly ellipsoid, not amyloid. | ++ | Contains muscarine, 0.0002% of fresh weight, and unknown principle(s) with atropine-like activity. Reported occurrences of bufotenine and hyoscyamine are doubtful. Amanita toxins absent. Acetylcholine and a quaternary compound, muscaridine, have been isolated, but physiological activity of latter is unknown. Indole compounds apparently present in traces. Illustration (M4, S10, S12). | C3, E5, E6, K5, K9, L1, M4, S10, S12, T3, W7 |
| A. *pantherina* (D.C. ex Fr.) Secr. | Gray-brown to yellow-brown pileus with whitish to cream warts. Narrow, free collarlike volva, sometimes inrolled. | ++ | Contains muscarine, but an unknown constituent with atropine-like activity appears to be the principal toxic agent. Similar in this, and other respects, to *A. muscaria*. Illustration (M4, S10, S12). | B7, C3, H8, L1, M4, S10, S12, T3, W7 |
| A. *parcivolvata* (Peck) Gilb. [*Amanitopsis parcivolvata* Peck] | Similar to *A. muscaria* except pileus has strongly striate margin, flesh beneath cuticle is red, and annulus is absent. Volva consists of fragile, disappearing particles at base of stipe. | ++? | Poisonous. Probably quite similar to *A. muscaria* because of close botanical relationship. | H4 |
| A. *peckiana* Kauff. | Pileus white with fringed margin, large two-layered volva, evanescent inner veil. | ? | Suspect, apparently on basis of botanical relationship. Singer believes this species | K1, S5 |

| Species | Description | | Remarks | References |
|---|---|---|---|---|
| | Innate fibrillose scales on cap and stem. Large subcylindric spores. | | probably identical with *A. agglutinata* (see above). Needs investigation. | |
| *A. phalloides* (Vaill. ex Fr.) Secr. | Greenish pileus with few whitish veil remnants (warts). Bulbous stipe base enclosed in sheathlike lobed volva which often remains in earth when carpophore is picked. | +++ | Old reports of this mushroom in the United States refer to *A. brunnescens* or other closely related species. Reliably reported only from California. Rare there, probably introduced. Deadly poisonous. Contains amanita toxins. Illustration (M4). | M4, S12, W8 |
| *A. porphyria* (A. & S. ex Fr.) Secr. | Dark gray-brown to purplish brown pileus with similarly colored annulus, lower stalk, and bulb. Occurs late summer to autumn in northern conifer and mixed conifer-hardwood forests. | + | Considered mildly toxic but is devoid of deadly amanita toxins. Injections of extract reported toxic to guinea pigs. Contains bufotenine. Illustration (M4, S12). | C3, F5, M4, S12, T4 |
| *A. silvicola* Kauff. | Most common pure white *Amanita* species in Pacific Northwest. Flat patches of veil tissue on pileus, never distinct warts. Evanescent annulus. Volva adnate to bulb. | ? | No data regarding toxicity in human beings. No amanita toxins. Preliminary experiments revealed lack of pronounced muscarinic activity. Illustration (S10). | C3, M3, S10 |
| *A. spissa* (Fr.) Quél. | Pileus gray with brown or sooty brown disc, covered with soft grayish scales or warts. Margin not striate. White pendant annulus may be grayish below. Gray volva is pulverulent, evanescent. | ? | Conflicting opinions. Listed as deadly poisonous and as edible. This species is rare in the United States, and there is considerable danger of erroneous identification. Mycologists disagree. Gilbert attributes Kauffman's description (here abstracted) to *A. morrisii* and considers both *A. excelsa* (see above) and *A. spissa* as conspecific with *A. ampla* Pers. Singer thinks *A. excelsa* and *A. spissa* not identical. Reinvestigation needed. Illustration (M4). | G1, K1, M4, S5 |

TABLE II (*Continued*)

| Species | Outstanding botanical characteristics | Relative toxicity | Comments | References |
|---|---|---|---|---|
| A. *spreta* Peck | Pale lead-colored glabrous pileus with striate margin in age. Stipe equal (no bulb), volva membranous. | ? | Considered deadly poisonous but reported eaten by some. Injections produced chronic toxicity in guinea pigs. Requires investigation. Illustration (S10). | C11, F5, K1, S10 |
| A. *tenuifolia* Murr. | Similar to A. *verna* but stipe shorter and spores cylindric, about $12 \times 5 \mu$. | +++ | Injection of extract fatal to mice. Amanita toxin ($\beta$-amanitin) detected chromatographically. Rare occurrence. | B4, M7 |
| A. *verna* (Lam. ex Fr.) Pers. ex Vitt. sensu Arcangeli, R. Maire, Heim | White pileus without universal-veil remnants, white gills and stipe. Annulus membranous, pendant, white. Volva membranous, splitting into lobes, forms true cup around bulb. Globose (spherical-ovate) spores. | +++ | Deadly poisonous. Amanita toxins ($\alpha$- and $\beta$-amanitin) detected chromatographically. Injection of extract fatal to mice and to guinea pigs. Illustration (M4, S12). | B4, C15, K1, M4, S12 |
| A. *verniformis* Murr. | Similar to A. *verna* but with ellipsoid spores, about $10 \times 6 \mu$. | +++ | Toxicity similar to A. *verna* in guinea pigs. | C15, M8 |
| A. *virosa* Lam. ex Secr. | Similar to A. *verna* except pileus conical when young, annulus rarely formed. Spores globose. | +++ | Deadly poisonous. Action of amanita toxins in guinea pigs. Illustration (M4). | F5, K1, M4, S12 |
| A. *virosiformis* Murr. | Similar to A. *virosa* but spores elongated oblong-ellipsoid, about $12 \times 6 \mu$. Distinct odor of chloride of lime. | +++ | Injection of extract fatal to guinea pigs. Symptoms suggested presence of amanita toxins and additional principle affecting central nervous system. | C15, M6 |

TABLE III

CHARACTERIZATION OF *Boletus* SPECIES

| Species | Outstanding botanical characteristics | Relative toxicity | Comments | References |
|---|---|---|---|---|
| *B. eastwoodiae* (Murr.) Sacc. & Trotter | Olivaceous-brown pileus contains tubes with brilliant scarlet mouths. Stipe red and yellow, reticulate. Broken flesh stains blue. | ? | Suspect, but toxicity needs verification. Probably similar to *B. luridus.* Illustration (S12). | S12 |
| *B. luridus* Schaeff. ex Fr. | Form is quite variable. Pileus dark yellow-brown. Tubes yellow-green with dark reddish openings. Yellow and reddish stipe, clearly reticulated. Flesh turns blue when damaged. | ± | Poisonous when raw. Unless well cooked, produces paralytic symptoms. Should be parboiled to eliminate any danger, although some persons more sensitive than others. Reported disulfiram-like activity not verified. Conditionally edible. Old report of muscarine content requires verification. Rare occurrence in United States. Illustration (M4). | B8, M4, S4, W5 |
| *B. miniatoolivaceus* Frost var. *sensibilis* Peck | Pileus reddish, tubes yellowish, stem thick, lemon yellow with red stains at base but devoid of reticulations. All parts change color instantly to dark blackish blue when touched or damaged. | + | Case of poisoning reported in 1899 was characterized by nausea, diarrhea, exhaustion, and myosis. Muscarine? Recovery was complete. Extracts fatal to guinea pigs but not to rabbits. | C10, F10, K8 |
| *B. satanas* Lenz | Similar to *B. eastwoodiae* but has a paler (whitish) cap. | + | Considered poisonous, particularly when eaten raw, but large quantities of cooked mushroom will produce gastrointestinal disturbances. Not as bad as its reputation. Probably similar to *B. luridus.* Illustration (M4). | M4, S12 |

TABLE IV

CHARACTERIZATION OF *Cantharellus* SPECIES

| Species | Outstanding botanical characteristics | Relative toxicity | Comments | References |
|---|---|---|---|---|
| *C. floccosus* Schw. | Pileus floccose-scaly, vase-shaped, with orange-red top. Undersurface pallid to buff, wrinkled to nearly poroid. | ± | Produces gastrointestinal upsets in some persons 8–14 hours after ingestion. Edible by others. Illustration (S12). | K1, S10, S12 |

TABLE V

CHARACTERIZATION OF *Clavaria* SPECIES

| Species | Outstanding botanical characteristics | Relative toxicity | Comments | References |
|---|---|---|---|---|
| *C. formosa* Pers. ex Fr. | Tips of clustered branches pale yellow, intermediate parts pinkish, underground portion white. Fades but does not stain with age. | + | May not be identical botanically with *C. formosa* of Europe, but toxic properties are probably similar. Produces, at least in certain individuals, stomach pain and diarrhea. Illustration (M4, P2, S12). | M4, P2, S12 |
| *C. gelatinosa* Coker | Similar to *C. formosa* but darker in color, light brown to pale orange depending on age. Easily distinguished by tough, gelatinous, translucent flesh and odor and taste of tobacco. | + | Poisonous to some. Illustration (C13, D5). | C13, D5, S10 |

TABLE VI

CHARACTERIZATION OF *Clitocybe* SPECIES

| Species | Outstanding botanical characteristics | Relative toxicity | Comments | References |
|---|---|---|---|---|
| C. cerussata var. difformis Schum. sensu Bres. | Shining white, plicate to lobed pileus often very irregular. Fruiting bodies grow in dense masses. Spores are not amyloid, 5–5.5 × 3 μ, ellipsoid, smooth, and hyaline. Clamp connections present. | + to ++ | Considered dangerous. One of a number of related species and varieties, most of which are difficult to distinguish. Illustration (S10). | S10 |
| C. dealbata (Sow. ex Fr.) Gill. Also varieties (minor differences) | White to somewhat yellowish, disc-shaped pileus with wavy margin. Stipe pale, short, tapering toward the base. Odor mealy or resembling freshly cut wood. Spores 5–6 × 3–4 μ. | + to ++ | The typically European species (here described) contains muscarine and is considered poisonous. Extracts of authenticated specimens of an American variety (*C. dealbata* var. *sudorifica* Peck) produced muscarinic effects in rabbits, guinea pigs, and on the frog's heart. The same variety was reported to exert a powerful sudorific effect in human beings. However, certain American authors report *C. dealbata* as edible. May be due to misidentification. Requires investigation. Illustration (M4). | F10, F11, J1, M2, M4, R3 |
| C. illudens (Schw.) Sacc.; C. subilludens Murr.; Pleurotus olearius (D.C. ex Fr.) Gill. | These three closely related species correspond to *Omphalotus olearius* (D.C. ex Fr.) Sing. Reddish orange to yellowish orange pileus with phosphorescent gills (glowing in the dark). Buff-colored stipe, tapered toward base where it may fuse with others. Spore size and shape distinguish these species. | + | All three species are mildly poisonous, causing violent vomiting following ingestion. Recovery is rapid. Physiological tests suggest the presence of muscarine in *C. illudens. C. subilludens* does not contain ergot alkaloids as had been reported. Illustration (H4, S10). | C8, F1, H4, S5, S10, T4 |
| C. rivulosa (Pers. ex Fr.) Quél. | Pileus dull pinkish to brownish, pruinose, concentrically furrowed. Stipe white to pinkish, short, often curved. Spores white, elliptical, 4.5 × 3 μ. | ++ | The typically European species (here described) contains muscarine and is considered extremely dangerous. Illustration (M4). | M4 |

TABLE VII

CHARACTERIZATION OF *Coprinus* SPECIES

| Species | Outstanding botanical characteristics | Relative toxicity | Comments | References |
|---|---|---|---|---|
| *C. atramentarius* (Bull. ex Fr.) Fr. | Gray to brownish, large pileus with smooth or slightly wrinkled surface, at first silvery from thin fibrillose coating. Grows in clusters. Many biotypes distinguished by constant minor characteristics. | ± | Produces disulfiram-like symptoms (at least in some persons) when ingested concomitantly with alcohol. Reaction may require previous sensitization. Presence of disulfiram reported but not verified by two independent investigations. Variations in response may be attributable to different biotypes. Needs investigation. Illustration (S10, T1). | C7, L4, S3, S10, T1, W9 |

TABLE VIII

CHARACTERIZATION OF *Galerina* SPECIES

| Species | Outstanding botanical characteristics | Relative toxicity | Comments | References |
|---|---|---|---|---|
| *G. venenata* A. H. Smith | Pileus cinnamon brown, fading, with crenate to lacerated margin. Taste bitter and disagreeable. Gills adnate, stipe enlarged toward base, often with thin, apical annulus. Spores $8–11 \times 6–6.5 \ \mu$, warty. Pleurocystidia and cheilocystidia present. | +++ | Extremely toxic. Contains a protoplasmic poison which produces symptoms in human beings similar to the amanita toxins. Little is known regarding the toxicity of related species of *Galerina*. *G. autumnalis* (Peck) A. H. Smith & Sing. [*Pholiota autumnalis* Peck] may be poisonous, but scientific investigation of authentic specimens is required. Illustration (G4). | F11, G4, S11 |

"inky caps." Some species are highly prized as edible mushrooms and much sought for by collectors (Table VII).

## 8. *Galerina* SPECIES

Typically small nondescript carpophores are characterized by yellowish brown spores. The margin of the pileus is appressed against the stipe in young stages; the stipe is slender and cartilaginous. The pileus cuticle is composed of narrow, appressed, filamentose hyphae. Species are distinguished principally on the basis of microscopic characteristics, especially of the spores and cystidia (Table VIII).

## 9. *Hebeloma* SPECIES

Carpophores of this species are characterized by ocher-brown spores, a fleshy central stipe continuous with the pileus, adnexed or emarginate gills, and a viscid to subviscid pileus. A volva and a true annulus are lacking. Species often possess a strong odor (radishes or sweet-aromatic). Their habitat is terrestrial. They are difficult to identify, and their intrageneric taxonomy is completely confused. At least three species occurring in the United States are either toxic or are edible only after special preparation. The question of *Hebeloma* poisoning cannot be resolved satisfactorily until *Hebeloma* taxonomy is revised (S5) (Table IX).

## 10. *Helvella* SPECIES

These nongilled fungi are characterized by a pileus surface which varies from nearly smooth to strongly convoluted but never pitted (distinction from *Morchella*). The pilei are nearly always lobed, usually more or less saddle-shaped. Mostly terrestrial in habitat, some of them occur on decaying wood. Certain species are undoubtedly toxic, but irregularly so, giving rise to numerous contradictory statements and much speculation (Table X).

## 11. *Inocybe* SPECIES

The pileus of members of this genus is fleshy, putrescent, subconic at first, then campanulate to subexpanded, silky, fibrillose or fibrillose-squamulose, usually dry. A more or less evanescent cortina is present. The gills are adnate or adnexed, and the stipe fleshy, central. Spores are brownish, pleurocystidia may be present, cheilocystidia are present on the sterile gill edges. Most species are some shade of brown; some are white, red, yellow, or lilac. The odors of some are very characteristic.

Recognition of a mushroom as an *Inocybe* is comparatively simple, but species identification is extremely difficult even when microscopic characteristics are considered. Not all species are toxic, but no author

TABLE IX

CHARACTERIZATION OF *Hebeloma* SPECIES

| Species | Outstanding botanical characteristics | Relative toxicity | Comments | References |
|---|---|---|---|---|
| *H. crustuliniforme* (Bull. ex Fr.) Quél. | Pileus pale, becoming brown to dark brown with age. Veil absent. Crushed flesh has odor of radishes. Spores rusty brown, $9\text{–}11.5 \times 5.5\text{–}7\ \mu$, inequilateral to almond-shaped. | ± | Probably contains some muscarine. Produces mild poisoning when eaten unless previously parboiled (discard water and juices). Illustration (M4, S10). | M4, S10 |
| *H. fastibile* (Fr.) Quél. | Pileus yellowish-ochraceous to alutaceous-whitish, margin pubescent. Gills emarginate, subdistant, stipe firm, white with remains of cortina above. Odor of radishes, taste disagreeable. Spores $10\text{–}12 \times 5\text{–}6\ \mu$. | ± | Contains muscarine-like poison according to older work. Probably similar to *H. crustuliniforme*. Illustration (K6). | F9, K1, K6 |
| *H. sinapizans* (Fr.) Gill. | Cinnamon-colored, viscid pileus and decidedly scaly stipe. No veil in button stage. Strong odor and taste of radishes. Spores $10\text{–}12.5 \times 6\text{–}7\ \mu$. | ± | Toxic according to certain authors. Probably similar to *H. crustuliniforme*. Illustration (R4). | R4, S10 |

TABLE X

CHARACTERIZATION OF *Helvella* SPECIES

| Species | Outstanding botanical characteristics | Relative toxicity | Comments | References |
|---|---|---|---|---|
| *H. esculenta* Fr. | Pileus dark red-brown to yellow-brown, wrinkled to convoluted. Stipe paler to whitish, typically round in section or flattened. Widespread in forests in northern United States, fruits in early spring. | +++ | Extremely poisonous, but irregular. Principally hepatotoxic with associated hematotoxicity and central neurotoxicity. Onset of symptoms is insidious, commencing about 8–24 hours after ingestion. Dried carpophores slowly lose their toxicity. A period of 6 months is required before they are completely safe. Parboiling twice (3–5 minutes) and discarding the cooking water apparently render this species edible for some persons, but not all. Illustration (M4, S10, S12). | D1, D2, F13, M4, S10, S12, S17 |
| *H. gigas* Krbh. | Similar to *H. esculenta*, but stipe is short, massive, irregular. Yellowish to dark brown pileus with very broad head. Commonly occurs near snow banks. | ++ ? | Smith reports no serious poisoning cases with this species in the Rocky Mountain area of the United States, but in Europe it is classified as a very poisonous species. Said to be rendered edible for most by parboiling. Probably similar to *H. esculenta*. Illustration (M4, S10, S12). | M4, S10, S12 |
| *H. underwoodii* Seaver | Edge of pileus curls away from stipe in distinctive manner. Stipe similar to that of *H. esculenta* but more massive. | + or ++ ? | Regarded as poisonous. Illustration (S12). | S12 |

recommends the collection of any of them for culinary purposes. Muscarine is the toxic principle found in all poisonous *Inocybe* species which have been examined. Although concentrations of this toxin vary in the different species, the type of poisoning is identical in all cases, obviating the necessity of species differentiation in this treatment.

The muscarine content of a number of species of *Inocybe* occurring in the United States has been determined chromatographically by Brown (B8). His findings are summarized in the following list in which the name of the species investigated is followed by the average determined percentage of muscarine, calculated on a dry weight basis:

*I. napipes* Lange, 0.73%; *I lilacina* (Boud.) Kauff., 0.38%; *I. agglutinata* Peck, 0.32%; *I. umbrina* Bres., 0.27%; *I. sororia* Kauff., 0.13–0.28%; *I. subdestricta* Kauff., 0.22%; *I. griseolilacina* Lange, 0.17%; *I. pudica* Kühn., 0.13–0.17%; *I. geophylla* (Fr.) Karst. var. *geophylla*, 0.16%; *I. pallidipes* Ellis & Everhart sensu Kauff., 0.16%; *I. mixtilis* (Britz.) Sacc. sensu Kühn., 0.10%; *I. lacera* (Fr.) Quél., 0.08%; *I. terrifera* Kühn., 0.08%; *I. cinnamomea* A. H. Smith, 0.03%.

Muscarine could not be detected by the same method in the following species:

*I. albodisca* Peck; *I. griseoscabrosa* (Peck) Earle; *I. hirsuta* var. *maxima* A. H. Smith; *I. nigrescens* Atk.; *I. picrosma* Stuntz; *I. subexilis* (Peck) Sacc.; *I. xanthomelas* Boursier & Kühn. in Kühn.

Species from which European investigators (E3, E6) have isolated muscarine and reported their results on a fresh weight basis include (*sic*) *I. patouillardi* (Bres.), 0.037%; *I. fastigiata* (Fr. ex Sch.) Quél., 0.01%; and *I. umbrina* (Bres.), 0.003%. Muscarine could not be detected in *I. bongardi* (Weinm.) Quél.

Loup (L6) had previously detected muscarine in more than twenty species of *Inocybe* by means of physiological tests.

### 12. *Lactarius* SPECIES

Relatively large, fleshy, often brittle plants which exude a mild or acrid latex (white or colored) when broken. The stipe is central, continuous with flesh of pileus. The spores are strongly amyloid, and sphaerocysts are present in the flesh of the stipe. Many species are recognizable in the field, since microscopic characteristics are usually nonessential. Most mild-tasting species are nonpoisonous, but a number of the acrid varieties are either poisonous, inedible, or edible only after special preparation during the cooking process. Several such acrid species are listed by various authors as poisonous or suspect but, since little specific information is available concerning them, they are not accorded tabular

TABLE XI

CHARACTERIZATION OF *Lactarius* SPECIES

| Species | Outstanding botanical characteristics | Relative toxicity | Comments | References |
|---|---|---|---|---|
| *L. glaucescens* Crossland | White pileus with extremely fine, crowded gills. Peppery latex turns green. | + to ++ | Cooked specimens produced severe gastro-intestinal disturbances resulting in death of child and extreme nausea and prolonged abdominal pain in adult. | C5, C12 |
| *L. helvus* (Fr.) Fr. | Tawny, buff-colored, dry floccose-squamulose, fragile pileus with aromatic odor which persists on drying. Watery, rarely white latex. | + | Weakly toxic. Eaten in quantity it produces nausea, diarrhea, and diaphoresis in 15–60 minutes following ingestion. Complications are ordinarily absent. The dried, powdered mushroom is used in small amounts as a condiment in Europe. Illustration (M4, P2). | C12, M4, P2 |
| *L. rufus* (Scop. ex Fr.) Fr. | Pileus bright red-brown, dry, umbonate, with very acrid, white latex. | + | Classified as a poisonous mushroom by most American authors. Apparently edible after special treatment (cut in small pieces, soak overnight in water, parboil, discard the cooking water, and rinse). Illustration (M4, P2). | K1, M4, P2, S10 |
| *L. torminosus* (Schaeff. ex Fr.) Gray | Pileus pinkish yellow or ochraceous, zoned on surface, with tomentose fringed margin. Acrid white latex does not change color. | + to ++ | Poisonous when raw but declared edible when prepared as described for *L. rufus*. Extracts of raw mushroom produced fatal acute intoxication in guinea pigs and rabbits. Boiling the extract destroyed its toxicity. Fatalities in children have been reported from ingestion of raw mushrooms. Illustration (M4, P2). | F6, K1, M4, P2 |
| *L. uvidus* (Fr. ex Fr.) Fr. | Viscid pileus, gray with black tinge or brownish gray. Flesh whitish, becoming lilac or violet when cut. Acrid white latex, rapidly changing to violet when in contact with flesh. | ± | Reported toxic to man. Extract acutely poisonous to guinea pigs but no effect upon rabbits. Illustration (R4). | F6, K1, R4 |

listing. These include *L. fuliginosus* (Fr. ex Fr.) Fr., *L. lignyotus* Fr.,
*L. pyrogalus* (Bull. ex Secr.) Fr., *L. scrobiculatus* (Scop. ex Fr.) Fr.,
*L. trivialis* (Fr. ex Fr.) Fr., and *L. vellereus* (Fr.) Fr. (Table XI).

## 13. *Lepiota* SPECIES

The mushrooms are characterized by a typically white (one exception) spore deposit, free gills, and central stipe. Members of this genus
possess an annulus but lack a volva. Many of the approximately 100
species which occur in the United States are edible and excellent. At
least one is poisonous to certain individuals. The chromatographic evidence for α-amanitin (B4) in *L. cretacea* (Bull.) Morg. [properly *L.
cepaestipes* (Sow. ex Fr.) Kummer (S13)] is not substantial and requires
verification. However, the genus is closely related botanically to *Amanita*,
and at least one European species (*L. helveola* Bres. sensu Joss.) produces poisoning similar to that of *A. phalloides* (J3) (Table XII).

## 14. *Panaeolus* SPECIES

Members of this genus are characterized by a black spore deposit and
attached, nondeliquescing gills which are often spotted by maturing
spores. The stipe is central; a veil may be present but is frequently
evanescent. Identification of the species is difficult for the specialist and
impossible for the layman.

Species of *Panaeolus* have long been thought to produce, on ingestion, a peculiar type of intoxication characterized by mental disturbances
(F8). Although Heim and Wasson (H2) have reported the isolation of
the psychotropic principle psilocybin from one species, *Panaeolus sphinctrinus* (Fr.) Quél., a chromatographic investigation of nine additional
species and varieties by Tyler and Smith (T6) failed to detect this compound or any known hallucinogenic principle in any of them. *Panaeolus*
species are characterized by the presence of relatively large amounts of
serotonin, its precursor 5-hydroxytryptophan, and related compounds,
but these cannot account for the reported cases of poisoning. A very
slight muscarinic activity has been found in extracts of *P. campanulatus*
(L. ex Fr.) Quél. (T5).

It seems probable to conclude that most of the psychotomimetic disturbances attributed to the ingestion of mushrooms of this species have
resulted from misidentifications and confusion with other dark-spored
agarics, particularly with species of the genus *Psilocybe*, section Caerulescentes, which are known to contain psilocybin.

Species of *Panaeolus* which may induce psychotropic manifestations
in the human being include:

*P. fimicola* (Fr.) Gill. (W3); *P. papilionaceus* (Bull. p. p. ex Fr. p. p.

TABLE XII

CHARACTERIZATION OF *Lepiota* SPECIES

| Species | Outstanding botanical characteristics | Relative toxicity | Comments | References |
|---|---|---|---|---|
| *L. molybdites* (Meyer ex Fr.) Sacc. [*L. morgani* (Peck) Sacc., *Chlorophyllum molybdites* (Meyer ex Fr.) Mass. (S5)] | Readily distinguished by unusual green color of spore deposit and by slate-green gills of mature specimens. | − to + + | Undoubtedly poisonous to some persons, producing mild to severe gastrointestinal disturbances characterized by emesis, diarrhea, and mental haziness. Eaten by others with impunity. Raw mushrooms reported fatal to child. Raw juice *per os* fatal to rabbit, but subcutaneous injection of extract into mice was without effect. Illustration (S12, T1). | B4, C6, G2, S10, S12, S16, T1 |

TABLE XIII

CHARACTERIZATION OF *Paxillus* SPECIES

| Species | Outstanding botanical characteristics | Relative toxicity | Comments | References |
|---|---|---|---|---|
| *P. involutus* (Batsch ex Fr.) Fr. | Broad brownish pileus with margin involute at first, then furrowed or ridged. Gills yellowish, decurrent, crowded, anastomosing or reticulated-porose on stem. Both gills and the yellow flesh become brownish when bruised. Stem centric or eccentric, enlarged at base. | ± | Poisonous when raw, produces gastric disturbances. Apparently edible after thorough cooking but of poor quality. Illustration (M4, P2). | K1, M4, P2 |

em. Fr. 1838) Quél. (N1); *P. retirugis* (Fr.) Quél. (D6); *P. subbalteatus* (Berk. & Br.) Sacc. [*P. venenosus* Murr.] (S14, S15) [but known psychotropic principles were not detected chromatographically in this species (T6)]; *P. sphinctrinus* (Fr.) Quél. (H2) (contains psilocybin).

## 15. *Paxillus* SPECIES

Species are characterized by a fleshy pileus with confluent stem tending to be eccentric or sometimes lacking. Gills are usually decurrent, anastomosing on the stem, and easily separable from the trama of the pileus. Spores are brownish (Table XIII).

## 16. *Psilocybe* SPECIES

The mushrooms are characterized by a dull-colored, convex to campanulate pileus with the margin incurved at first. Later the pileus may expand until it is quite plane. The gills are adnexed to adnate-subdecurrent; spores are purplish brown. The stipe is rigid-fragile or tough with a cartilaginous cortex. A veil is usually scarcely noticeable or lacking. Many of the toxic (hallucinogenic) species of *Psilocybe* belong to the section Caerulescentes and are characterized by the formation of a bluish color when wounded, in age, or on drying (S8). Species differentiation requires expert knowledge, but it is not necessary to present the details here since the active principles of all investigated species are similar.

Interest in the hallucinogenic fungi of Mexico (W2) culminated with the isolation of the 4-substituted tryptamines psilocybin and psilocin from *Psilocybe mexicana* Heim in 1958 (H5). Since that time, a number of species of the genus, mostly of Mexican origin but some occurring in the United States, have been reported to possess psychotomimetic activity. All species subjected to chemical studies have been found to contain psilocybin and/or psilocin.

Wasson has enumerated the *Psilocybe* species employed as hallucinogens by the Mexican Indians (W3): *P. acutissima* Heim; *P. aztecorum* Heim; *P. caerulescens* Murr., four varieties and forms; *P. caerulipes* (Peck) Sacc. var. *gastonii* Sing. & A. H. Smith; *P. candidipes* Sing. & A. H. Smith; *P. cordispora* Heim; *P. cubensis* (Earle) Sing.; *P. fagicola* Heim & Cailleux; *P. hoogshagenii* Heim; *P. isauri* Sing., *P. mexicana* Heim; *P. mixaeensis* Heim; *P. semperviva* Heim & Cailleux; *P. wassonii* Heim; *P. yungensis* Sing. & A. H. Smith; *P. zapotecorum* Heim and its var. *elongata* Heim.

In addition, *Psilocybe pelliculosa* A. H. Smith has been found to contain psilocybin (T4). There are several species of genera other than *Psilocybe* which possess similar psychotropic activity and which may contain the same active principles. These include certain *Panaeolus* species which have been treated previously, *Conocybe siligineoides* Heim, *Psathyrella sepulchralis* Sing., A. H. Smith & Guzmán, and *Russula nondorbingi* Sing.

Because of the relatively small size and unappetizing appearance of most hallucinogenic *Psilocybe* species, cases of accidental poisoning by them are not as common as the rather appreciable number of such species might seem to warrant.

## 17. *Rhodophyllus* Species

Members of this genus are characterized principally by flesh-colored angular spores and the lack of both an annulus and a volva. The genus includes the genera *Eccilia, Entoloma, Leptonia, Nolanea,* and the angular-spored species of *Claudopus* and *Clitopilus* of the Friesian classification. Species identification in this genus is very difficult for the professional mycologist. Many species are suspected to be poisonous; at least one is very toxic (Table XIV).

## 18. *Russula* Species

These are typically fragile or hard, thick-stemmed mushrooms with strongly amyloid, verrucose to reticulate spores. Their flesh is composed of nests of sphaerocysts and connective tissue. Latex is absent, as is a pronounced veil in all American species. Recognition of the genus is comparatively simple, but exact identification of its species is difficult. All mild-tasting *Russula* species are probably edible. Those with bitter or acrid tastes should be avoided. One tropical species, *R. nondorbingi* Sing., is said to be employed by the natives of New Guinea as an inebriant (S7), but this activity has not been reported in any North American species (Table XV).

## 19. *Tricholoma* Species

Species of this genus have white spores, a central fleshy stipe which is confluent with the pileus, and adnexed to sinuate gills. Both a volva and a membranous annulus are lacking. *Tricholoma* species are difficult to recognize, and a number are either poisonous (gastrointestinal disturbances) or suspect (Table XVI).

Varro E. Tyler, Jr.

TABLE XIV

CHARACTERIZATION OF *Rhodophyllus* SPECIES

| Species | Outstanding botanical characteristics | Relative toxicity | Comments | References |
|---|---|---|---|---|
| *R. murraii* (Berk. & Curt.) Sing. [*Entoloma cuspidatum* (Peck) Sacc.] | Broad, conical, pale yellow pileus bearing an elongated papilla at apex. Narrowly adnate gills, pale yellow at first, then turning flesh color. Thick, hollow, pale yellow stipe. | ? | Injection of extract killed guinea pig in 12 days but had no action on rabbits. Reported edible for man but needs further study. Illustration (K1). | F6, K1 |
| *R. nidorosus* (Fr.) Quél. | Broad, grayish brown, hygrophanous pileus with fragile white flesh. Flesh-colored gills are broad, subdistant, and adnexed to whitish stipe. Odor strongly acid or alkaline. | ? | Injection of extract fatal to guinea pigs after 6–15 days but had no effect upon rabbits. Edibility for man is unknown. Illustration (R4). | F6, K1, R4 |
| *R. rhodopolius* (Fr.) Quél. | Pileus campanulate, firm, hygrophanous, umber to fuscous, with pale livid-gray glabrous cuticle. Flesh watery, then white. Broad, subdistant rose-colored gills are adnate, becoming emarginate. Stipe glabrous, pure white. No odor or taste. | ? | Injection of extract slowly fatal to guinea pigs but had no effect upon rabbits. Reported edible for human beings. Needs investigation. Illustration (K1). | F6, K1 |
| *R. salmoneus* (Peck) Sing. | Pileus broad, conic-papillate, orange-salmon with (at times) greenish disc. Broad adnexed gills are salmon-colored as is the long stipe (often tinged with green). Odor and taste are mild. May be a color variety of *R. murraii.* | ? | Injection of extract fatal to guinea pig in 3 days. No effect upon rabbits. Edibility for man is unknown. Illustration (H4) as *Entoloma salmoneum.* | F6, H4, K1 |
| *R. sinuatus* (Bull. ex Fr.) Sing. [*R. lividus* (Bull. | Yellowish brown pileus is lubricous to subviscid, losing water very slowly, not typically hygrophanous. Gills adnexed. | ++ | Produces violent gastrointestinal upsets following ingestion by human beings. Vomiting, diarrhea, abdominal pains, | F6, J3, K1, M4, P2, R4, S10 |

| Species | Outstanding botanical characteristics | Relative toxicity | Comments | References |
|---|---|---|---|---|
| ex Fr.) Quél., *Entoloma sinuatum* Fr., *E. lividum* Quél.] | Stipe white, glabrous. Odor faint. Taste strongly farinaceous. | | headache, thirst, and great weakness commence within 1 hour and subside slowly over a period of several days. Some liver damage may result. Death is infrequent but has been observed, especially in children. Injection of extract fatal to guinea pig after 12 days but had no effect on rabbits. Chemical nature of toxic principle(s) unknown. Illustration (M4, P2, R4). | |
| *R. strictior* (Peck) Sing. [*Entoloma strictius* (Peck) Sacc.] | Pileus broad, more or less umbonate, hygrophanous, olive-buff to brown. Broad ventricose gills, pallid, becoming rosy-incarnate. Stipe dingy, usually twisted, splits easily. Odor farinaceous, slight. | ? | Injections of extract fatal to both guinea pigs and rabbits. Edibility for human beings is unknown. Illustration (K1, M4). | F6, K1, M4 |

TABLE XV

CHARACTERIZATION OF *Russula* SPECIES

| Species | Outstanding botanical characteristics | Relative toxicity | Comments | References |
|---|---|---|---|---|
| *R. emetica* Schaeff. ex S. F. Gray (G3) | Pileus fleshy, fragile, rosy to blood-red, margin strongly tubercular-striate. Flesh white but red under cuticle. Gills pure white, narrowly adnexed or free. Stipe white or slightly reddish. Spores white. Taste very acrid. | + | Muscarinic activity detected in extract. Ingestion of raw mushroom causes prompt gastrointestinal upsets (emesis). Supposedly edible after parboiling. Caution. Illustration (M4). | B1, F9, G3, K1, M4, S10 |

TABLE XVI

CHARACTERIZATION OF *Tricholoma* SPECIES

| Species | Outstanding botanical characteristics | Relative toxicity | Comments | References |
|---|---|---|---|---|
| *T. album* (Schaeff. ex Fr.) Quél. | Pileus glabrous, entirely white or sometimes yellowish. Flesh tough, gills white, unchanging. Stem thick, solid, elastic. No odor but acrid taste. | ? | Inedible or toxic, needs investigation. Illustration (P3). | J3, K1, P3 |
| *T. pardinum* Quél. | Grayish, fine fibrillose squamules on pileus. Flesh white, stipe white, smooth. | ++ | Produces violent gastrointestinal disturbances similar to those caused by *Rhodophyllus sinuatus*. Illustration (M4, S12). | M4, S12 |
| *T. saponaceum* (Fr.) Quél. | Pileus brown to grayish, often olive-tinged. Flesh white, becoming pinkish. Gills distant, whitish. Stipe white, becoming pink within. Odor and taste strongly soapy. | + | Practically inedible (distasteful) but harmless in small quantities. Ingestion of larger amounts produces nausea and vomiting. Illustration (M4). | K1, M4 |
| *T. sulphureum* (Bull. ex Fr.) Quél. | Pileus at first sulfur-yellow, later brownish red over disc. Gills rather distant, sulfur-yellow. Stipe same color. Odor and taste strong, repulsive. | + | Assumed mildly toxic, certainly inedible. Illustration (M4). | J3, M4 |
| *T. venenatum* Atk. | Pileus pale buff to clay-color, minutely scaly. Flesh white, gills whitish, dull clay-color when bruised. Stipe subbulbous, whitish, becoming darker when bruised. Odor and taste mild. | ++ | Produces rather violent poisoning. Gastrointestinal symptoms, characterized by vomiting, retching, and some prostration, occur 1 hour after ingestion. | F2, K1 |
| *T. virgatum* (Fr.) Gill. | Grayish streaked, conic pileus. Flesh white, becoming ash-color. Gills close, whitish, becoming grayish. Stipe whitish. Odor earthy, taste slowly but strongly acrid. | + | Assumed mildly toxic, certainly inedible. Illustration (M4). | M4, S10 |

REFERENCES

(A1) Ahronheim, J. H. *J. Michigan State Med. Soc.* **37**, 921 (1938).
(A2) Alder, A. E. *Schweiz. Z. Pilzkunde* **26**, 17 (1948).
(A3) Alder, A. E. *Schweiz. Z. Pilzkunde* **38**, 65 (1960).
(A4) Alder, A. E. *Deut. Med. Wochschr.* **86**, 1121 (1961).
(A5) Atkinson, G. F. "Mushrooms Edible, Poisonous, Etc." Andrus & Church, Ithaca, New York, 1900.
(B1) Balenović, K., Cerar, D., Pučar, Z., and Škarić, V. *Arhiv Kem.* **27**, 15 (1955).
(B2) Birch, C. A. *Practitioner* **157**, 135 (1946).
(B3) Block, S. S., Stephens, R. L., Barreto, A., and Murrill, W. A. *Science* **121**, 505 (1955).
(B4) Block, S. S., Stephens, R. L., and Murrill, W. A. *J. Agr. Food Chem.* **3**, 584 (1955).
(B5) Boehm, R. *Arch. Exptl. Pathol. Pharmakol.* **19**, 60 (1885).
(B6) Boehm, R., and Külz, E. *Arch. Exptl. Pathol. Pharmakol.* **19**, 403 (1885).
(B7) Brady, L. R., and Tyler, V. E., Jr. *J. Am. Pharm. Assoc. Sci. Ed.* **48**, 417 (1959).
(B8) Brown, J. K. "An Investigation of the Muscarine Content of *Inocybe* Species." M.S. Thesis, University of Washington, Seattle, Washington, 1962.
(B9) Buck, R. W. *New Engl. J. Med.* **265**, 681 (1961).
(C1) Caglieri, G. E. *Med. Record* **52**, 298 (1897).
(C2) Cann, H. M., and Verhulst, H. L. *Am. J. Diseases Children* **101**, 128 (1961).
(C3) Catalfomo, P., and Tyler, V. E., Jr. *J. Pharm. Sci.* **50**, 689 (1961).
(C4) Cerletti, E. *Deut. Med. Wochschr.* **84**, 2317 (1959).
(C5) Charles, V. K. *Mycologia* **34**, 112 (1942).
(C6) Chestnut, V. K. *Asa Gray Bull.* **8**, 87 (1900).
(C7) Child, G. F. *Mycologia* **44**, 200 (1952).
(C8) Clark, E. D., and Smith, C. S. *Mycologia* **5**, 224 (1913).
(C9) Clark, M., Marshall, E. K., Jr., and Rowntree, L. G. *J. Am. Med. Assoc.* **64**, 1230 (1915).
(C10) Collins, F. S. *Rhodora* **1**, 21 (1899).
(C11) Coker, W. C. *J. Elisha Mitchell Sci. Soc.* **33**, 3 (1917).
(C12) Coker, W. C. *J. Elisha Mitchell Sci. Soc.* **34**, 1 (1918).
(C13) Coker, W. C. "The Clavarias of the United States and Canada." Univ. of North Carolina Press, Chapel Hill, North Carolina, 1923.
(C14) Cook, C. D., and Haggerty, R. J. *New Engl. J. Med.* **262**, 832 (1960).
(C15) Cook, K. F. *Mycologia* **46**, 24 (1954).
(C16) Costa, P. J., and Dews, M. J. *Am. J. Nursing* **56**, 998 (1956).
(D1) Dearness, J. *Mycologia* **3**, 75 (1911).
(D2) Dearness, J. *Mycologia* **16**, 199 (1924).
(D3) Dearness, J. *Mycologia* **27**, 85 (1935).
(D4) Denis, A. *Bull. Trimestr. Soc. Mycol. France* **77**, 64 (1961).
(D5) Doty, M. S. "Clavaria, the Species Known From Oregon and the Pacific Northwest." Oregon State College Press, Corvallis, Oregon, 1944.
(D6) Douglass, B. *Torreya* **17**, 171 (1917).
(D7) Dubash, J., and Teare, D. *Brit. Med. J.* **1**, 45 (1946).
(D8) Dujarric de la Rivière, R., and Heim, R. "Les Champignons Toxiques." Encyclopédie Medico-Chirurgicale, Paris, France, 1938.

(E1) Elliott, W., Hall, M., Kerr, D. N. S., Rolland, C. F., Smart, G. A., and Swinney, J. *Lancet* **281**, 630 (1961).
(E2) Eugster, C. H. *Helv. Chim. Acta* **39**, 1002 (1956).
(E3) Eugster, C. H. *Helv. Chim. Acta* **40**, 886 (1957).
(E4) Eugster, C. H. *Helv. Chim. Acta* **40**, 2562 (1957).
(E5) Eugster, C. H. *Rev. Mycol.* **24**, 369 (1959).
(E6) Eugster, C. H., and Müller, G. *Helv. Chim. Acta* **42**, 1189 (1959).
(E7) Eugster, C. H., and Waser, P. G. *Experientia* **10**, 298 (1954).
(F1) Farlow, W. G. *Rhodora* **1**, 43 (1899).
(F2) Fischer, O. E. *In* "The Agaricaceae of Michigan" (C. H. Kauffman, ed.), Vol. 1, p. 825. Michigan Geol. and Biol. Survey, Publ. 26, Biol. Ser. 5, Lansing, Michigan, 1918.
(F3) Ford, W. W. *Bull. Johns Hopkins Hosp.* **18**, 123 (1907).
(F4) Ford, W. W. *Science* **30**, 97 (1909).
(F5) Ford, W. W. *J. Pharmacol. Exptl. Therap.* **1**, 275 (1909).
(F6) Ford, W. W. *J. Pharmacol. Exptl. Therap.* **2**, 285 (1911).
(F7) Ford, W. W. *In* "Legal Medicine and Toxicology" (F. Peterson, W. S. Haines, and R. W. Webster, eds.), 2nd ed., Vol. II, p. 817. Saunders, Philadelphia, Pennsylvania, 1923.
(F8) Ford, W. W. *J. Pharmacol. Exptl. Therap.* **29**, 305 (1926).
(F9) Ford, W. W., and Clark, E. D. *Mycologia* **6**, 167 (1914).
(F10) Ford, W. W., and Sherrick, J. L. *J. Pharmacol. Exptl. Therap.* **2**, 549 (1911).
(F11) Ford, W. W., and Sherrick, J. L. *J. Pharmacol. Exptl. Therap.* **4**, 321 (1913).
(F12) Forster, E. *J. Boston Med. Surg. J.* **123**, 267 (1890).
(F13) Friese, W. *Pharm. Zentralhalle* **89**, 37 (1950).
(G1) Gilbert, E. J. *Iconographia Mycol.* **27**, 1 (1940).
(G2) Graff, P. W. *Mycologia* **19**, 322 (1927).
(G3) Gray, S. F. "A Natural Arrangement of British Plants," Vol. I, p. 618. Baldwin, Cradock, and Joy, London, 1821.
(G4) Grossman, C. M., and Malbin, B. *Ann. Internal Med.* **40**, 249 (1954).
(H1) Heim, R., and Hofmann, A. *Compt. Rend. Acad. Sci.* **247**, 557 (1958).
(H2) Heim, R., and Wasson, R. G. "Les Champignons Hallucinogènes du Mexique." Muséum National d'Histoire Naturelle, Paris, France, 1958.
(H3) Hendricks, H. V. *J. Am. Med. Assoc.* **114**, 1625 (1940).
(H4) Hesler, L. R. "Mushrooms of the Great Smokies." Univ. of Tennessee Press, Knoxville, Tennessee, 1960.
(H5) Hofmann, A., Heim, R., Brack, A., and Kobel, H. *Experientia* **14**, 107 (1958).
(H6) Hofmann, A., Heim, R., Brack, A., Kobel, H., Frey, A., Ott, H., Petrzilka, T., and Troxler, F. *Helv. Chim. Acta* **42**, 1557 (1959).
(H7) Horita, A., and Weber, L. *J. Biochem. Pharmacol.* **7**, 47 (1961).
(H8) Hotson, J. W. *Mycologia* **26**, 194 (1934).
(J1) Jelliffe, S. E. *N. Y. State J. Med.* **37**, 1357 (1937).
(J2) Jenkins, A. E. *Mycologia* **52**, 521 (1960).
(J3) Jahn, H. "Pilze rundum." Park-Verlag, Hamburg, Germany, 1949.
(K1) Kauffman, C. H. "The Agaricaceae of Michigan," Vols. I and II. Michigan Geol. and Biol. Survey, Publ. 26, Biol. Ser. 5, Lansing, Michigan, 1918.
(K2) Kessler, A. *Am. J. Med. Sci.* **80**, 393 (1880).
(K3) Kögl, F., Cox, H. C., and Salemink, C. A. *Ann. Chem.* **608**, 81 (1957).
(K4) Kögl, F., Salemink, C. A., Schouten, H., and Jellinek, F. *Rec. Trav. Chim.* **76**, 109 (1957).

(K5) Kögl, F., Salemink, C. A., and Schuller, P. L. *Rec. Trav. Chim.* **79**, 278 (1960).
(K6) Konrad, P., and Maublanc, A. "Icones selectae Fungorum," Vol. 1. Paul Lechevalier, Paris, 1924–1930.
(K7) Krieger, L. C. C. *Mycologia* **3**, 200 (1911).
(K8) Krieger, L. C. C. "The Mushroom Handbook." Macmillan, New York, 1936.
(K9) Kwasniewski, V. *Deut. Apotheker Ztg.* **94**, 1177 (1954).
(L1) Lewis, B. S. *African Med. J.* **29**, 262 (1955).
(L2) Limousin, H., and Petit, G. *Bull. Acad. Natl. Med. (Paris)* **107**, 698 (1932).
(L3) List, P. H. *Planta Med.* **8**, 383 (1960).
(L4) List, P. H. *Arzneimittel-Forsch.* **10**, 34 (1960).
(L5) Locket, S. "Clinical Toxicology." Mosby, St. Louis, Missouri, 1957.
(L6) Loup, C. "Contribution a l'Étude Toxicologique de Trente-Trois Inocybe de la Région de Genève." Thesis, Docteur en Médecine-Dentaire, University of Geneva, Geneva, Switzerland, 1938.
(M1) McIlvaine, C. *Med. Surg. Reptr.* **53**, 684, 713 (1885).
(M2) McIlvaine, C., Macadam, R. K., and Millspaugh, C. F. "One Thousand American Fungi," new ed. Bobbs-Merrill, Indianapolis, Indiana, 1912.
(M3) Malone, M. Personal communication (1961).
(M4) Michael, E., and Hennig, B. "Handbuch für Pilzfreunde," Vols. I and II. Fischer, Jena, Germany, 1958–1960.
(M5) Murrill, W. A. *Mycologia* **1**, 211 (1909).
(M6) Murrill, W. A. *Mycologia* **33**, 434 (1941).
(M7) Murrill, W. A. *Mycologia* **37**, 270 (1945).
(M8) Murrill, W. A. *Quart. J. Florida Acad. Sci.* **8**, 175 (1945).
(M9) Murrill, W. A. *Mycologia* **45**, 794 (1953).
(N1) Neuhoff, W. *Z. Pilzkunde* **24**, 87 (1958).
(P1) Peck, C. H. *Mycologia* **5**, 67 (1913).
(P2) Pilát, A., and Ušák, O. "Mushrooms." H. W. Bijl, Amsterdam, 1954.
(P3) Pilát, A., and Ušák, O. "Naše Houby II." Nakladatelství Československé Akademie věd, Prague, Czechoslovakia, 1959.
(P4) Porcher, F. P. *Trans. Am. Med. Assoc.* **7**, 167 (1854).
(P5) Prentiss, D. W. *Phil. Med. J.* **2**, 607 (1898).
(R1) Ramsbottom, J. "Mushrooms and Toadstools." Collins, London, 1954.
(R2) Ridgway, R. "Color Standards and Color Nomenclature." Published by the Author, Washington, D. C., 1912.
(R3) Roberts, J. W. *Mycologia* **13**, 42 (1921).
(R4) Romagnesi, H. "Nouvel Atlas des Champignons," Vols. I–III. Bordas, Paris, 1956–1961.
(S1) Sartory, A., and Maire, L. "Les Champignons Vénéneux." Librairie le François, Paris, France, 1921.
(S2) Schmiedeberg, O., and Koppe, R. "Das Muscarin." Vogel, Leipzig, Germany, 1869.
(S3) Simandl, J., and Franc, J. *Chem. Listy* **50**, 1862 (1956).
(S4) Singer, R. *Mycologia* **48**, 768 (1945).
(S5) Singer, R. *Lilloa* **22**, 5 (1949).
(S6) Singer, R. *Mycologia* **50**, 239 (1958).
(S7) Singer, R. *Mycopathol. Mycol. Appl.* **9**, 275 (1958).
(S8) Singer, R., and Smith, A. H. *Mycologia* **50**, 262 (1958).
(S9) Smith, A. H. *Papers Mich. Acad. Sci.* **24**, 107 (1939).

(S10) Smith, A. H. "Mushrooms in Their Natural Habitats." Sawyer's, Portland, Oregon, 1949.
(S11) Smith, A. H. *Mycologia* **45,** 892 (1953).
(S12) Smith, A. H. "The Mushroom Hunter's Field Guide." Univ. of Michigan Press, Ann Arbor, Michigan, 1958.
(S13) Smith, H. V. *Lloydia* **17,** 307 (1954).
(S14) Stein, S. I. *Mycologia* **51,** 49 (1959).
(S15) Stein, S. I., Closs, G. L., and Gabel, N. W. *Mycopathol. Mycol. Appl.* **11,** 205 (1959).
(S16) Stevens, F. L. *J. Mycol.* **9,** 220 (1903).
(S17) Stuhlfauth, K., and Jung, F. *Arch. Toxicol.* **14,** 86 (1952).
(T1) Thomas, W. S. "Field Book of Common Mushrooms," 3rd ed. Putnam, New York, 1948.
(T2) Trask, J. D. *Am. J. Med. Sci.* **85,** 358 (1883).
(T3) Tyler, V. E., Jr. *Am. J. Pharm.* **130,** 264 (1958).
(T4) Tyler, V. E., Jr. *Lloydia* **24,** 71 (1961).
(T5) Tyler, V. E., Jr., and Malone, M. H. *J. Am. Pharm. Assoc. Sci. Ed.* **49,** 23 (1960).
(T6) Tyler, V. E., Jr., and Smith, A. H. In press.
(V1) Vander Veer, J. B., and Farley, D. L. *A.M.A. Arch. Internal Med.* **55,** 773 (1935).
(V2) Verhulst, H. L. Personal communication (1961).
(W1) Waser, P. G. *Experientia* **11,** 452 (1955).
(W2) Wasson, R. G. *Trans. N. Y. Acad. Sci.* Ser. II, **21,** 325 (1959).
(W3) Wasson, R. G. *Botan. Museum Leaflets, Harvard Univ.* **19,** 137 (1961).
(W4) Wasson, V. P., and Wasson, R. G. "Mushrooms, Russia and History," Vols. I and II. Pantheon, New York, 1957.
(W5) Weber, F. C. *Schweiz. Z. Pilzkunde* **38,** 20 (1960).
(W6) Wieland, T. *Helv. Chim. Acta* **44,** 919 (1961).
(W7) Wieland, T., and Motzel, W. *Ann. Chem.* **581,** 10 (1953).
(W8) Wieland, T., and Wieland, O. *Pharmacol. Revs.* **11,** 87 (1959).
(W9) Wier, J. K., and Tyler, V. E., Jr. *J. Am. Pharm. Assoc. Sci. Ed.* **49,** 426 (1960).
(W10) Wilkinson, S. *Quart. Revs.* (*London*) **15,** 153 (1961).
(Z1) Zeller, S. M. *Mycologia* **30,** 468 (1938).
(Z2) Zellner, J. "Chemie der höheren Pilze." Engelmann, Leipzig, Germany, 1907.

# Poisonous Seeds and Fruits

by Arthur E. Schwarting

*School of Pharmacy, University of Connecticut, Storrs, Connecticut*

## I. Introduction

Plants which are poisonous are so qualified because some or all parts of their structure have accumulated one or more poisonous chemical substances. A variety of seeds and fruits are common entries in lists of poisonous plants and, in terms of frequency of cause of human poisoning, these parts are cited more often than other parts. This frequency is accountable and several reasons are worthy of consideration.

Seeds and fruits represent a virtual storehouse for a number of primary (carbohydrate, protein, lipid) and secondary (alkaloid, glycoside, volatile terpenoid) constituents, generally reaching levels of accumulation higher than those in other tissues. In a few instances a poisonous principle is essentially localized in these parts (ricin in *Ricinus communis*, coniine in *Conium maculatum*). More generally, however, a toxic component of a fruit or seed is also found in other organs of the plant (atropine in *Datura* spp., hydrocyanic acid in *Prunus* spp.). Although the absolute quantities, in such diversification, may be in favor of the leaf, root, bark, etc., the percentage concentration is usually higher in the seed or fruit.

This differential accumulation is acknowledged in agricultural practices involving the harvest of forage crops. A harvest is usually made in advance of fruit maturation of "weeds" in the crop, the herbage of such plants being regarded as nonpoisonous. Certain weed seeds associated

385

with cultivated grains have been shown to be toxic to domestic animals (T2).

Fruits, with their component seeds, are frequently colorful and attractive. Fruits frequently persist and become manifest structures on leafless stems. These features are of some significance in assessing a reason for poisoning of children and novices. The brilliant red "berry" of ornamental *Taxus* spp. contains the poisonous alkaloid complex, taxine, in the seed; poisonous grapelike seeds of *Caulophyllum thalictroides* appear in woodlands in the season when wild grapes are collected.

Occasionally succulent fruits or seed coats serve as a "decoy" for poison-containing seeds. The nonseed component, being edible and on occasion tasty and nutritious, harbors the lethal seed. The cyanide-containing embryo of the seed of the fruit of *Prunus* spp. (almond, wild cherry, etc.) and the edible red aril of yew (*Taxus spp.*) seed are examples of such structures.

The collection of "edible" foods from woodland plants is a primary cause of accidental poisoning. Although the taste sensation of the majority of poisonous seeds or fruits is that of bitterness, acridness, or astringency, children appear to be not particularly fastidious in their taste discrimination.

Among the numerous fruits and seeds regarded as poisonous, a considerable number are rendered innocuous upon cooking and roasting. Others, particularly seeds, do not readily liberate their toxic components in the digestive tract—in normal passage—unless they are chewed or otherwise broken. The testa of deadly nightshade seed (*Atropa belladonna*) and jequirity (*Abrus precatorius*) are highly impermeable.

## II. Definitions and Distinctions

The fruit is a matured ovary containing the seed. This organ includes such diverse structures as a peapod, corn grain, banana, tomato, and watermelon. Common usage of the term is in conflict with the technical definition; peas are vegetables not fruits—only sweet pulpy fruits are such by popular usage of the term.

Many kinds of fruits exist. The basic classification includes soft pulpy (*fleshy*) or papery hard (*dry*) structures. *Berries* (grapes, oranges) and *drupes* (peaches, olives) are common fleshy fruits while *achenes* (sunflower), *grains* (cereal "seeds"), *nuts* (walnut, hazelnut), *legumes* (pea, bean), and *capsules* (poppy, iris) are examples of dry fruits. Fruits are also classified according to the number and origin of ovaries and on the basis of adhering or enclosed accessory parts of the ovary.

The *sclereid* or the lignified sclerenchyma tissue of the *pericarp* is a significant characteristic cell structure of most fruit tissues. Stomata, papilla, and cell inclusions offer additional characteristics useful in distinguishing fruit tissues by histological features.

The seed is a matured ovule: an undeveloped plant (*embryo*), usually with a food storage tissue (*endosperm*) and a coat (*testa* and, in some, an additional layer, the *tegmen*). In some seeds (bean, sunflower) the endosperm is absorbed and is lacking in the mature tissue (*exalbuminous* seed); in others (cereal grains, castor) the endosperm is present (*albuminous seeds*). A small scar (*hilum*) on the seed coat is the attachment site; the pollen grain entrance pore (*micropyle*) is visible in some seeds.

The characteristic features of a seed are found in the histological details of the testa including such layers as the *palisade* (polygonal cells), *sclereid* (thick-walled, sometimes lignified cells), *nucilage* (lumina, filled with polysaccharide), and a *testa* containing hairs or stomata.

Among poisonous plants the characteristic hairs of the seeds of *Strychnos* spp., the palisade of *Ricinus communis,* and the sclereids of solanaceous seeds are features of definitive character in either intact or disintegrated specimens. In addition, the color of the testa tissue and the cell contents (starch, aleurone) of the endosperm and embryo cells may offer clues for qualification.

## III. Toxic Components

The poisonous property of a seed or fruit is due to a single component or more generally to a group of chemically related compounds. It is rare that widely different toxic chemical components are found in the same seed or fruit. In many instances, however, the identity of the toxic component is unknown. The following classes of components are prominent ingredients of toxic fruits and seeds.

### A. Alkaloids

These nitrogen bases, biosynthetically derived (H3) from amino acids (lysine, ornithine, phenylalanine) and from nicotinic acid, anthranilic acid, or mevalonic acid (isoprenoid), are found throughout the plant kingdom. Although systematic position is definable for some alkaloids, the lack of total knowledge of the chemistry of the plant kingdom denies accuracy in establishing limits. Certain families (Ranunculaceae, Liliaceae, Apocynaceae, Rutaceae, Solanaceae, Papaveraceae, Menispermaceae, Berberidaceae, etc.) are alkaloid-rich while others contain alkaloids only in one or several genera (Erythroxylaceae, Crassulaceae, Caricaceae, Rhamnaceae, etc.). Some families (Labiatae, Salicaceae) are essentially alkaloid-free.

## B. Steroids and Triterpenoids

These compounds either as glycosides (saponins, steroidal glycosides, sterolins) or as the free or liberated nonsugar compound (genins, aglycons) are of frequent occurrence in seeds and fruits. Certain of the toxic compounds in this group are known as sapotoxins. The majority are gastrointestinal irritants particularly abundant among species of Dioscoraceae, Amaryllidaceae, and Liliaceae; toxic saponins appear not to have phylogenetic limitations. Cardiotoxic steroid glycosides found in the seeds of several *Strophanthus* spp. (Apocynaceae) and the gastrointestinal irritant, githagin, in seeds of *Agrostemma githago* (Caryophyllaceae) are examples of toxic steroids. Those sapotoxins which cause hemolysis act by forming a complex with cholesterol in a manner analogous to digitonide formation.

## C. Toxalbumins

The toxic proteins of plants are largely seed components. These substances are proteolytic (ricin, curcin), hemolytic (ricin), or hypoglycemic (hypoglycin). The inadequacy of present knowledge concerning this group is examplified by the assessment of the toxicity of the *Abrus precatorius seed*. Abrin is reported to be composed of two fractions: a globulin, the most toxic, and albumose (E1). Abrin, is regarded by some as a singular substance while others have concluded that abraline is an added toxic component.

## D. Hydrocyanic Acid

Cyanogenetic glycosides are common components of seeds. Amygdalin occurs in *Prunus amygdalus, Pygeum parviflorum*, and *Pyrus cydonia* while other glycosides (phaseolunatin in *Phaseolus lunatus*) also yield hydrocyanic acid upon hydrolysis. The lethal potentiality of such tissues is to be doubted. One of the richest sources of amygdalin is the bitter almond seed. The content is variable but has never been shown to be >3.0%. The HCN content of amygdalin is slightly less than 6.0%. Thus several hundred grams of seed would be required to provide a toxic dose. It has been estimated (K3) that forty to sixty seeds, yielding 70 mg HCN, may result in severe toxicity or death.

## IV. Toxic Fruits and Seeds

The following list, with the associate descriptive detail, is of those seeds and fruits regarded as toxic and which have been and are currently of importance in this respect. The list is arranged alphabetically by common name. The scientific name (genus and species) and family are recorded and the toxic action is listed. The description of each seed and fruit and its occurrence is followed, in each monograph, by a presentation of certain facts concerning the toxic components (maximum concentration is listed) and, when describable, the prognosis of the toxicity. Toxic components are arranged alphabetically in Table I; pathology is outlined in Table II.

**Baneberry;** *Actaea alba* Mill. (Ranunculaceae); gastrointestinal irritant.

Both the red (*A. rubra* Willd.) and the white (*A. alba*) baneberry fruit contain principles which cause gastrointestinal distress. These perennial herbs of rich woods in the north temperate zones probably contain saponins.

The white berries are globular-ovoid while those of the red-berried species are ovoid-ellipsoid. The fruits are smooth and contain seeds in two rows.

**Bitter almond;** *Prunus amygdalus* Batsch var. *amara* (Rosaceae); asphyxia, dyspnea.

The seeds of bitter almond are somewhat smaller than those of sweet almond, being shorter and proportionally broader. They are also distinguished by their bitter taste and by the characteristic odor of benzaldehyde which is evident when the seed is bruised and moistened.

Bitter almond seeds contain 1819 ppm of cyanide (W3) and as few as a dozen seeds have caused the death of a child (C1). The seeds of other *Prunus* species (peach, *P. persica,* choke cherry, *P. serotina*) also contain amygdalin. This glycoside liberates HCN and benzaldehyde upon hydrolysis.

**Bittersweet, black nightshade;** *Solanum dulcamara* L. (Solanaceae); stupefaction, convulsions.

The green unripe globular berries of this species and *S. nigrum,* up to 1 cm in diameter, are generally regarded as toxic. Yet the ripe fruit is used in the preparation of edible food products. Saponins have been isolated and the toxicity of one of these, solanine, has been shown (T1). It is probable that the solanine content may be greater in the unripe fruit or that it is destroyed in the process of cooking the ripe berries.

The species, *S. pseudocapsicum* L. (Jerusalem cherry), is widely cultivated for house decoration purposes. The orange-red berries have been fatal (W4); the toxicity of a leaf alkaloid has been shown (W2).

The reported toxicity of these fruits cannot be explained on the basis of solanine content. It is a nauseant whereas sedative-convulsant symptoms are typically reported following ingestion by man and animals. The toxicity of *Solanum nigrum* has been attributed to atropine and related alkaloids (T3).

TABLE I

TOXIC COMPONENTS OF SEEDS AND FRUITS

| Compound | Source | |
|---|---|---|
| | Common name | Botanical name |
| Abrin | Jequirity | *Abrus precatorius* |
| Agrostemmic acid | Githago | *Agrostemma githago* |
| Anacardic acid | Cashew nut | *Anacardium occidentale* |
| Atropine | Datura | *Datura* spp. |
| Colocynthin | Colocynth | *Citrullus colocynthis* |
| Coniine | Poison hemlock | *Conium maculatum* |
| Curcin | Jatropha | *Jatropha curcas* |
| Cyanide | Bitter almond | *Prunus amygdalus amara* |
| Cytisine | Laburnum | *Cytisus laburnum* |
| Delphinine | Delphinium | *Delphinium ajacis* |
| α-Elaterin | Bitter apple | *Citrullus colocynthis* |
| Eserine (see physostigmine) | | |
| Euonymin | Euonymus | *Euonymus atropurpurea* |
| | | *Euonymus europaeus* |
| | | *Euonymus americanus* |
| Ginkgolic acid | Ginkgo | *Ginkgo biloba* |
| Githagenin | Githago | *Agrostemma githago* |
| β-(N-γ-L-glutamyl)-aminopropionitrile | Vetch | *Lathyrus* spp. |
| Mucunian | Cowhage | *Mucuna pruriens* |
| Myristicin | Nutmeg | *Myristica fragans* |
| Ouabain | Strophanthus | *Strophanthus* spp. |
| 3-Pentadecylcatechol | Poison ivy | *Toxicodendron radicans* |
| Physostigmine | Calabar bean | *Physostigma venenosum* |
| Picrotoxin | Cocculus | *Anamirta paniculata* |
| Ricin | Castor bean | *Ricinus communis* |
| Saponin (Sapotoxin) | Baneberry | *Actaea alba* |
| | | *Actaea rubra* |
| | Poke | *Phytolacca americana* |
| | Tung | *Aleurites fordii* |
| Solanine | Black nightshade | *Solanum dulcamara* |
| | | *Solanum nigrum* |
| Strophanthidin | Strophanthus | *Strophanthus* spp. |
| Strychnine | Nux vomica | *Strychnos nux-vomica* |
| Taxine | Yew | *Taxus* spp. |
| Toxalbumin | Broad bean | *Vicia faba* |
| | Castor bean | *Ricinus communis* |
| | Jatropha | *Jatropha curcas* |
| | Jequirity | *Abrus precatorius* |
| Thevetin | Yellow oleander | *Thevetia peruviana* |
| Wistarin | Wisteria | *Wisteria sinensis* |

**Broad bean**; *Vicia faba* L. (Leguminosae); favism.

This bean when ingested as the green, undried fruit or when inadequately cooked causes favism. The toxicity, prevalent in Mediterranean countries is characterized by icterus, hemoglobinuria, and severe anemia. Dizziness, an early manifestation, is followed by vomiting, diarrhea, and prostration (H5, R1).

An acute toxicity has also been described. It is regarded as an allergy, caused by the seed protein.

**Calabar bean**; *Physostigma venenosum* Bal. (Leguminosae); cholinesterase inhibitor, motor depressant.

The seed of this vinelike legume is oblong, up to 30 mm in length, brown to reddish brown, with a groove along the convex edge. The plant is indigenous to Africa but is cultivated in India, Brazil, and other countries.

The toxicity of the bean is due to physostigmine (eserine) which is present up to 0.25%. Total alkaloids occur up to 0.3%. Symptoms of toxicity include salivation, nausea, lacrimation, and excessive perspiration.

**Cashew nut**; *Anacardium occidentale* L. (Anacardiaceae); vesicant, allergen causing dermatitis.

The pericarp (shell) is a by-product of the production of the edible seed. The entire fruit is a fleshy, pear-shaped receptacle, supporting a hard, shiny, ash-colored, kidney-shaped nut, 2.5 cm or more in length and 1.0–1.5 cm broad. The pericarp possesses large balsam canals; the edible receptacle is red or yellow. The tree occurs widely in tropical lands.

The pericarp contains the phenols anacardic acid and cardol (B1); the roasted kernel is edible. The toxic components of the raw pericarp and the expressed oil cause acute dermatitis similar to that of poison ivy. The shell oil is a commercial product used as a plasticizer and as an ingredient in insecticide products. Vanilla beans are sometimes painted with the oil.

**Castor bean**; *Ricinus communis* L. (Euphorbiaceae); purgative, allergen, produces hemagglutination.

The fruit, a soft spiny three-celled capsule, contains the ovoid albuminous seeds. The latter are 8–18 mm in length with a wartlike caruncle covering the micropyle. The testa is smooth, brittle, mottled gray, brown, red, or black. The cotyledons are oily. The plant is extensively cultivated and is grown as an ornamental.

Ricin (0.2%), a toxalbumin, accounts for the severe toxicity following seed ingestion. One or two seeds (beans) produce distressing symptoms

(K3) and have been fatal. Nausea, within a few moments of ingestion, is followed by abdominal pain and vascular collapse. In rabbits, 0.75 mg/kg ricin is lethal in 72 hours. Kidney damage is known to result from seed ingestion.

An allergenic principle, which appears to be a mucoprotein (W1), has been isolated. Severe allergy—dermatic and asthmatic—is exhibited by workers involved with the harvest and processing of the seed.

**Cocculus**; *Anamirta paniculata* Colebrooke (Menispermaceae); central stimulant, gastrointestinal irritant.

The red, kidney-shaped drupe becomes brown and slightly wrinkled when dry. The plant is native to tropical asiatic areas and is cultivated in other lands.

The toxic component, picrotoxin (up to 5.0%), causes salivation, vomiting, diarrhea. Severe toxicity shows anxiety, narcosis, and convulsions. Death is by asphyxia (B2).

**Colocynth, bitter apple**; *Citrullus colocynthis* (L.) Schrad. (Cucurbitaceae); purgative.

The pulp of the unripe fruit of this creeping vine is toxic. The plant, native to Asia and Mediterranean countries, is frequently cultivated. The plant and its fruit resemble the common watermelon in growth features and other detail; the fruit is smaller and is yellow when ripe.

The toxic components include colocynthin and $\alpha$-elaterin (0.2%). They are a drastic hydragogue cathartic. The toxicity has been described (H1); it resembles ricin.

**Cowhage**; *Mucuna pruriens* DC. (Leguminosae); local irritant.

The fruit of this leguminous tropical vine is a pod covered with hairs. When handled, the barbed hairs cling to the fingers and produce an intense itching sensation and erythema.

A proteolytic enzyme, mucunian (S4), and serotonin (B4) have been isolated from the hairs. The presence of a histamine liberator has been shown.

**Croton**; *Croton tiglium* L. (Euphorbiaceae); purgative, vesicant.

The fruit is a smooth capsule containing three anatropous seeds. The seeds resemble castor beans, being oblong. The "shell" is covered with a soft yellow-brown epidermis beneath which the surface is black mottled. The endosperm is oily. The tropical plant is grown for the production of the oil.

The seed contains a resin with a multiplicity of components (D3, S5). The resin is responsible for the vesicant action and in part for the purgative action of the seed and its expressed oil. Death results from circulatory or respiratory failure.

**Daphne;** *Daphne mezereum* L. (Thymelaeaceae); local irritant, gastrointestinal irritant.

The fruit of several species of *Daphne* (*D. gnidium, D. laureola*) also are toxic. The fruit is oval, fleshy, red, with a single seed. The plant is native to Europe and western Asia and is cultivated.

The acrid resin, mezerin, which contains mezereic acid (mezereinic acid anhydride) is the toxic component. The symptoms of toxicity, following skin absorption of the juice or ingestion of the berries, are headache, vomiting, diarrhea, and delirium. The latent action includes albuminuria and narcosis (G1).

**Delphinium, larkspur;** *Delphinium ajacis* L. (Ranunculaceae); hypotensive action, prostration, hypothermia.

The brownish black to yellow-brown seed is irregularly tetrahedral, about 2 mm in length, and possesses eight to twelve ridges transversely encircling the seed. This species and other cultivated species contain toxic alkaloids. *D. requienii* and *D. staphisagria* both contain alkaloids (e.g., delphinine) resembling aconitine and are thus somewhat different toxicologically.

*D. ajacis* seed contain alkaloids (ajacine and ajaconine). These and other alkaloids effect the heart and respiration causing a slow pulse and labored respiration. Stiffness of the facial muscles and irregular muscle twitchings are responses to severe toxicity.

The seed, in the form of the tincture, has been used to rid the body of lice. Repeated application results in dermatitis in some individuals.

**Erythrina;** *Erythrina abyssinica* Lam. ex DC. (Leguminosae); paralyzing effect similar to curare.

The spiny two-valved fruit of this and several related species of tropical trees have yielded a number of convulsive and paralyzing alkaloids. Fifty-one of one hundred and five species (F2) of *Erythrina* collected in Africa, Asia, and the Western hemisphere contain curarelike alkaloids.

The plant is frequently grown as a household ornamental. The highly colored seeds are attractive.

**Euonymus, burning bush;** *Euonymus atropurpureus* Jacq. (Celastraceae); cardiotoxic.

The plants of this genus are cultivated shrubs and small trees. This species and others (*E. europaeus, E. americanus*) yield an attractive

TABLE II

PATHOLOGICAL CHANGES CAUSED BY TOXIC SEEDS AND FRUITS

| Pathology | Seed or fruit | |
|---|---|---|
| Collapse | Bitter almond | Laburnum |
| | Bitter apple | Nutmeg |
| | Bittersweet | Poison hemlock |
| | Calabar bean | Poke |
| | Castor bean | Strophanthus |
| | Delphinium | Yellow oleander |
| | Euonymus | Yew |
| Convulsions | Calabar bean | Mistletoe |
| | Castor bean | Nux-vomica |
| | Cocculus | Poke |
| | Erythrina | |
| Cyanosis | Bitter almond | Strophanthus |
| | Datura | Yellow oleander |
| | Ricin | |
| Delirium | Bittersweet | Datura |
| | Cocculus | Euonymus |
| | Daphne | Laburnum |
| Dermatitis (including vesication) | Cashew nut | Ginkgo |
| | Cowhage | Osage orange |
| | Croton | Poison ivy |
| | Daphne | Tung |
| | Delphinium | |
| Diarrhea | Bittersweet | Githago |
| | Broad bean | Jatropha |
| | Castor bean | Jequirity |
| | Cocculus | Laburnum |
| | Colocynth | Poison hemlock |
| | Croton | Poke |
| | Daphne | Tung |
| | Euonymus | Wisteria |
| | Ginkgo | Yew |
| Dyspnea | Castor bean | Nutmeg |
| | Jatropha | |
| Lassitude | Bitter almond | Euonymus |
| | Bittersweet | Fasle pepper |
| | Castor bean | Jequirity |
| | Croton | Nutmeg |
| | Datura | Poke |
| | Delphinium | |

TABLE II (*Continued*)

| Pathology | Seed or fruit | |
|---|---|---|
| Nausea | Baneberry | Githago |
| | Broad bean | Jatropha |
| | Calabar bean | Laburnum |
| | Castor bean | Mistletoe |
| | Cocculus | Poison hemlock |
| | Colocynth | Poke |
| | Corn cockle | Strophanthus |
| | Croton | Tung |
| | Datura | Yellow oleander |
| | Euonymus | Yew |
| | False pepper | |
| Prostration | Bitter almond | Githago |
| | Broad bean | Laburnum |
| | Croton | Poke |
| | Delphinium | Tung |
| | Erythrina | |
| Visual disturbances | Calabar bean | Finger cherry |
| | Castor bean | Laburnum |
| | Datura | Strophanthus |
| | Delphinium | |

fruit. The fruit is three- to four-lobed, crimson to orange, enclosing seeds, each covered by a succulent aril. The seeds contain digitalislike substances. Euonymin is the major toxic component.

Ingestion of the fruit or seed is followed by diarrhea, vomiting, and coma. The toxicity has been described (H4, U1).

**False pepper;** *Schinus molle* L. (Anacardiaceae); gastrointestinal irritant, produces headache and lassitude.

The immature green berry becomes red when ripe. A cultivated ornamental, the fruit shows toxicity when eaten in quantity (B7, C1). Native to South America, the species is cultivated as an ornamental evergreen. The toxic components are not present in the volatile oil and are unknown.

**Finger cherry, loquat;** *Rhodomyrtus macrocarpa* Benth. (Myrtaceae); blindness.

The unripe fruit of this shrub, native to Australia, has been reported to produce blindness (F3). Contradictory accounts indicate the fruit can be eaten without ill effect.

The guava-like fruit is 1–1.5 cm in diameter. The fruit of a related species (*R. tomentosa*) is edible.

The poisonous principle has been described (B5) as a saponin or as a product of the fungus *Gleosporium periculosum* which attacks the ripe fruit. The optic nerve is damaged and the toxicity occurs shortly after ingestion of the fruit.

**Ginkgo;** *Ginkgo biloba* L. (Ginkgoaceae); local irritant and gastrointestinal irritant.

The fruit is a yellow-orange drupe which resembles the persimmon. The ill-smelling pulp surrounds a thin-shelled, two-angled, creamy white nut. The kernel is sweet and edible.

The juice of the fruit pulp contains substances irritating (S1) to the epidermis. When ingested the fruit produces gastroenteritis and nephritis. A hemolytic substance has been isolated. It resembles cantharidin in action (S2) but appears to be a mixture of triterpenes (F3) including ginkgolic acid and bilobol.

**Githago, corn cockle;** *Agrostemma githago* L. (Caryophyllaceae); gastrointestinal irritant, githagism.

The seed, a contaminant in cereal grains, contains toxic saponins; agrostemmic acid and githagenin have been isolated. Both chronic and acute (G2, M1) toxicity have been described. Vertigo, vomiting, diarrhea, paralysis, and coma are reported toxicity symptoms.

**Jatropha, purging nut;** *Jatropha curcas* L. (Euphorbiaceae); gastrointestinal irritant.

The fruit, a capsule, contains three seeds. The latter are black mottled with white, oval, 1.5–2.0 cm long. The plant and related species are widely cultivated in tropical lands.

The seed contains a toxalbumin and curcin (D2), which together with resinous components are responsible for the varied toxic actions. The action of curcin(e) resembles that of ricin and the resin resembles that of croton seed.

**Jequirity, prayer bead;** *Abrus precatorius* L. (Leguminosae); hemorrhagic, gastrointestinal irritant, allergen.

The licorice bush which bears the seed known also as love pea, crab's eye, and jumble bead grows in tropical and semitropical areas throughout the world. The seeds are ovoid, 5–8 mm in length, shiny smooth, and are brilliant red-colored with a black spot at the hilum. The seeds are attractive and throughout recent history have been involved in innumerable poisonings, both willful and accidental. The seed is occasionally a part of costume jewelry (A1).

The toxic albumin abrin is not to be confused with N-methyltryptophan. The latter is variously titled abrine or abrin and the use of the seed as an oral contraceptive (K1) has been related to this component.

The powdered seed and the isolated toxalbumin are highly toxic. The lethal dose is 0.01 mg/kg (W5). Toxic symptoms include purging, lassitude, and incoordinant movements. The toxic reaction may occur 1–3 days following ingestion. Repeated inhalation of the powder of the seed produces asthmatic reactions.

**Laburnum, golden chain;** *Cytisus laburnum* L. (Leguminosae); respiratory paralysis.

The seeds of the 2.5–8 cm long pod of this cultivated shrub contain cytisine (laburnine) and related alkaloids. The symptoms include salivation, nausea, diarrhea, and delirium. Respiration is of the Cheyne–Stokes type and death is due to respiratory paralysis.

**Mistletoe;** *Phoradendron flavescens* (Pursh) Nutt. (Loranthaceae); gastrointestinal irritant, prostration, coma, convulsive.

The one-seeded white berries of the American mistletoe and the European mistletoe (*Viscum album* L.) contain toxic principles. The toxic components of each appear to be different but choline is present in both. The European species contain a hypotensive principle while the American species contain principles which are hypertensive.

**Nutmeg;** *Myristica fragrans Houttuyn* (Myristicaceae); circulatory collapse.

The ripe seed is a common household spice. Both the seed and its aril, mace, contain a volatile oil. The toxic principle is probably myristicin, a phenol. Frequent toxicities develop from the lay use of the seed to induce menses.

The ingestion of one or several nutmegs has caused distressing symptoms and has been fatal (G3, O1). The toxicity symptoms are dyspnea, tremors, and unconsciousness.

A related genus, *Virola*, yields fruit similar to the nutmeg and it is regarded as narcotic.

**Nux vomica, poison nut;** *Strychnos nux-vomica* L. (Loganaceae); paralysis, convulsions.

The seed, an item of commerce for the isolation of strychnine, is orbicular, flat, up to 30 mm in diameter, gray to olive, and is covered with hair. The seed is hard and intensely bitter. The tree is a native of India but is cultivated in other lands.

Strychnine, up to 2.0%, is the toxic component. All aspects of toxicity are strychnine-related.

Osage orange; *Maclura pomifera* (Raf.) Schneid. (Moraceae); dermatitis.

The tree, native to Arkansas and Texas and adjoining area, is much planted for hedges. The fruit is a syncarp formed of the enlarged fleshy perianths embodying the drupelets.

A few individuals show hypersensitivity to the latex of the fruit.

Poison hemlock; *Conium maculatum* L. (Umbelliferae); paralysis, asphyxia.

The fruit—sometimes called conium seed—is an ovoid cremocarp, about 3 mm long and somewhat curved. The convex side has five pale yellow ribs and the flattened side is marked with a deep groove. The plant, native to Europe, is naturalized in the United States and possesses a fetid odor. The fruit resembles anise and has been mistaken for that fruit.

The fruit contains coniine (up to 3.0%); 120 mg of coniine is fatal. The essential effect is paralysis of the motor nerves. Death due to asphyxia is a result of the effect on the action of the diaphragm (K4). Other toxicity symptoms are salivation, nausea, and irritation of the pharynx.

Poison ivy; *Toxicodendron radicans* Ktze. (Anacardiaceae); allergen causing dermatitis.

The toxic principles of the leaf, stem, and root are present in the fruit. The fruit is a globular, glabrous, grayish drupe which persists on the vines after leaves have fallen.

The basic moiety of the major toxic principles of poison ivy is 3-pentadecylcatechol (L1). The chemistry of poison ivy has been presented (D1).

Ingestion of the plant parts, containing these principles, produces gastrointestinal distress. Large doses cause mydriasis, delirium, and convulsions.

Poke; *Phytolacca americana* L. (Phytolaccaceae); gastrointestinal irritant, respiratory paralysis.

The green unripe fruit, occuring as a cluster of berries, each flattened, divided into ten loculi and containing one seed, becomes dark purple when ripe.

The unripe fruits contain saponins and other components which account for the emetic and cathartic action. Death by respiratory paralysis has been described (G4) but the precise toxic components have not been shown.

Strophanthus; *Strophanthus kombe* Oliv. (Apocynaceae); cardiotoxic.

The seed of this and other species (*S. hispidus, S. emini,* etc.) found in Africa and Asia contain toxic steroidal glycosides and genins. The seeds are oblong-lanceolate, up to 25 mm in length, pale yellow to green or brown, and covered with hairs. Used for centuries as an arrow poison, the extracts and isolated components have a digitalislike action.

Ingestion causes increased peristalsis and on occasion intestinal spasm.

The components include strophanthidin, ouabain, cymarin, strophanthidiol, and periplogenin. Seeds of *Acokanthera schimperi* (A. DC.) Schwf. contain ouabain.

**Thorn apple**; *Datura stramonium* L. (Solanaceae); depressant, mydriatic, parasympatholytic action.

The green fruit is a nodding, subglobular, spiny, four-valved capsule. The brown to black seeds are flattened reniform structures up to 3 mm long.

The seeds of *Datura* species (*D. metel, D. arborea, D. ferox, D. innoxia, D. fastuosa*, etc.) contain atropine (*d,l*-hyoscyamine) and hyoscine (scopolamine) and other tropane alkaloids. The alkaloid concentration (up to 0.8%) is generally higher in seeds than other plant parts.

Poisoning is most common among children (H2, J1) but the seeds have been cited as the cause of toxicity in contaminated foods. Twenty seeds have been known (O1) to be lethal.

Whereas *Datura stramonium* is a weed in Europe and North America, species such as *D. metel* and its forms are widely cultivated as ornamentals. The appellations angel trumpet and moonflower are applied to this flowering plant.

**Tung**; *Aleurites fordii* Hemsl. (Euphorbiaceae); gastrointestinal irritant, dermatitis.

The brown ripe fruit, 5.0–7.5 cm in diameter, contains three or more broadly obovoid seeds. The seed contains sapotoxins, retained in the expressed seed, which act as a drastic purgative (E2). The seed cake also produces dermatitis.

**White vetch, vetchling**; *Larthyrus sativus* L. (Leguminosae); lathyragenic.

This pea is a food in Europe and Asia and together with related species (*L. cicera, L. odoratus, Vicia sativa*, etc.) is the cause of lathyrism and cicerism. The incidence of lathyrism in certain areas of India has been estimated (S6) as high as 7% of the population. Lathyrism toxicity is characterized by spastic paraplegia, tremor, osteoporosis, and skeletal changes.

Osteolathyrism is caused by the component $\beta$-($N$-$\gamma$-L glutamyl)-aminopropionitrile (S3). The causative agent of neurolathyrism is unknown.

Wisteria;[1] *Wisteria sinensis* Sweet (Leguminosae); gastrointestinal irritant.

Wisteria is a woody vine widely used as an ornamental for covering arbors. The fruit is a pubescent flattened two-valved pod, 10–15 cm long.

The seeds of cultivated species of *Wisteria* contain sapotoxins which cause nausea, diarrhea, abdominal swelling, and collapse. The name wistarin has been assigned to one of the toxic components (O2) and a toxic resin has been isolated (K2).

Yellow oleander, yccotli; *Thevetia peruviana* Schum. (Apocynaceae); cardiotoxic.

The kernel of the fruit of this species and *T. yccotli* A.DC., native to Central America and South America, contains thevetin and related glycosides. The plant is extensively cultivated as an ornamental.

Thevetin toxicity parallels that of strophanthus glycosides; Mexican species paralyze the sympathetic nerves.

Yew; *Taxus baccata* L. (Taxaceae); gastrointestinal irritant, cardiac failure.

The ripe scarlet fruit, a globose disk, in which is contained an ellipsoidal brown seed, is present in both native and cultivated yew.

The alkaloid complex, taxine (0.92%), is responsible for the toxic character of the seed; the red aril is edible. The chemical nature of taxine has been partially elucidated (B3) and the toxic action has been described (B6). The essential toxic action is cardiac depression.

## REFERENCES

(A1) Anonymous. *J. Am. Med. Assoc.* **157,** 779 (1955).
(B1) Backer, H. J., and Haack, N. H. *Rec. Trav. Chim.* **60,** 661 (1941).
(B2) Baer, A. W. *J. Am. Med. Assoc.* **43,** 341 (1904).
(B3) Baxter, J. N., Lythgoe, B., Scales, B., and Trippett, S. *Proc. Chem. Soc.* p. 9 (1958); Baxter, J. N., Lythgoe, B., Scales, B., Scrowton, R. M., and Trippett, S. *J. Chem. Soc.* p. 2964 (1962).
(B4) Bowden, K., Brown, B. G., and Batty, J. E. *Nature* **174,** 925 (1954).
(B5) Brunnich, J. C. *Ann. Rept. Dept. Agr. Stock* (*Queensland*) **1914–15,** 37 (1915).
(B6) Bryan-Brown, T. *Quart. J. Pharm. Pharmacol.* **5,** 205 (1932).
(B7) Burtt Davy, J. *Ann. Rept. Transvaal. Dept. Agr.* **No. 261** (1903).
(C1) Cleland, J. B. *Australian Med. Gaz.* **35,** (1914); *Med. J. Australia* **2,** 775 (1931).
(D1) Dawson, C. R. *Trans. N. Y. Acad. Sci.* **18,** 427 (1956).
(D2) Droit, S. *Bull. Mat. Grasses Inst. Colonial Marseille* **16,** 270 (1932).
(D3) von Duuren, A. J. *Chronica Naturae* **106,** 466 (1950).

---

[1] Also known as *Wistaria* [after Dr. C. Wistar (1760–1818)]. The name *Wisteria* is accepted by most botanists, however.

(E1) Edmunds, C. W., and Gunn, J. "Cushny's Pharmacology and Therapeutics," 11th ed., p. 788. Lea & Febiger, Philadelphia, Pennsylvania, 1936.

(E2) Erickson, J. E., and Brown, J. H., Jr. *J. Pharmacol. Exptl. Therap.* **74,** 114 (1942).

(F1) Flecker, H. *Med. J. Australia* **2,** 183 (1944).

(F2) Folkers, K., and Una, K. *J. Am. Pharm. Assoc.* **28,** 1019 (1939).

(F3) Furukawa, S. *Sci. Papers Inst. Phys. Chem. Res. (Tokyo)* **26,** 178 (1935).

(G1) Gessner, O. *Samml. Vergiftungsfällen* **6,** 165 (1935).

(G2) Gessner, O. "Die Gift- und Arzneipflanzen von Mitteleuropa," p. 242. Winter, Heidelberg, Germany, 1953.

(G3) Green, R. C. *J. Am. Med. Assoc.* **171,** 1342 (1959).

(G4) Gress, G. *Repts. Penn. Dept. Agr. Bull.* **531,** 1935.

(H1) Hammarstan, G., and Lindgren, G. *Samml. Vergiftungsfällen* **12,** 107 (1941).

(H2) Hansen, A. A. *Purdue Univ. Agr. Expt. Sta. Circ.* No. **175** (1930).

(H3) Hegnauer, R. *Planta Med.* **6,** 1 (1958).

(H4) Hermkes, L. *Münch. Med. Wochschr.* **83,** 1011 (1941).

(H5) Hutton, J. E. *J. Am. Med. Assoc.* **109,** 1618 (1937).

(J1) Jennings, R. E. *J. Pediat.* **6,** 657 (1935).

(K1) Karrer, P. "Organic Chemistry," 4th ed. Am. Elesevier, New York, 1950.

(K2) Kobert, R. "Lehrbuch der Intoxikationen," 2nd ed. Enke, Stuttgart, Germany, 1902–1906.

(K3) Koch, L. A., and Caplan, J. *Am. J. Diseases Children* **64,** 485 (1942).

(K4) Krayer, O. *Arch. Exptl. Pathol. Pharmakol.* **162,** 342 (1931).

(L1) Loev, B., and Dawson, C. R. *J. Am. Chem. Soc.* **78,** 1180 (1956).

(M1) Muenscher, W. C. "Poisonous Plants of the United States," revised ed., p. 75. Macmillan, New York, 1951.

(O1) von Oettingen, W. F. *Natl. Insts. Health Bull.* **190,** 325 (1949).

(O2) Otto, R. *Nieuw. Tijdschr.* **19,** 207 (1886); *Arch. Pharm.* **225,** 455 (1887).

(Q1) Quarre, P., and Mols, A. "Plantes toxique du Katanga." Comité Special du Katanga, Elisabethville, Congo, 1945.

(R1) Rosen, A. P., and Scanlan, J. J. *New Engl. J. Med.* **239,** 367 (1948).

(S1) Saito, J. *Japan. J. Dermatol. Urol.* **29,** 1930 (1929).

(S2) Saito, J. *Tohoku J. Exptl. Med.* **16,** 385 (1930).

(S3) Selye, H. *Arch. Exptl. Pathol. Pharmakol.* **230,** 155 (1957).

(S4) Shelley, W. B., and Arthur, R. P. *Arch. Dermatol.* **72,** 399 (1955).

(S5) Spies, J. R., and Coulson, E. J. *J. Am. Chem. Soc.* **65,** 1720 (1943).

(S6) Stockman, R. *J. Pharmacol. Exptl. Therap.* **37,** 43 (1929).

(T1) Terbrüggen, A. *Samml. Vergiftungsfällen* **7,** 101 (1936).

(T2) Thompson, R. B., and Sifton, H. B. "A Guide to the Poisonous Plants and Weed Seeds of Canada and the Northern United States." Univ. of Toronto Press, Toronto, Canada, 1922.

(T3) Towers, R. P. *Irish J. Med. Sci.* **326,** 77 (1953).

(U1) Urban, G. *Samml. Vergiftungsfällen* **13,** 27 (1944).

(W1) Waler, G. R., and Negi, S. S. *J. Am. Oil Chemist's Soc.* **35,** 409 (1958).

(W2) Watt, J. M., and Meltzer, E. *Quart. J. Pharm. Pharmacol.* **5,** 649 (1932).

(W3) Wokes, F., and Willimott, S. G. *J. Pharm. Pharmacol.* **3,** 905 (1951).

(W4) Wood, H. C., and Osol, A. "The Dispensatory of the United States of America," 23rd ed., p. 1527. Lippincott, Philadelphia, Pennsylvania, 1943.

(W5) Wood, H. C., and Osol, A. "The Dispensatory of the United States of America," 23rd ed., p. 1237. Lippincott, Philadelphia, Pennsylvania, 1943.

# AUTHOR INDEX

Numbers in parentheses are reference numbers and are included to assist in locating references in which authors' names are not mentioned in the text. Numbers in italics refer to pages on which the references are listed.

# SUBJECT INDEX

## A

Abrin
  botanical source, 396
Acetaldehyde
  after alcohol ingestion, 84
  gas chromatography, (Table V) 36
  normal blood levels, 84
Acetate, amyl
  gas chromatography, (Table V) 36
Acetate, ethyl
  gas chromatography, (Table V) 36
Acetate, propyl
  gas chromatography, (Table V) 36
Acetates
  chromatographic columns for, (Table
    III) 15
Acetoketobemidone
  paper chromatography, (Table XX)
    266
Acetone
  gas chromatography, (Table V) 36
Acetylanileridine
  determination of, 226
Acetylanileridine acid
  determination of, 226
Acetyldihydrocodeine
  paper chromatography, (Table XX)
    266
Acetylmethadols
  determination of, 226
  metabolism of, 227
  paper chromatography, (Table XIX)
    264, (Table XX) 266
  tissue distribution, 226
Acetylmorphenol
  paper chromatography, (Table XX)
    266
Acidic and Neutral drugs, 136
  extraction with special solvents, 136
  gas chromatography, 141
  infra-red spectroscopy, 143
  modified extraction procedure, 137
  paper chromatography, 8, (Table
    VIII) 44, (Table IX) 46, 140

  paper chromatography multiple sprays,
    140
  purification procedures, 138
  scheme of extraction, 8
  thin layer chromatography, 141, 210
Aconitine
  paper chromatography, (Table XXI)
    270
Agrostemmic acid
  botanical source, 396
Air pollutants, 297ff
  analytical methods, 317
  classes of, (Table I) 298, 318
  continuous automatic measurements of,
    335
  occupational exposures to, 304
  threshold limits of, (Table III) 306
  toxicity of, 304
Air pollution, *see* Air pollutants
Ajamaline
  paper chromatography, (Table XXI)
    270
Alcohol, abnormal changes, 99
  diffusion from stomach, 100
  effect of burning, 104
  effect of drowning, 104
  effect of putrefaction, 103
  post-mortem changes, 100
  stability of stored blood, 99
Alcohol absorption, 57
  by inhalation, 60
  dilution effect, 59
  effect of exercise, 59
  effect of food, 57
  effect of stress, 59
  habituation effect, 59
  through the skin, 60
Alcohol, analytical methods, 107ff
  accuracy of, 117
  acetaldehyde-thiosemicarbazone
    method, 113
  acid permanganate methods, 109
  alcohol dehydrogenase methods, 110
  alcohol dehydrogenase plus Diaphor-
    ase, 111

422